Spectral Domain
Optical Coherence Tomography
A Practical Guide

Louise Nicklin

Spectral Domain
Optical Coherence Tomography
A Practical Guide

Second Edition

Shaun Dacosta MS
Assistant Director - Research
The Eye Research Foundation
Vijaya Hospital, 180 Arcot Road
Chennai, Tamil Nadu, India
shaundacosta@yahoo.com

Babu Rajendran MS FACS
Medical Director and Vice President
The Eye Research Foundation
Vijaya Hospital, 180 Arcot Road
Chennai, Tamil Nadu, India
drbabu@eth.net

P Janakiraman MS DOMS
Joint Medical Director
The Eye Research Foundation
Vijaya Hospital, 180 Arcot Road
Chennai, Tamil Nadu, India
janakiraman@vsnl.in

JAYPEE - HIGHLIGHTS
MEDICAL PUBLISHERS, INC.

Published by
Jaypee Brothers Medical Publishers (P) Ltd

Corporate Office
4838/24, Ansari Road, Daryaganj, **New Delhi** 110 002, India
Phone: +91-11-43574357, Fax: +91-11-43574314
www.jaypeebrothers.com

Offices in India

- **Ahmedabad**, e-mail: ahmedabad@jaypeebrothers.com
- **Bengaluru**, e-mail: bangalore@jaypeebrothers.com
- **Chennai**, e-mail: chennai@jaypeebrothers.com
- **Delhi**, e-mail: jaypee@jaypeebrothers.com
- **Hyderabad**, e-mail: hyderabad@jaypeebrothers.com
- **Kochi**, e-mail: kochi@jaypeebrothers.com
- **Kolkata**, e-mail: kolkata@jaypeebrothers.com
- **Lucknow**, e-mail: lucknow@jaypeebrothers.com
- **Mumbai**, e-mail: mumbai@jaypeebrothers.com
- **Nagpur**, e-mail: nagpur@jaypeebrothers.com

Overseas Offices

- **Central America Office, Panama City, Panama**, Ph: 001-507-317-0160
  e-mail: cservice@jphmedical.com, Website: www.jphmedical.com
- **Europe Office, UK**, Ph: +44 (0) 2031708910
  e-mail: info@jpmedpub.com

Spectral Domain Optical Coherence Tomography: A Practical Guide

First Edition: 2008

Second Edition: 2011

ISBN 978-93-5025-387-8

Typeset at JPBMP typesetting unit

Printed in India

To

Our Parents, Teachers, Families and Patients,
who made us what we are today

PREFACE TO THE SECOND EDITION

The most important thing in science is not so much to obtain new facts, as to discover new ways of thinking about them.

—Sir William Bragg
Australian Physicist
1915 Nobel Prize in Physics

The Spectral Domain OCT gave us so much new facts about retinal disease that we wonder how we ever practiced as Vitreoretinal Consultants all these years. The last two years have been indeed an eye opener for us in this field. Apart from admiring the several new facts and enjoying trying to correlate them to and with associated investigations and the disease process it certainly has made us discover new ways of thinking about them as well.

We did not realize that TWO years had indeed flown by with the Topcon 1000 machine and since our First Edition came out until the Topcon 2000 along with its upgraded software landed on our doorstep. With its improved and enhanced speed of 27,000 A scans/sec, improved software algorithms and additional facilities for anterior segment imaging, we thought it was time and justified to write this second edition.

We have attempted to highlight all these features and added newer chapters in keeping with the newer features. Images from the previous edition have been updated with the latest pictures with the series 2000.

We are greatly appreciative of the continued support and guidance we have received from the Singapore office of Topcon as well as the Service Engineers and Support Staff of M/s Mehra Eye Tech, the local distributors of the equipment in India.

We are sure you will enjoy this book as much as we have enjoyed putting this edition together. Not only did we enjoy ourselves, but we have learnt a great deal in the process.

Shaun Dacosta
Babu Rajendran
P Janakiraman

By learning you will teach, by teaching you will learn.

—Latin Proverb

PREFACE TO THE FIRST EDITION

Technology feeds on itself. Technology makes more technology possible.

—Alvin Toffler

Just as we were getting used to Optical Coherence Tomography, and began raving about its wonderful potential and its many uses, comes an enhanced and more precise technology called Spectral Domain OCT. It enhances the wide potential of 2D-OCT and is more precise with less interpolation in the interpretation of results.

Several companies manufacture different types of machines using the principle of Spectral Domain OCT. The TOPCON 3D-OCT-1000 is inbuilt with a nonmydriatic fundus camera and therefore has the unique ability of capturing the color picture and the OCT in one sitting and rather quickly making it comfortable for both patient and doctor.

While several books are available on OCT and its interpretation, this is possibly one of the early ones to be a practical guide to the beginner to this new and exciting technology.

We have attempted to outline a step-by-step approach to image capturing, analysis and interpretation with a large collection of selected cases.

We hope this book will generate the excitement in the reader enough to want to delve into this new 3D domain as much as it did in all of us when we were first exposed to it.

Before long this technology will be enhanced with the addition of Adaptive Optics to the OCT technology. This will enable cellular level resolution rather than the present-day tissue level pictures. Till that time enjoy the present and the book.

Shaun Dacosta
Babu Rajendran
P Janakiraman

Many a time, the reading of a book has made the future of a man.

—Ralph Waldo Emerson

CONTENTS

Section 1: Introduction to Spectral Domain OCT

Section 2: OCT Patterns in Various Diseases

Section 1

Introduction to Spectral Domain OCT

1 An Overview of Optical Coherence Tomography

Optical Coherence Tomography (OCT) is a noninvasive, noncontact imaging technique which produces cross-sectional images with millimeter penetration (approximately 2-3 mm in tissue) and micrometer scale axial and transverse resolution of not only the retina and optic nerve but also the anterior segment of the eye. The technique was first demonstrated in 1991 with ~30 μm axial resolution. With advancement in technology, today we have the conventional OCT with an axial resolution of ≤10 μm and the 3D OCT with a much higher resolution of 5 μm.

The working principle of OCT is similar to ultrasound, which uses echoes to locate structures within the body. The speed of light being almost a million times faster than sound allows measurement of structures with a resolution of ≤10 microns as compared to 100 micron scale for ultrasound.

OCT works through the magic of low-coherence interferometry. Broad bandwidth near infrared light (820 nm) generated by using a superluminescent diode is projected on the retina. The light is then broken into two arms—a sample arm (containing the item of interest) and a reference arm (usually from a mirror). The combination of reflected light from the sample arm and light from the reference arm gives rise to an interference pattern. By scanning the mirror in the reference arm, a reflectivity profile of the sample can be obtained (this is time domain OCT). This reflectivity profile, called an **A-scan** contains information about the spatial dimensions and location of structures within the item of interest. A cross-sectional tomograph **(B-scan)** may be achieved by laterally combining a series of these axial depth scans **(A-scan)**.

OCT can clearly image the cornea, sclera, iris, and lens in the anterior segment using infrared light having a wavelength of 1310 nm (Figure 1.1).

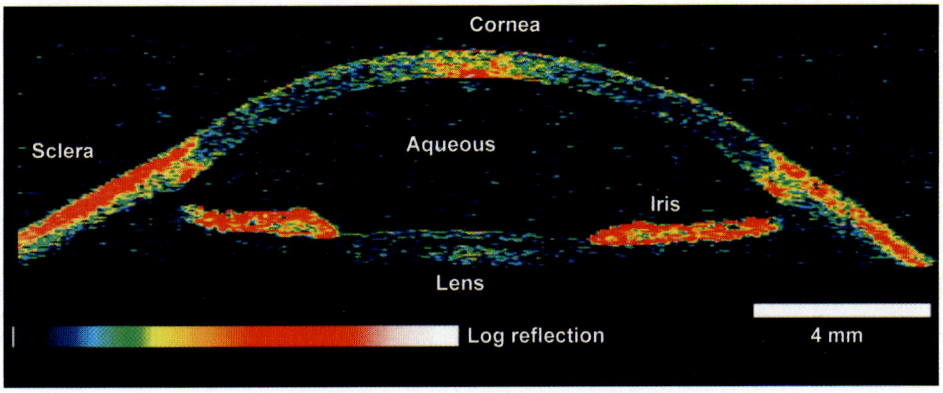

Figure 1.1: OCT of the anterior segment

OCT is the only technique which resolves the substructure of the retina in living eyes. It has, therefore, developed into an indispensable diagnostic tool for managing patients with vitreoretinal diseases. Figure 1.2 illustrates the capability of OCT to detect subsurface microscopic tissue layers *in vivo*.

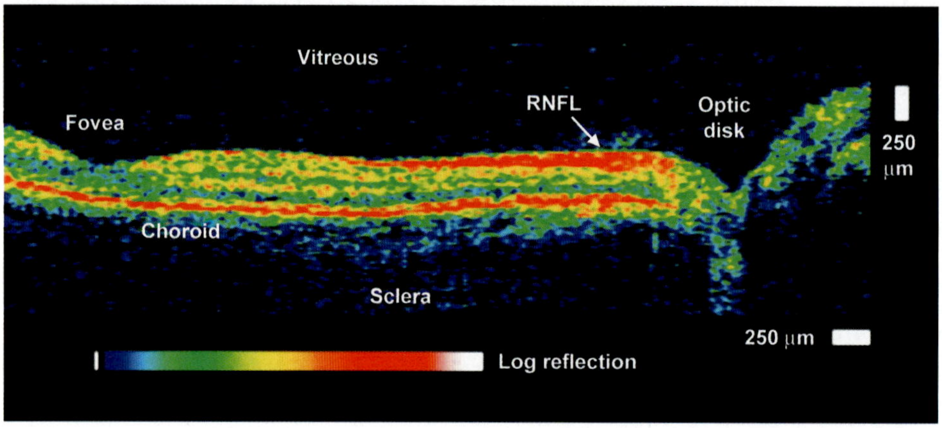

Figure 1.2: OCT along the papillomacular axis connecting the fovea and optic nerve head.

New three-dimensional optical coherence tomography (3D OCT) instruments developed by companies such as Topcon, Inc. are cutting-edge ophthalmic imaging solutions that merge technology, speed, quality, and clinical versatility. These devices are up to 50 times faster and 25% more accurate than conventional OCT.

Using higher speeds, 3D OCT acquires more data in less time easing the scanning process for both patients and technicians. 3D OCT provides unparalleled views of retinal and subretinal structures with the best resolution available in any commercial device. Capturing, viewing, and analyzing images are easier with the software improvements. Integration with a non-mydriatic retinal camera as in the Topcon 3D OCT allows for a direct comparison between the raster scans on the retinal image to the corresponding OCT tomographic layers.

3D OCT based on spectral domain technology (SD-OCT) replaces the moving parts found in conventional OCT instruments with a stationary spectrometer. By using mathematical calculations, an SD-OCT instrument can capture scans very quickly-before the patient shifts his or her gaze. The faster speed, higher resolution and improved signal-to-noise ratio of SD-OCT systems may ultimately improve the detection of the true outer retinal boundary and retinal layers, and enable the detection and quantification of clinically relevant disease features, such as subretinal fluid.

One of the distinguishing features of the 3D OCT device is that it can capture 256 B-scans in rapid succession, resulting in a dense three-dimensional cube of OCT information. This 3-D data can then be viewed en face as a 'C-scan', or in an infinite number of orientations and directions to visualize specific regions of the fundus.

Despite numerous, rapid technological advances in the last decade, conventional time domain OCT devices have many hardware and software limitations. Because these instruments rely on mechanical movements of internal components to make thickness measurements, their image acquisition speed is limited. This restricts the number of scans that can be acquired before a patient looks away from the fixation point. For instance, current time domain OCT instruments construct a high-resolution retinal thickness map using 6 radially oriented B-scans captured in 8-10 seconds. In this mode, however, the instrument measures less than 5 percent of the total macular area and must approximate more than 95 percent of the output data. Therefore, the device may incorrectly estimate retinal thickness, and may miss small lesions that fall between the radial-line scans (Figures 1.3A to C).

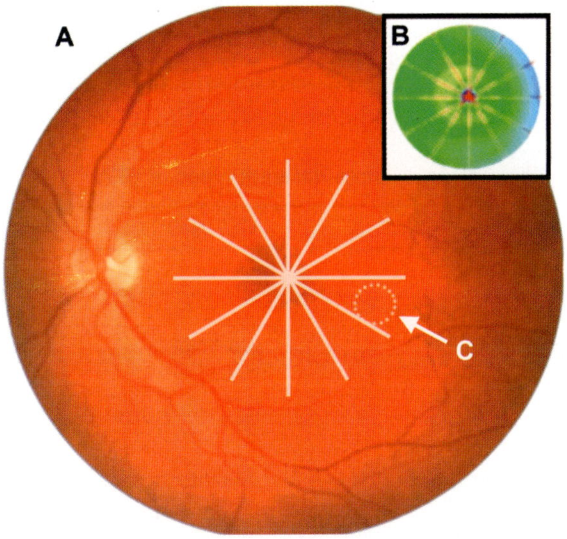

Figure 1.3: (A) The white lines on this fundus image indicate the locations of the six radial line B-scans performed by Stratus OCT. (B) Red lines show points measured by Stratus OCT, and non-red points are estimated. (C) Example of a focal lesion that could be missed by the radial-line protocol

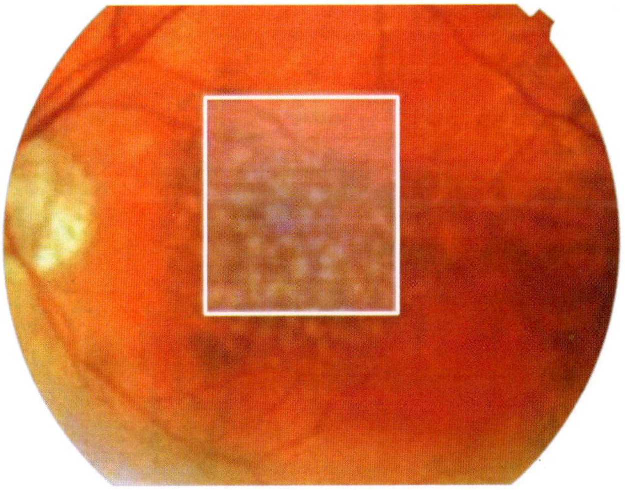

Figure 1.4: Examples of data from the Topcon 3D OCT-1000 instrument showing: Dense grid of B-scans (from the area with the soft drusen) (Courtesy: Yijun Huang, Topcon Medical Systems, Inc.)

In contrast, 3D OCT captures a dense, uniform grid of data that is unlikely to miss small, focal lesions (Figure 1.4). Furthermore, the consistency of the information allows blood vessels on the scans to be aligned between patient visits, and comparison of scans to other diagnostic imaging modalities, such as fluorescein angiograms.

ROLE OF OCT IMAGING

OCT is useful in the diagnoses of diseases, staging of diseases which help in their management, assessing the response of disease to treatment and in monitoring the progress of the disease.

Comparison of three different types of OCT

Features	*Conventional OCT*	*UHR-OCT**	*3D OCT*
Measurement principle	Time Domain	Time Domain	Spectral Domain
Measurement capabilities	A-scan B-scan	A-scan B-scan	A-scan B-scan C-scan 3D-scan
Light source	Superluminescent diode laser	Femtosecond Sapphire laser	Superluminescent diode laser
Wavelength	820 nm	815 nm	840 nm
Bandwidth	25 nm	125 nm	50 nm
Axial resolution	10 μm	3 μm	5 μm
Transverse resolution	20 μm	15-20 μm	<20 μm
Scanning speed	1.3 sec	4 sec	0.05 sec
Dilatation	Required	Required	Not required
Macular scan	6 radial scans	6 radial scans	Raster scan

* *Ultra High Resolution*

Various types of Spectral/Fourier Domain OCT are commercially available:

1. TOPCON - 3D OCT-1000
2. TOPCON - 3D OCT-2000
3. OTI - OCT/SLO
4. OPTOVUE - RTVue-100
5. OPTOPOL - SOCT COPERNICUS
6. HEIDELBERG - SPECTRALIS HRA + OCT
7. CARL ZEISS MEDITEC - CIRRUS HD-OCT

SUGGESTED READING

1. Sunitha R, Andrew MR, Jonathan ER, Siavash Y, Volker W, David SB, et al. Real-time optical coherence tomography of the anterior segment at 1310. Arch Ophthalmol. 2001;119:1179-85.
2. Tony H Ko, Andre J Witkin, James G Fujimoto, Annie Chan, Adam H Rogers, Caroline R Baumal, et al. Ultrahigh-Resolution Optical Coherence Tomography of Surgically Closed Macular Holes. Arch Ophthalmol. 2006 June; 124(6): 827-36.

2 3D OCT-1000

HOW 3D OCT-1000 WORKS

Optical coherence tomography (OCT) is a method by which light from a defined light source (typically a super luminescent diode [SLD] producing light at approximately 850 nanometer wavelength) is split into two separate beams. One of the two beams is passed over the surface of a tissue being analyzed, such as the retina, before being

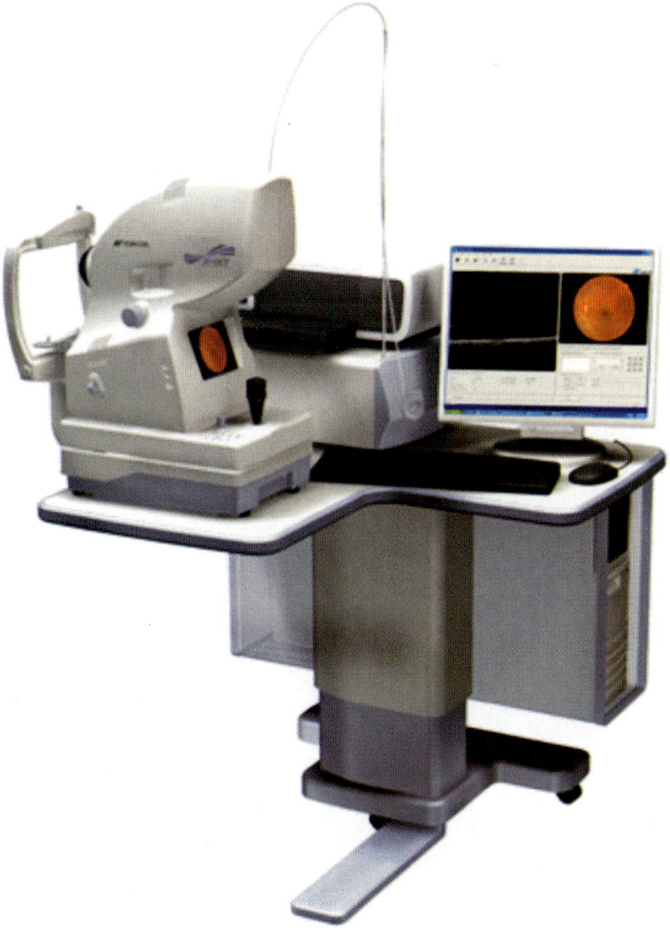

Figure 2.1: Topcon 3D OCT-1000

reflected back to a light sensor. The second half of the original beam, known as the reference beam, is reflected off a mirror rather than the retina before returning to the same light sensor. By adjusting the distance of the reference mirror (and thus the time it takes for the reflected light to reach the sensor) and comparing the two light beams, time domain OCT devices measure the optical backscattering of light, and describe a pixel representation of the anatomic layers within the retina.

Instead of adjusting the position of the reference mirror, the TOPCON 3D OCT-1000 (Figure 2.1) optical coherence tomography system records the interferometric information using a Fourier domain spectrometric method, allowing for an increase in the scanning speed (~18,000 A-scan/sec). Through an integration with the TOPCON non-mydriatic retinal camera, 3D OCT-1000 provides high-resolution cross-sectional B-scan OCT images (up to 4096 resolution) and three-dimensional volumetric images to cover up to 6 × 6 mm of the retinal area. The acquired 3D OCT data are further viewed and analyzed by this software (Figures 2.2 and 2.3).

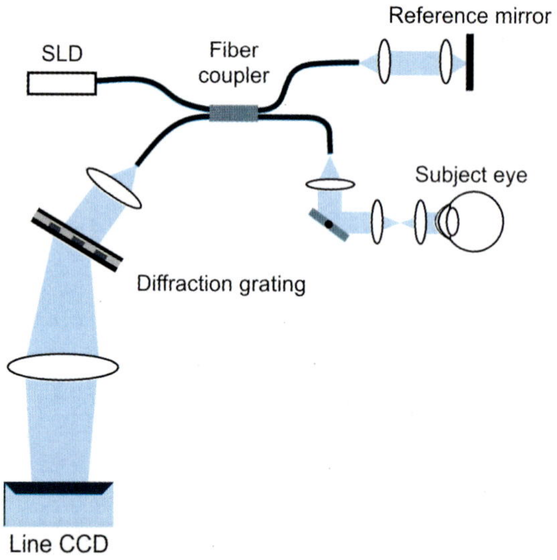

Figure 2.2: Diagrammatic representation of principle of OCT imaging

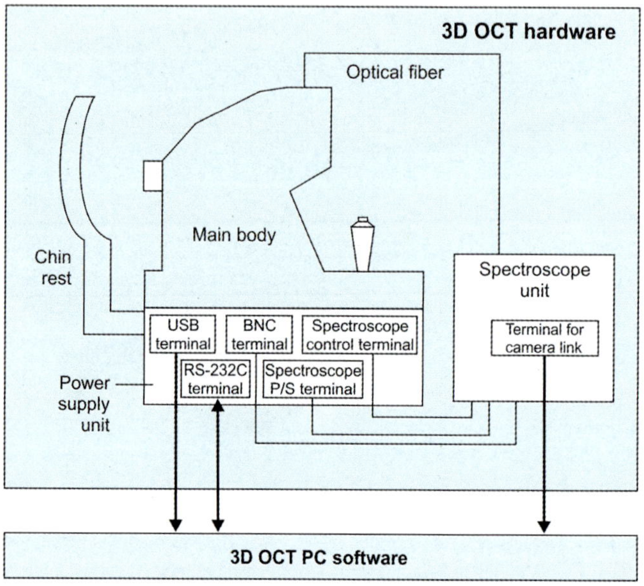

Figure 2.3: Diagrammatic cross-section of 3D-OCT

The 3D-OCT-1000 is composed of four main components:

- Main body
- Chin rest unit
- Power supply unit
- Spectroscope unit

The specifications for the 3D-OCT-1000 optical systems for observing and photographing the fundus are as follows:

- Angle of view for photographing: 45° ± 7% or less. Digital zoom available: 2X and 4X
- Photographable diameter of pupil: 45° (φ 4.0 mm or more)

Digital zoom	:	φ 3.7 mm or more
Scanning range on fundus	:	6 × 6 mm ± 5%
		4.5 × 4.5 mm ± 5%
		3 × 3 mm ± 5%
Frame rate - B-scanning mode	:	5 Hz or more (variable)
Frame rate - 3D-scanning mode	:	0.2 Hz or more (variable)
Lateral resolution	:	20 μm or less
In-depth resolution	:	6 μm or less

NAVIGATING THE 3D OCT-1000 PROGRAM

Start and Exit the 3D OCT-1000 Program

To Start 3D OCT-1000:

1. Click the start button to open the Start menu on the taskbar.
2. Choose Programs and then choose TOPCON → 3D OCT-1000 → 3D OCT-1000 from the sub-menu. The 3D OCT-1000 PC software main window will be displayed (Figure 2.4).

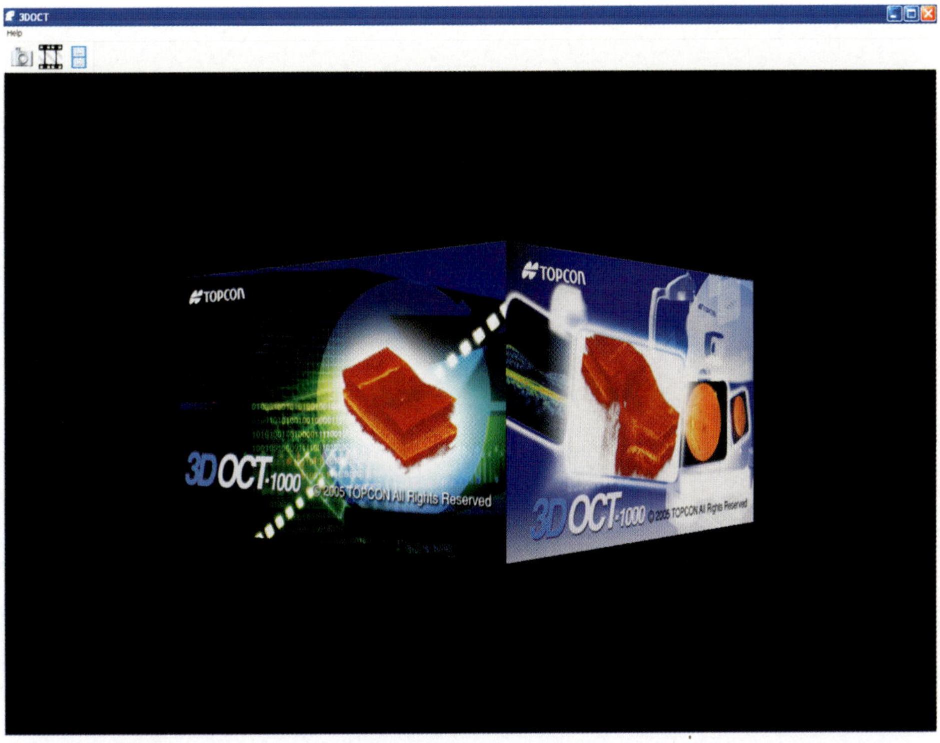

Figure 2.4: Opening screen

To Exit 3D OCT-1000:

Click the Close icon 

The 3D OCT-1000 program is organized in the following three categories: Capture, Analyze and Data Management. The user can select the desired operation by clicking on the respective icon on the tool bar.

3 Capturing and Analyzing 3D OCT Scans

Capturing images in 3D OCT-1000 usually requires the following steps:

1. Prepare the patient.
2. Enter patient information.
3. Select OCT scan pattern (in live mode).
4. Align and optimize OCT scans (in live mode).
5. Capture.
6. Review (playback) captured scans.
7. Save or delete captured scans.

PREPARE THE PATIENT

The 3D OCT examination is very similar to a nonmydriatic retinal camera screening, and is usually short in duration and comfortable for the patient. The patient is usually required to maintain the best fixation possible to capture the best OCT images. Therefore, a brief orientation to the patient as to what he or she is expected to "look at" and when to "blink" and "don't blink" is usually helpful to start the capture session.

3D OCT-1000 is capable of capturing both OCT and fundus images with pupils as small as 4 mm in diameter. Thus, pupil dilation using a mydriatic agent is optional. On the other hand, it is generally easier to obtain images of adequate signal strength through a larger pupil. If no mydriatic agent is applied, it is recommended to dim the room lights so that the pupil will naturally dilate slightly.

To Start the Capture Session

1. Click the Capture icon 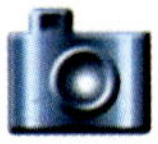 on the toolbar.
2. The Register Patient dialog appears (Figure 3.1).

To Register a New Patient

1. Fill in the patient information fields in the dialog box.
2. Click the OK button.
3. You may add additional information by clicking the More... button (Figure 3.2).
4. If the patient information already exists in the database, click the Select Patient... button and choose the corresponding patient from the patient list.

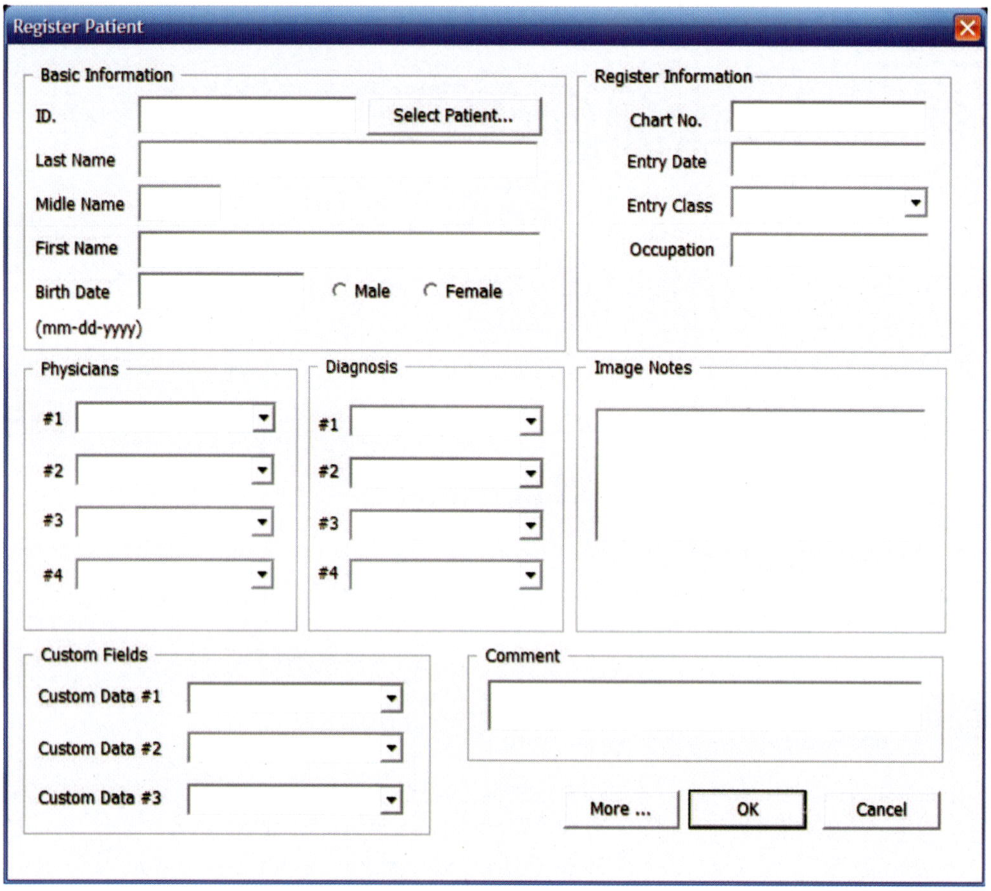

Figure 3.1: Registration screen

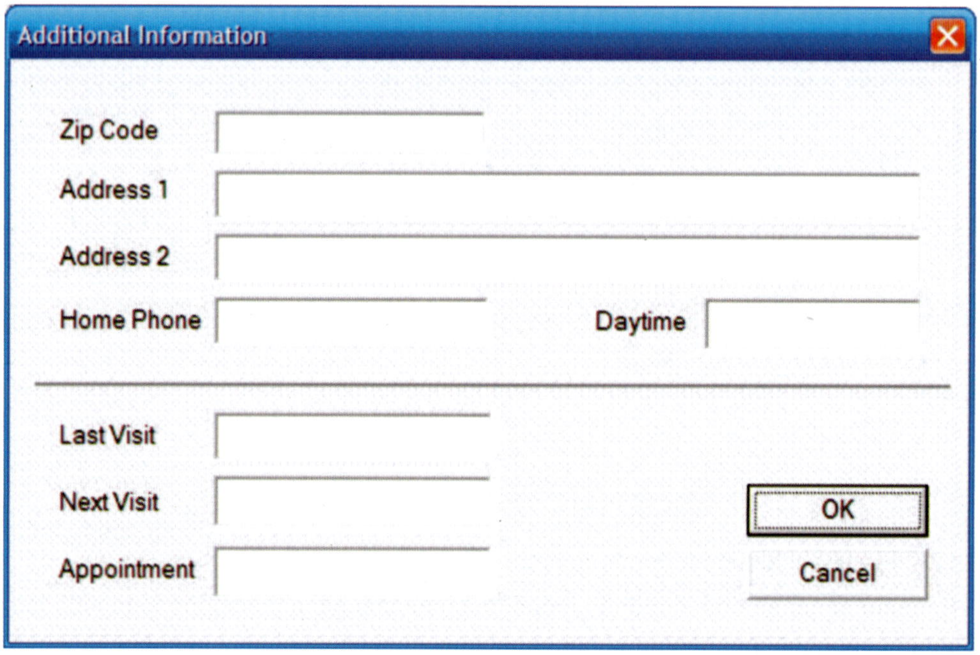

Figure 3.2: Additional registration screen

The Patient ID code and name must be specified. Other information fields may be optional. Date of birth and gender information may be required, should the user make them mandatory. In addition, except for the Patient ID, all fields are editable.

After the patient information is entered, 3D OCT-1000 PC software will automatically enter the "Live" mode (Figure 3.3).

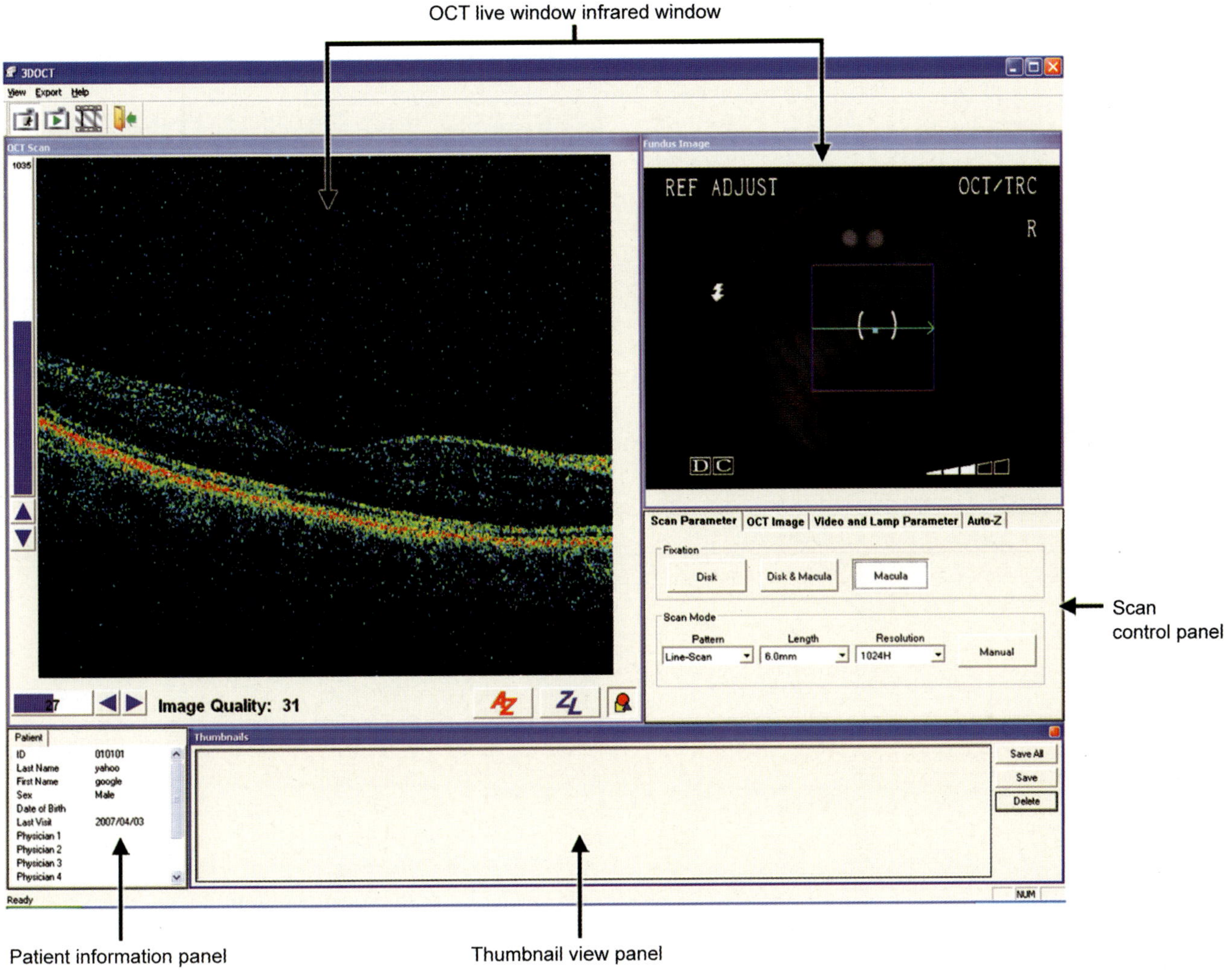

Figure 3.3: Live window in capture mode

The OCT data is usually represented by a thumbnail, which consists of two parts. For a regular B-scan, the top is the miniature OCT B-scan and the bottom is the associated miniature color fundus photo. For a 3D-scan, the top is the miniature OCT B-scan at the center location and the bottom is the miniature projection image. These are the thumbnails for a Line-scan and a 3D-scan (Figure 3.4).

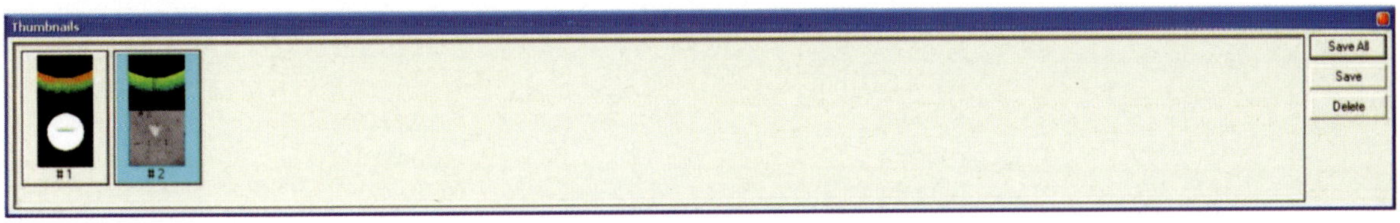

Figure 3.4: Thumbnails display

Once the Capture window is live, the first step is to select the proper OCT scan protocol for data acquisition. The operator chooses the desired scanning protocol from the Scan Mode drop-down menus in the Scan Parameter tab (Figure 3.5).

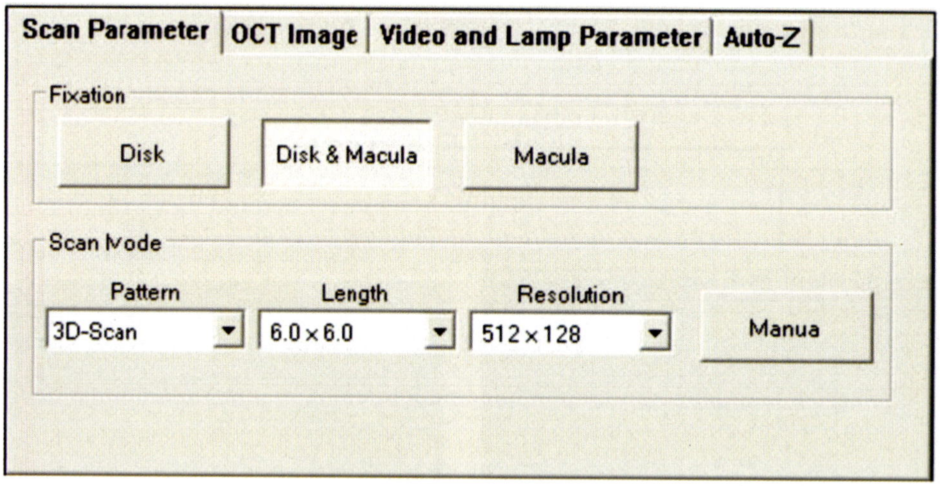

Figure 3.5: Scanning protocol window

3D OCT-1000 is capable of scanning the retina in a number of predefined scan patterns, areas and densities, as listed in the following table.

Type of scan	*Scan area*	*Scan density*
3D	6.0 × 6.0 mm	256 × 256 512 × 128 512 × 64 512 × 32
3D	4.5 × 4.5 mm 3.0 × 3.0 mm	256 × 256 256 × 128 256 × 64 256 × 32
Line Scan	6 mm	1024H – H = Horizontal 2048H 4096H 1024V – V = Vertical 2048V 4096V
Line Scan	4.5 mm	1024H – H = Horizontal 2048H 1024V – V = Vertical 2048V
Line Scan	3 mm	1024H – H = Horizontal 1024V – V = Vertical
Circle Scan	3.0 mm 2.4 mm	
Cross Scan	6.0 × 6.0 mm 4.5 × 4.5 mm 3.0 × 3.0 mm	1024 2048
Radial Scan	6.0 mm 4.5 mm 3.0 mm	1024 2048

Next, the operator selects the proper fixation method for patients. 3D OCT-1000 has both internal fixation and external fixation. The operator chooses the desired fixation protocol from the Fixation buttons (Disc, Disc and Macula, and Macula) in the Scan Parameter tab based upon the section of the patient's retina that needs to be scanned. These steps are performed to setup the patient for the examination:

1. Seat the patient comfortably on an exam stool or exam chair.
2. Adjust the table height or chair height so the patient can relax with their chin placed centrally on the chin rest and forehead against the forehead rest.
3. Adjust the height of the chin rest so the outside corner of the patient's eye is level with the Canthus marker on the chin rest post (Figure 3.6).
4. Use the joystick to pull the instrument backwards toward the operator. For optimal results, the patient should focus on the internal green fixation target in the center of the display.
5. Move the instrument in all directions until the patient's eye is in the center of the monitor.

ALIGN AND OPTIMIZE OCT SCANS

These steps need to be performed to align the retinal image.

1. On the video monitor, bring the ( ) (Figure 3.7) scale towards the patient's pupil. Make sure the patient's pupil is larger than the ( ) scale. Comparison of the ( ) scale and the eye determine whether the pupil is large enough for retinal photography.
2. The Z offset has to be adjusted in order to align the retinal image within the display. This may be accomplished by two methods. Each method should be performed separately:
   a. Turn the lower set of left and right knobs on the 3D OCT-1000 to adjust the two white curved lines so they are synchronized.
   b. Select the up and down arrows on the left side of the display by clicking and holding the left mouse button. Turn the knobs or hold the mouse button until the retinal image is displayed. Adjust as necessary to achieve the optimum image.

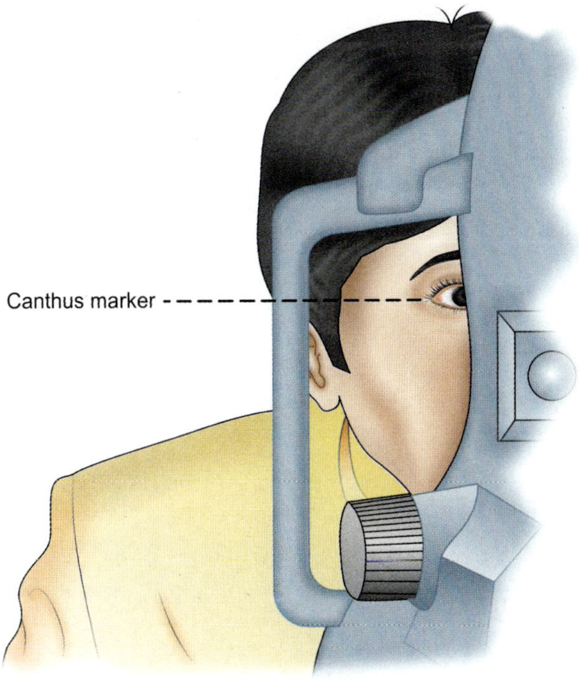

Figure 3.6: Patient position

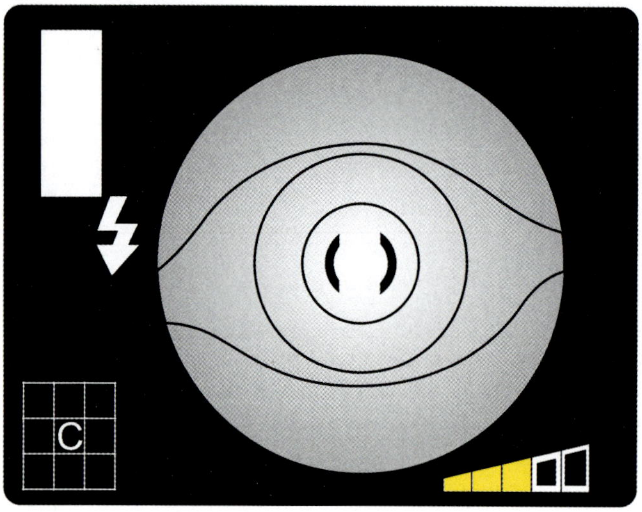

Figure 3.7: Bracket for alignment

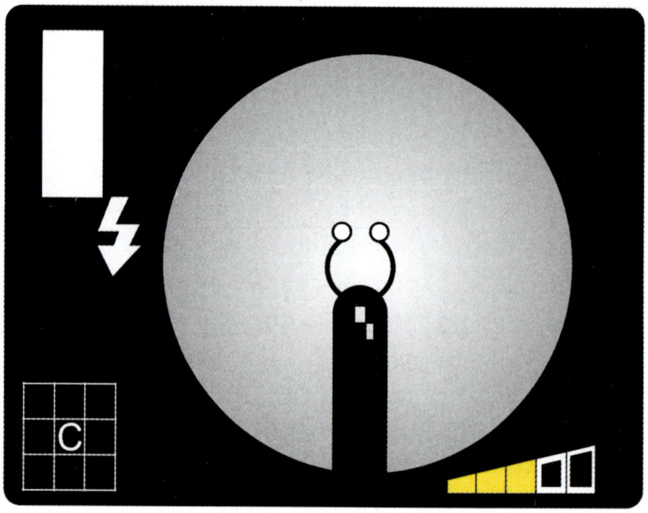

Figure 3.8: Bright spots

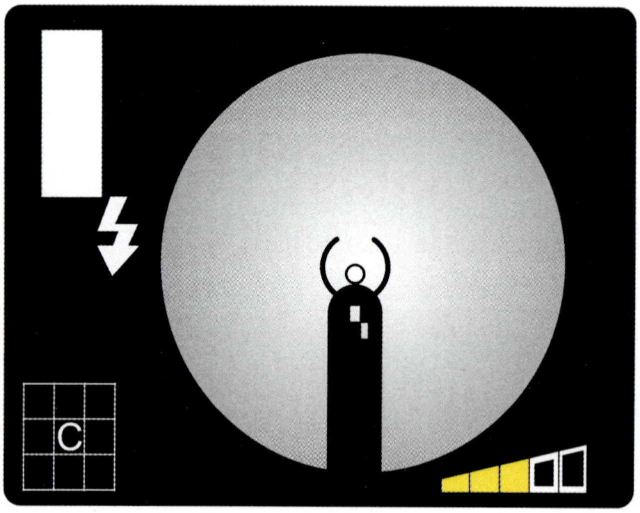

Figure 3.9: Proper alignment

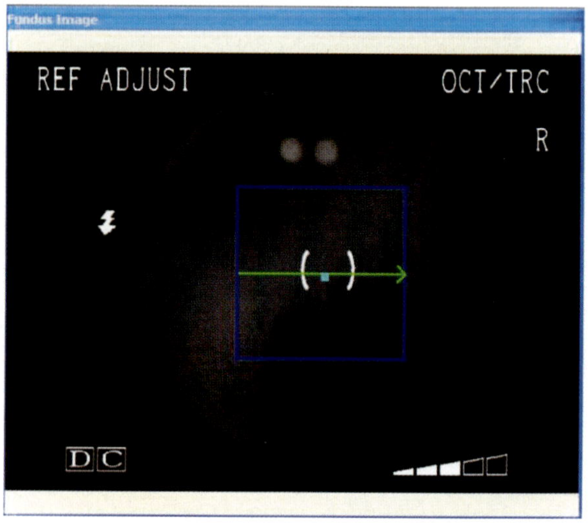

Figure 3.10: Screen view of fundus image

3. Bring the 3D OCT-1000 closer to the patient until two bright spots become visible (Figure 3.8).
4. These two bright spots need to be aligned by moving or twisting the joy stick to form one dot. This dot is referred to as the Focus Dot.
5. Align the Focus Dot within the ( ) scale on the video monitor (Figure 3.9).
6. The Focus Bar is a vertical line in the center of the image on the 3D OCT-1000. Use the focusing knob to align it with the retinal image.
7. The final focus is achieved by turning the upper set of left and right focusing knobs on the 3D OCT-1000 to adjust the retinal image (Figure 3.10).

CAPTURE

To capture an image, click the button on the joystick or the Capture button in the Auto-Z tab and create a Thumbnail View.

The patient is asked to try not to blink while the image is being captured. (Figures 3.11 and 3.12)

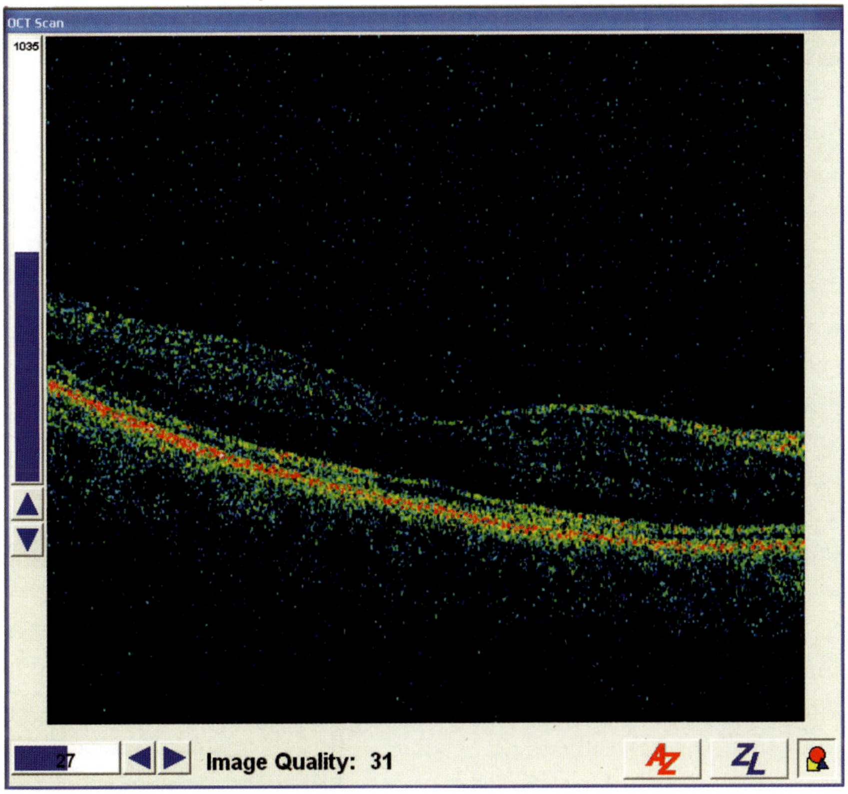

Figure 3.11: 2D image in capture mode

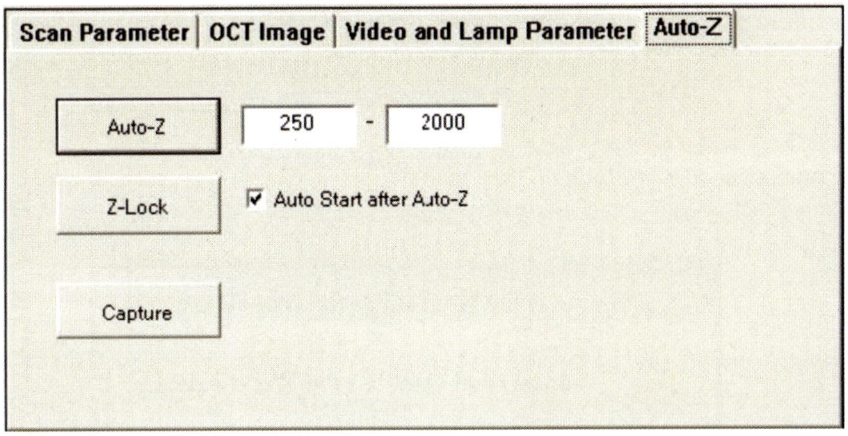

Figure 3.12: Scan parameter

The OCT data is captured and saved temporarily in the hardware following image downloading and processing. A thumbnail of OCT data will be added to the Thumbnail View panel, and the Live Capture window will automatically start again (Figure 3.4).

After the OCT scans are captured, the quality of the captured data can be evaluated by immediately entering the playback mode. Double click on a thumbnail in the Thumbnail View panel or click the Playback icon on the tool bar.

To Evaluate a B-scan

1. A B-scan has no scroll bar.
2. Zoom in and out with the right mouse button.
3. Drag the scan with the middle mouse button.
4. Once the scan is saved, it can be analyzed by clicking the Analyze icon on the tool-bar. However, the analysis will be limited to only a 2D view.

To Evaluate a 3D Scan

1. A 3D-scan has a scroll bar. Therefore, the scroll bar can be used to view different portions of the scan.
2. Zoom in and out with the right mouse button.
3. Drag the scan with the middle mouse button.
4. Once the scan is saved, it can be analyzed by clicking on the Analyze icon on the toolbar. The scan can be analyzed in both 2D and 3D.

Once the captured OCT scans are reviewed, the user determines if they should be deleted or saved to the database.

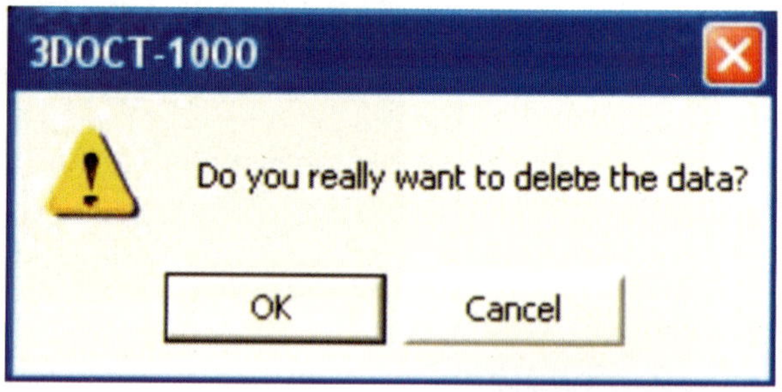

To Delete a Scan

1. Highlight the thumbnail in the Thumbnail View panel.
2. Click the Delete button in the Thumbnail View panel.
3. Confirm the deletion. Click the OK button.

To Save a Scan

1. Highlight the thumbnail in the Thumbnail View panel.
2. Click the Save button in the Thumbnail View panel. The label on the thumbnail will change to "Saved".

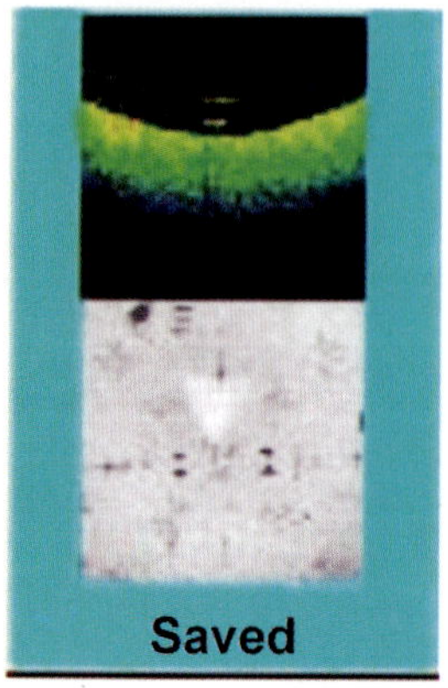

To Save all Scans

1. Click the Save All button in the Thumbnail View panel.
2. Confirm the choice to "Save All". Click the OK button.

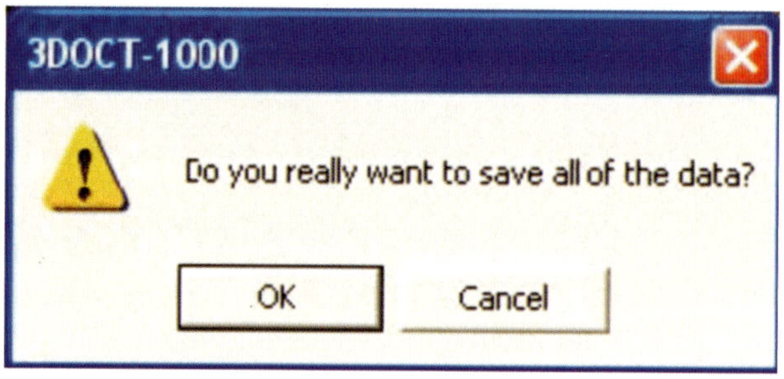

ANALYZING 3D OCT SCANS

Once the OCT scan is selected, the user automatically enters the View mode for data evaluation. In most cases, users are more familiar with OCT B-scan images than OCT 3D images. To facilitate a user's transition from conventional B-scan images to 3D image analysis, the 3D-OCT viewing window has 2D and 3D tabs available for 3D scans. By default, the Viewing mode always starts with 2D mode.

If the OCT data record is a conventional B-scan (line scan), cross scan, or circle scan, it is only displayed in 2D mode.

The 3D OCT viewing window consists of the following five sub-windows (Figure 3.13):

1. Primary OCT Viewing Area... (Window A)
2. En face Image Viewing Area... (Window B)
3. Auxiliary OCT Viewing Area... (Window C)
4. Patient and Scan Information... (Window D)
5. Image Processing Controls... (Window E)

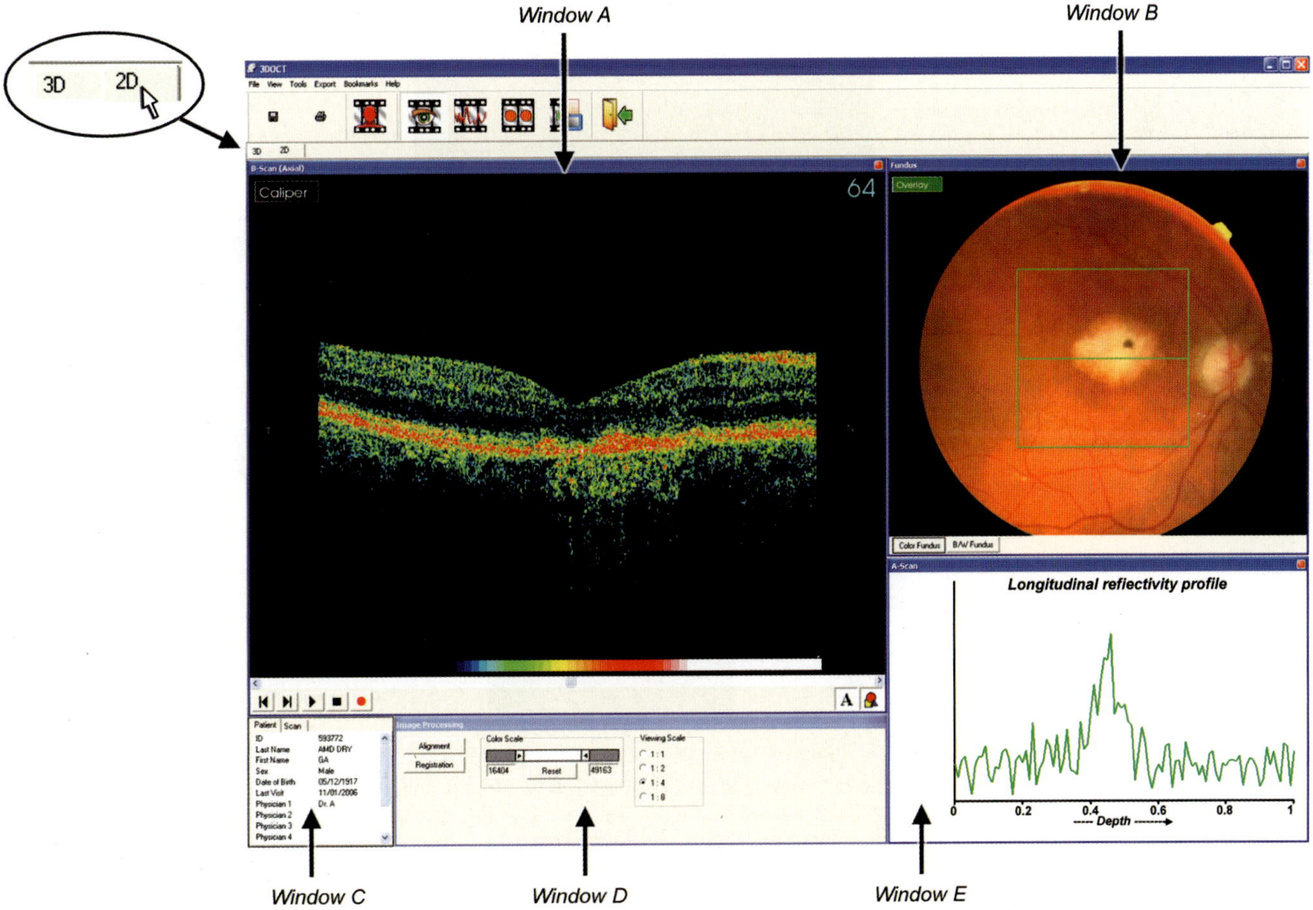

Figure 3.13: Viewing window

One of the powerful features of the 3D OCT software is the tight interaction between OCT data and en face fundus images (Windows A, B and C).

One of the significant features in 3D OCT Software is to provide direct correlation between OCT scans with the corresponding en face retinal images, which are shown in Window B (Figure 3.14). There are four types of retinal images for OCT correlation:

- Nonmydriatic color fundus image
- B/W infrared image
- Projection image
- Reference image

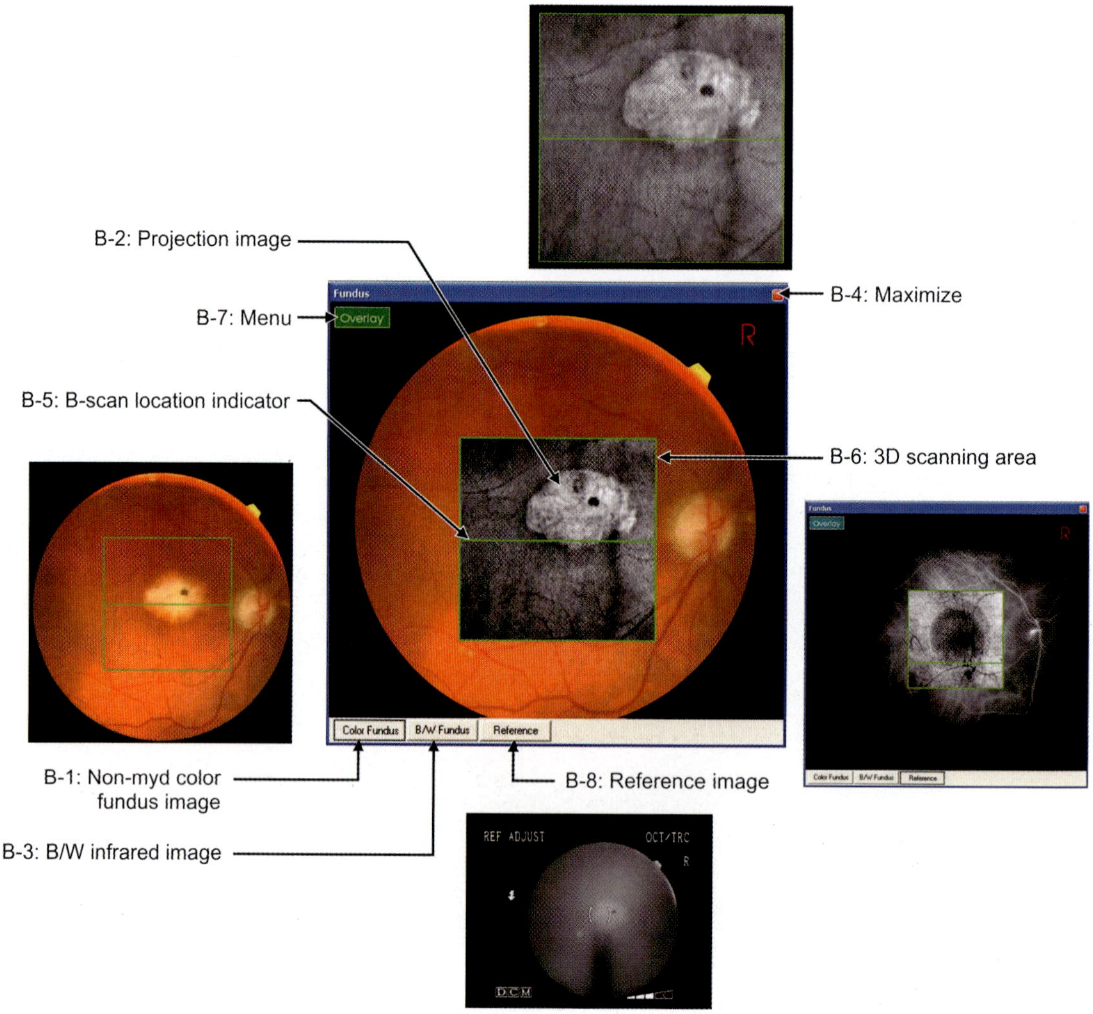

Figure 3.14: En face image viewing area

B-1: Nonmydriatic color fundus image B-2: Projection image of 3D OCT data B-3: B/W infrared fundus image B-4: Maximize this sub-window or return to its original size. B-5: B-scan location indicator shows where the B-scan image is acquired. B-6: 3D scanning area B-7: Menu button (Overlay -Projection and Reposition are sub-menus for Overlay.) B-8: Reference image

Pin-Point Registration™

In conventional OCT examination, the patient is requested to fixate on the fixation LED target for a period of a few seconds. Small eye movements are, however, difficult to prevent during this short duration. This reduces the confidence in data analysis as where in the retina the OCT scans were obtained, and consequently reduces the confidence to associate the pathology seen in OCT scans with the pathology seen in en face retinal images.

Projection Image (Figure 3.15)

3D-OCT provides a unique opportunity to solve this particular problem, with the introduction of the "projection image". A projection image is created by summing all data points in the 3D OCT data longitudinally, and is usually displayed as a B/W image. Interestingly, the retinal features (for example, blood vessel pattern) are visible in the projection image, while mathematically there is a pixel-to-pixel correspondence between the projection image and a 3D OCT A-scan.

3D OCT software takes advantage of this unique characteristic of the projection image and applies advanced computer algorithms to achieve a clinically-useful operation called Pin-point Registration™.

Automatic Registration

3D OCT software uses advanced pattern recognition algorithms to register the "projection image" with the accompanying fundus photos.

To Perform Automatic Registration

1. Click the Registration button in the Image Processing window (Window E).
2. A projection image will appear within the boundary in the Fundus window (Window B), as shown below. If the automatic registration algorithm is successful, a letter "R" is also displayed at the upper right corner in the Fundus window. The projection image in the boundary should also look properly aligned with the fundus image (Figure 3.16).

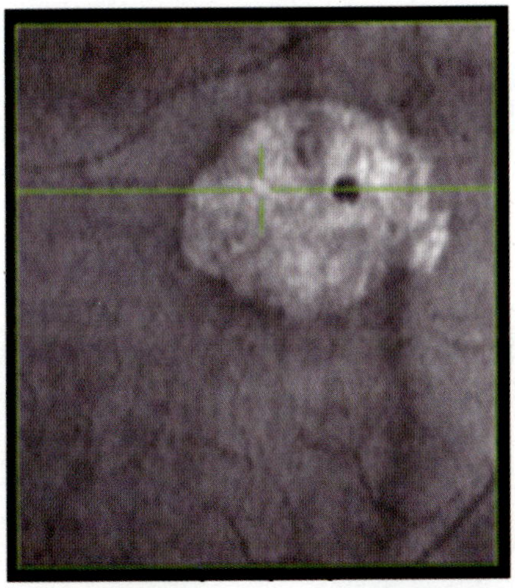

Figure 3.15: Projection image

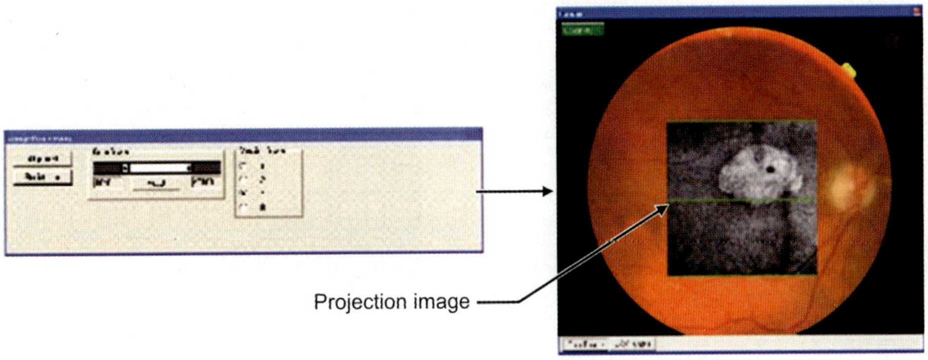

Figure 3.16: Automatic registration

The automatic registration may fail when the projection image does not provide enough features for registering. In this case, the "R" letter will not be displayed. The user may choose to register the projection image manually.

To Perform Manual Registration

1. Hold down the <Shift> key on the keyboard and drag the middle mouse button at the same time.
2. The projection image will become transparent to allow the user to move and align to the appropriate position of the fundus image (Figures 3.17 and 3.18).

Corresponding Locations (Figure 3.19)

Once the projection image is registered properly with the fundus image, the 3D OCT data is linked with the fundus image with pin-point proximity. 3D-OCT software provides a user-friendly interface to enable the user to gain additional insight on the intrinsic correspondence between the features seen in fundus images and features seen in OCT scans at any given locations, by simple mouse clicks.

In Fundus Window B, double click on a specific point of interest. The point location is shown as a green line with cross hash-mark, where the green line corresponds to the location of the resultant B-scan, Also, the center of the cross hash-mark corresponds to the location of the white line on the B-scan and the A-scan shown on the Auxiliary OCT Window (Window C).

Alternatively, the user can also double click on the any locations in the B-scan image, and the corresponding points will be marked on the fundus image.

The quality and precision of pin-point registration™ depends on the quality of the projection image. When blink, saccade, and other large eye movements occur during the image capture, the confidence of determining the exact correspondence between OCT and fundus images may be compromised.

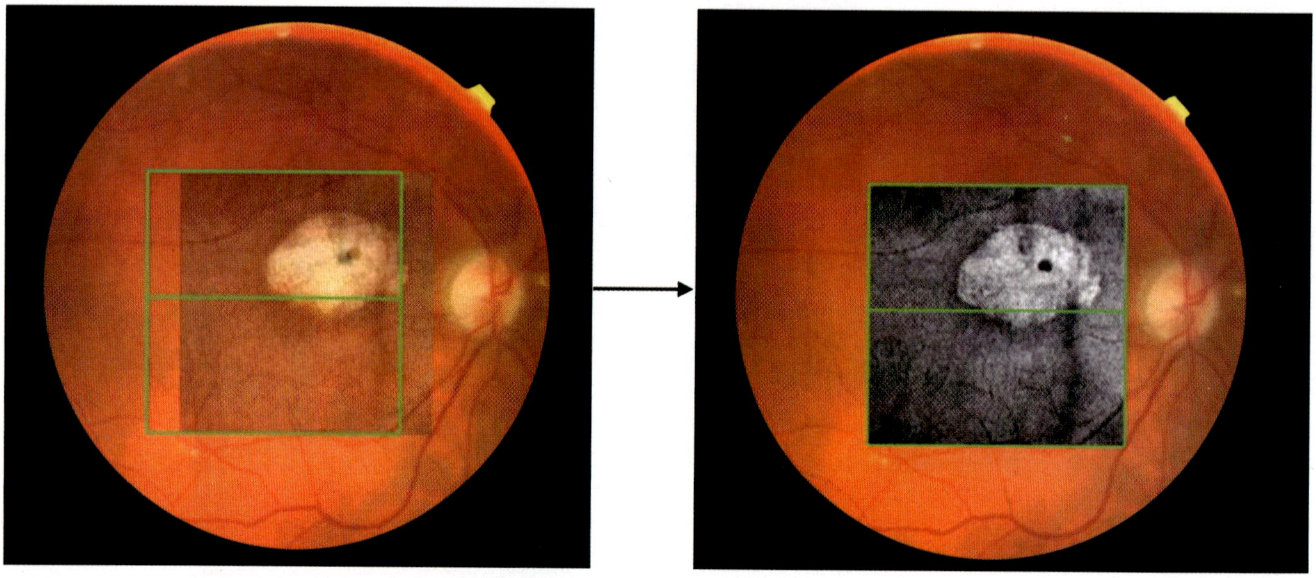

Figures 3.17 and 3.18: Manual registration

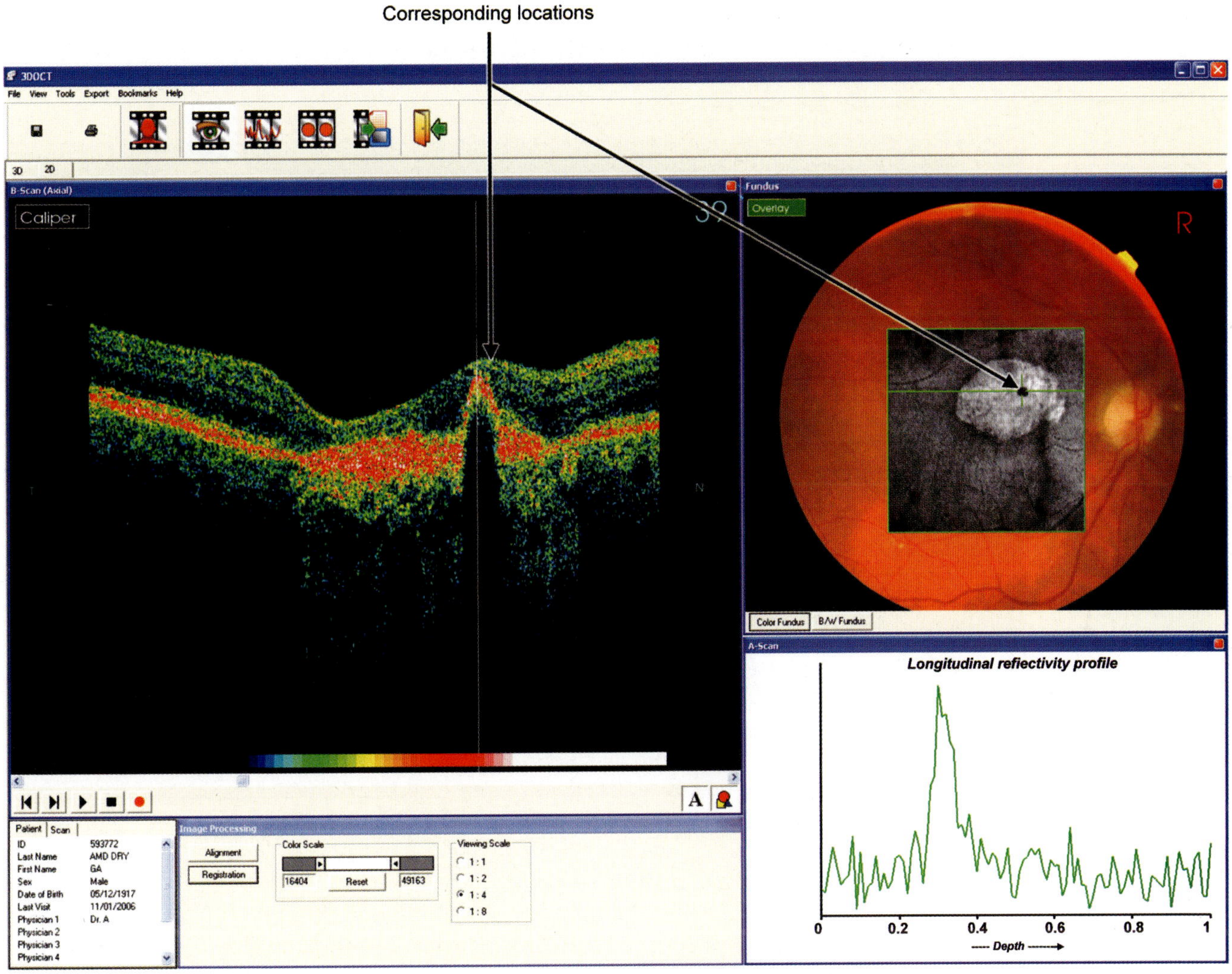

Figure 3.19: Viewing window showing correlation

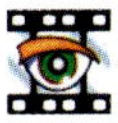 3D OCT Software also provides the user 3D volumetric rendering capability for in-depth analysis of 3D OCT data. This 3D mode can be initiated by selecting the 3D tab in the 3D OCT Viewing window (Figure 3.20).

If the OCT data record is a Radial or Volume window, the record is displayed in 2D mode. However, the 3D and 2D tabs are both available. This allows the user to view the record in both 2D and 3D modes.

For a 3D scan, the 3D mode is similar to the 2D mode, except that the volumetric rendering image is now shown in the Primary OCT Viewing Area (Window A) and 2D images are shown in the Auxiliary OCT Viewing Area (Window C).

However, for a radial scan, the radial rendering image is now shown in the Primary OCT Viewing Area (Window A) and 2D images are shown in the Auxiliary OCT Viewing Area (Window C). The radial rendering has no Volume menu, it only has a Slicing menu, and the Slicing menu has no submenus.

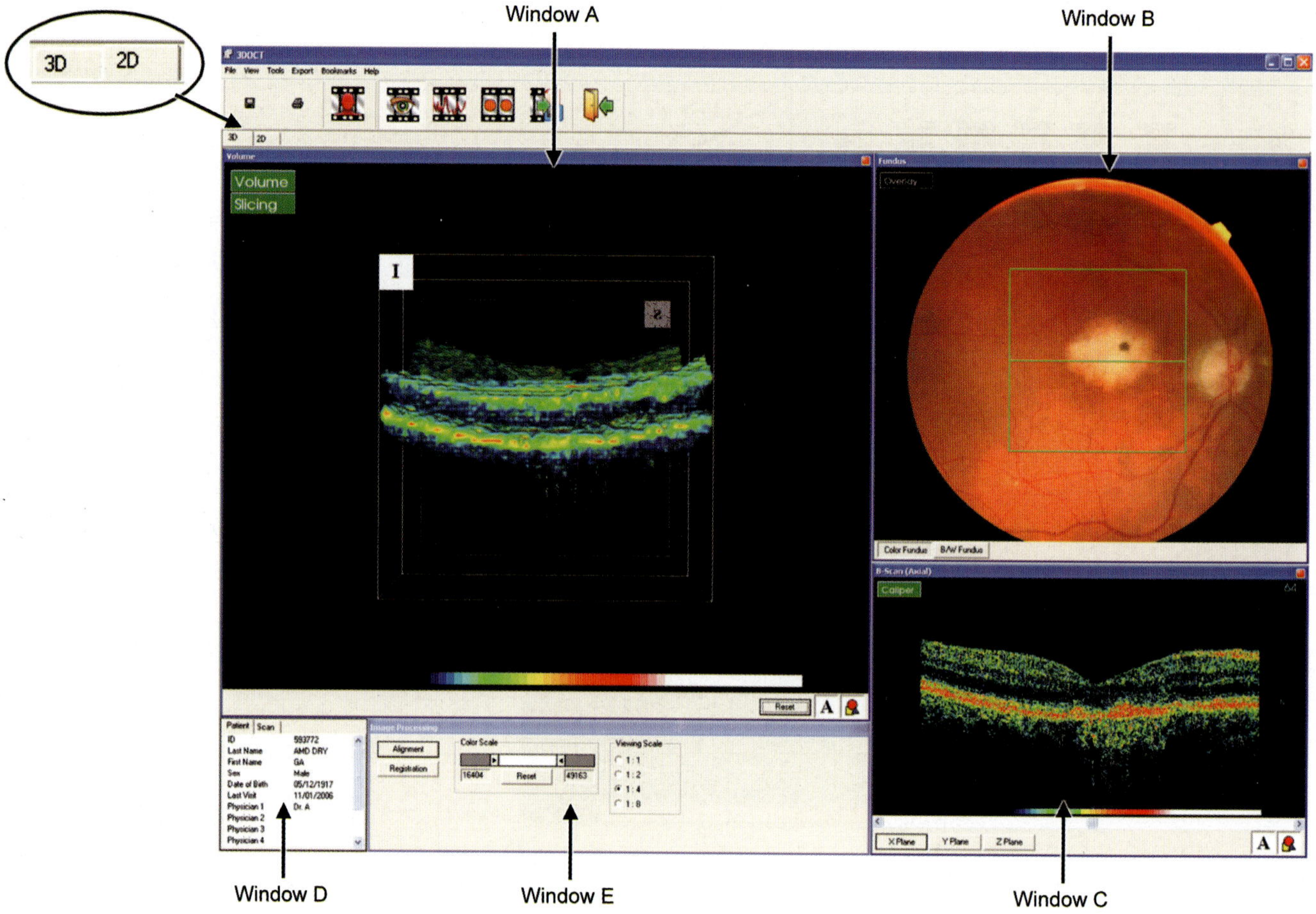

Figure 3.20: Analysis window

X-, Y-, Z-planes and Slicing

The 3D OCT volumetric data is created by obtaining horizontal sequential B-scans in a raster pattern. Naturally, the X-, Y- and Z-planes are defined in the following fashion:

X- plane—the horizontal B-scan as it is acquired. Note that the anatomical OCT features shown in the X-plane are "real" since the eye movement is negligible. Y-plane—the vertical "reconstructed" B-scan. The eye movement in this "reconstructed" B-scan is quite noticeable. Z-plane—also called Coronal scan, or C-scan. This is a reconstructed en face image.

The relationship among the X-, Y-and Z-plane images with the 3D volumetric rendering is best viewed by turning on "Slicing" (Figure 3.21).

Cropping

In order to visualize the pathology located inside the 3D rendered image, the user may need to crop off portions of the 3D rendered image (Figure 3.22). 3D-OCT Software provides an easy-to-use tool to accomplish this task.

Click the Volume—Cropping buttons and the "Cropping" handles will appear as shown. The user will use the mouse to select the desired "cropping" handle and drag it to push/pull the corresponding surface. The underlying 3D rendered image will change accordingly.

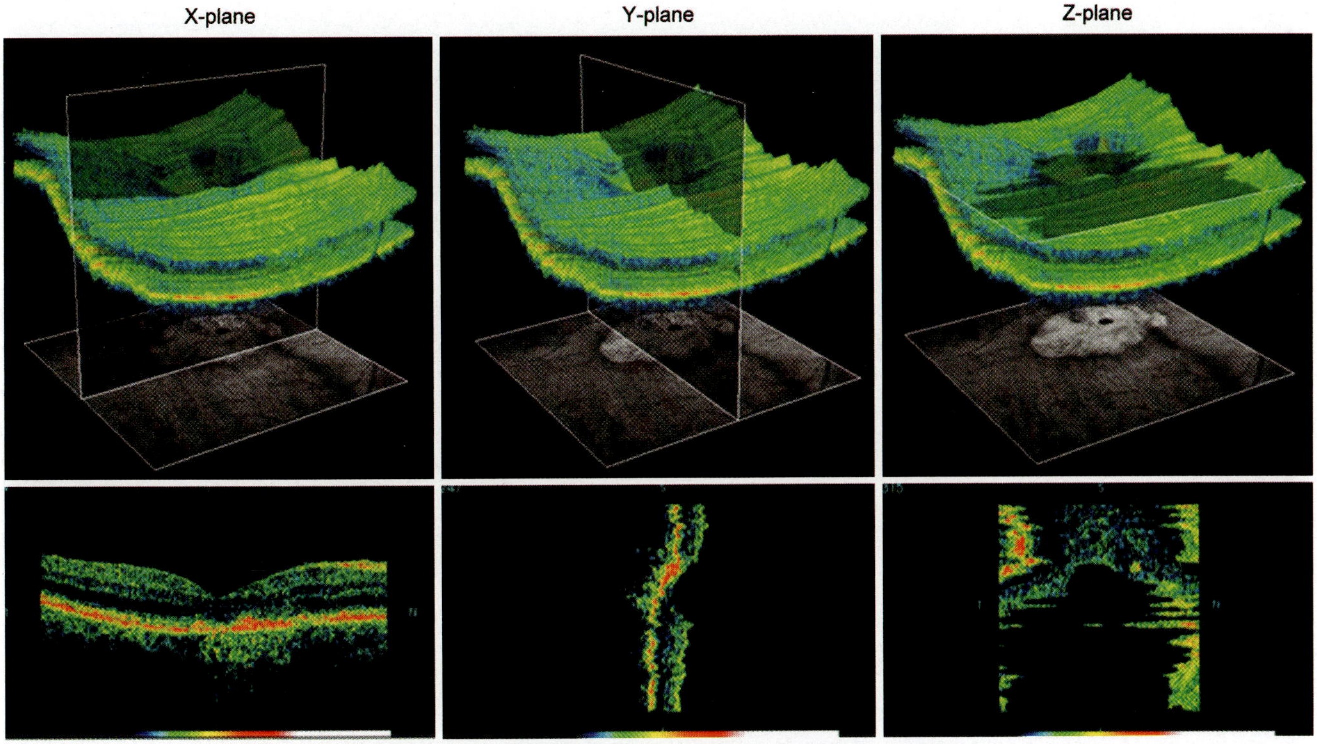

Figure 3.21: Slicing in various planes

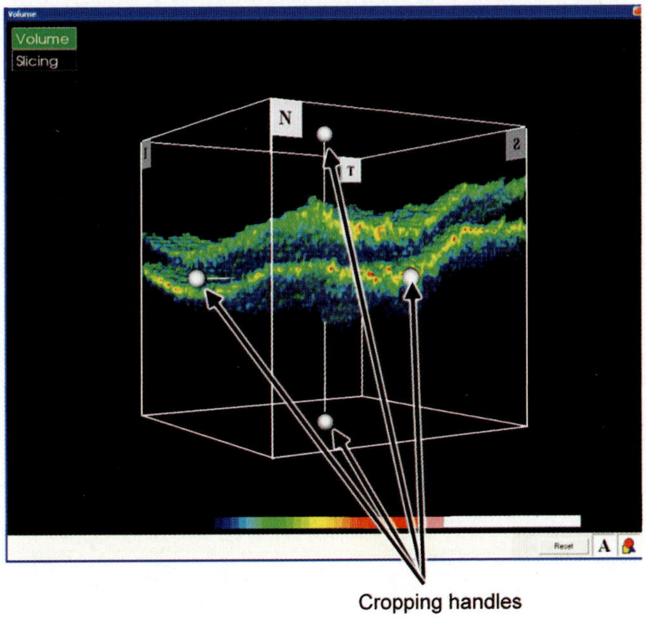

Figure 3.22: Cropping handles

Peeling and Layer Separation options are additional functions that can be found in the Volume window. These functions are performed mainly in the 3D mode. A user can utilize these options to investigate and separate layers of the 3D image view (Figure 3.23). These layers are analogous to the white outline boundary layers in the 2D mode.

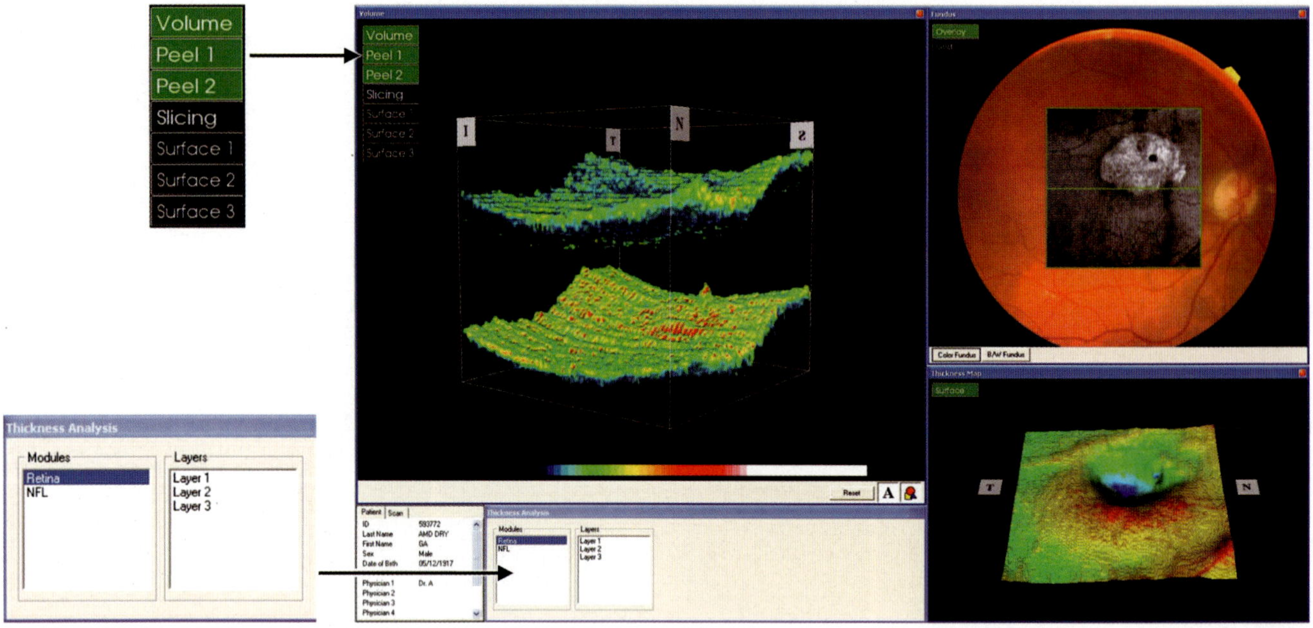

Figure 3.23: Peeling window

First, select 3D mode viewing from top-left menu bar. Keeping all other options deselected, select the Volume → Peeling buttons in the 3D Volume window. The Peel 1 and Peel 2 buttons are now available.

To "peel" layers: Select either the Peel 1 or Peel 2 button to peel away the desired layer.

To separate layers: Select either the Peel 1 → Move or Peel 2 → Move buttons to separate the desired layer. Move the selected layer by scrolling with the middle mouse button until the desired separation distance has been achieved.

To reset "Peeling" and Layer Separation process: Repeat the separation process in reverse to return to the original shape.

Compare Results (Optional) 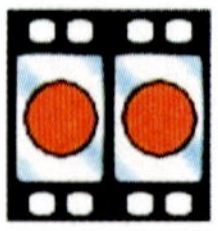

If applicable, a user can compare scan results of different sessions for each patient.

First, select the Compare ("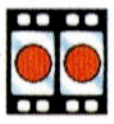") button from the top menu bar. In the generated Compare Image windows, Fundus and 2D scan image views are displayed as an overview.

A new Compare window is displayed at the bottom of the Compare Image windows, as pictured right. A user can utilize these window functions to upload record data and sychronize data for comparison. (Figure 3.24)

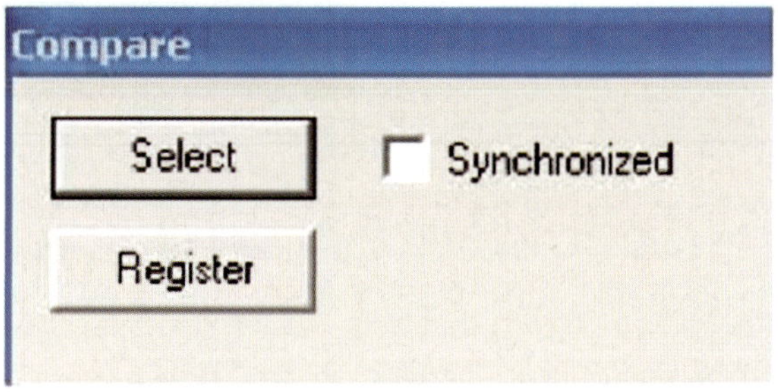

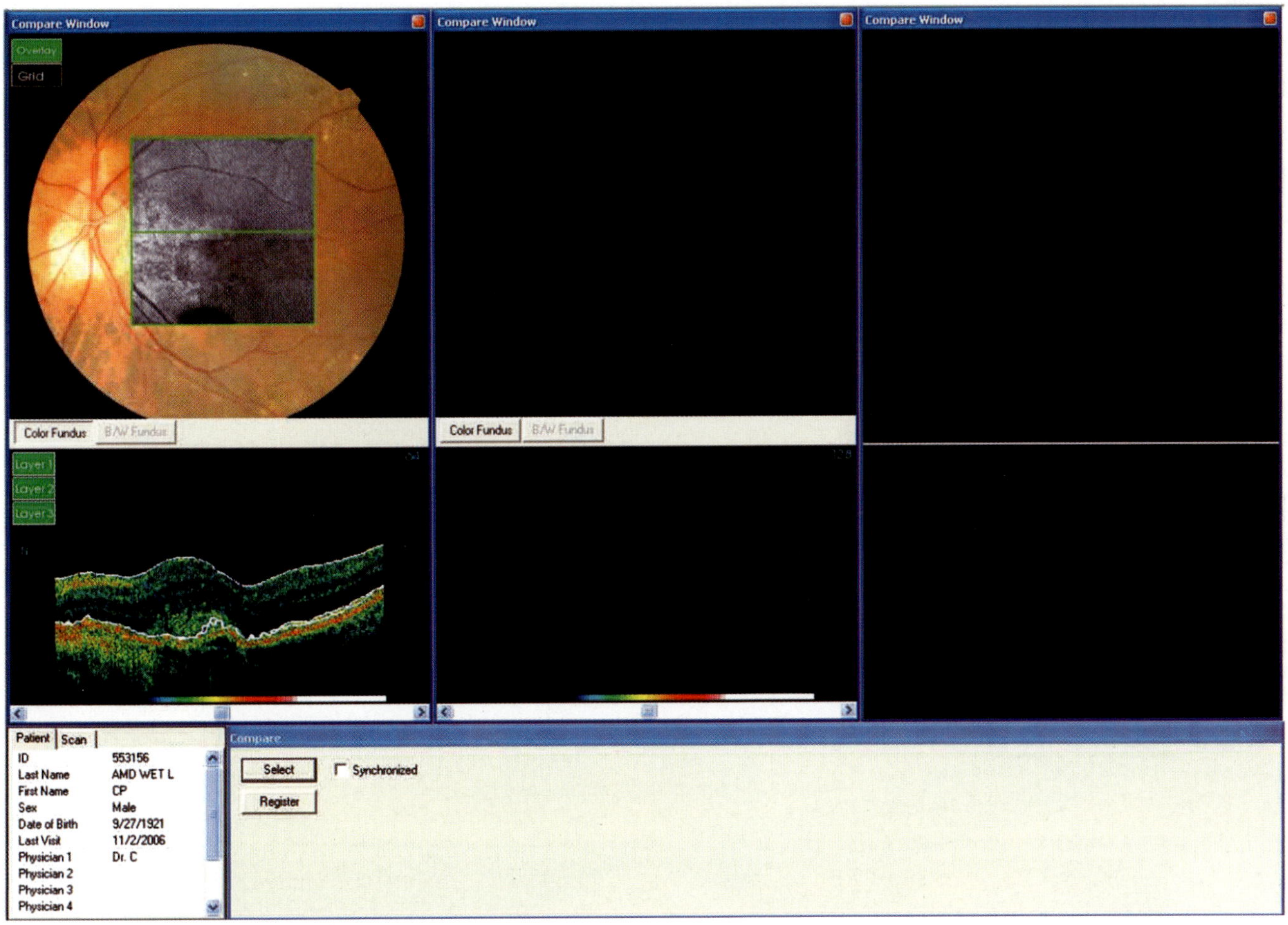

Figure 3.24: Comparison window

> ⚠ *Caution:* When you use "Compare" function, you have to use a pair of data for same condition in order to take an image.

1. Press the Select button in the Compare window. This launches a pop-up Select Record window, which displays all other analysis records performed for this patient (Figure 3.25).

To Perform Results Comparison

1. Check the synchronized checkbox to enable the Pin-point Registration™ application and to display interlinked images for comparison (Figure 3.26).
2. There are additional options in the Compare Image window. Users have the same options as in the Fundus window:

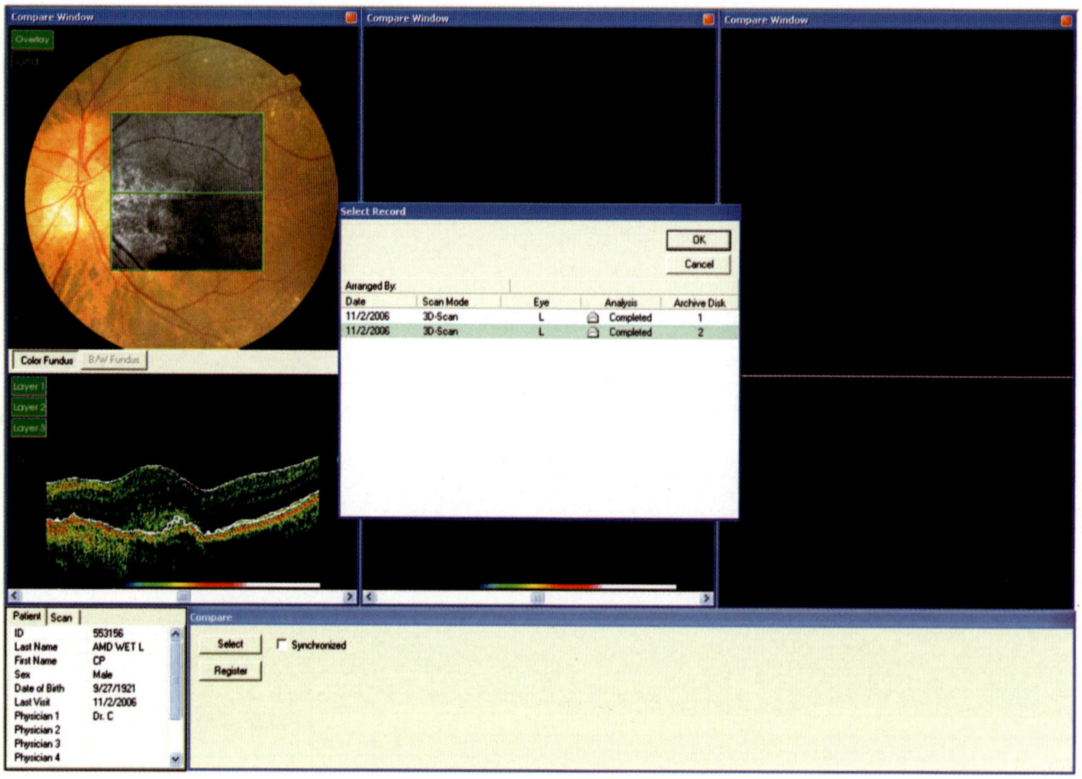

Figure 3.25: Comparison window add record

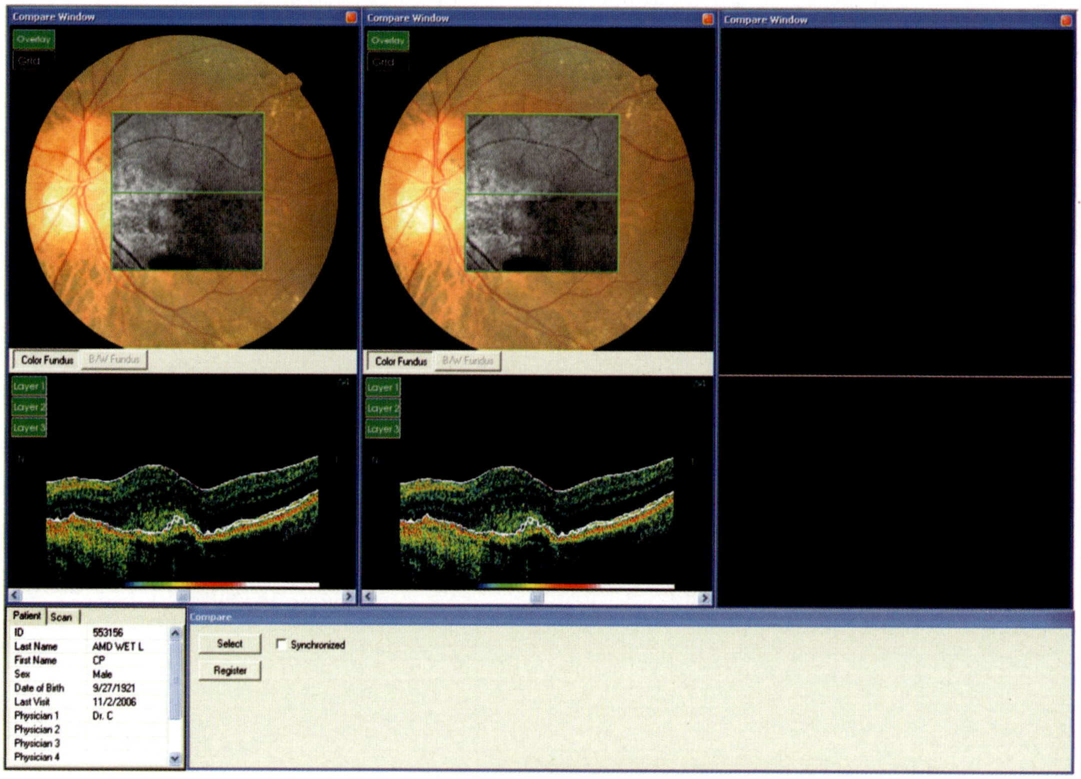

Figure 3.26: Compared image

Overlay

1. Projection (default)
2. Shadowgram
3. Thickness map
4. Reposition

Grid

1. Rectangular (Figure 3.27)
2. ETDRS

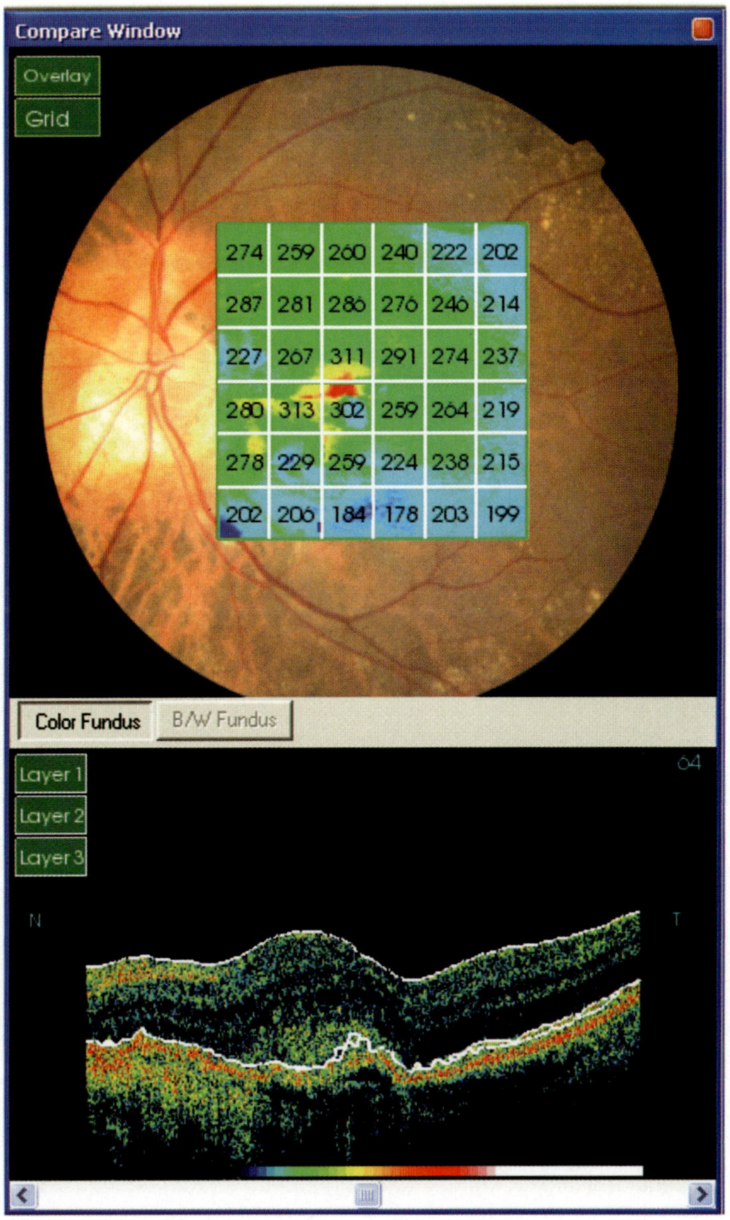

Figure 3.27: Rectangular grid overlay

Make Movies

Select Movies tab on the top-left menu bar. Three windows are generated as follows (Figure 3.28):

a. 3D volume image
b. Movie control menu
c. Patient and scan information

> *Caution:* Make sure that no other windows or images are blocking or placed over the volume window during the movie-saving/recording procedure.

The volume image window is displayed on the right side, with its different display parameters (Cropping, Peeling, Slicing, Surface 1-3 and Volume).

For a radial scan, cropping and peeling are disabled since these functions are not applicable to this type of scan.

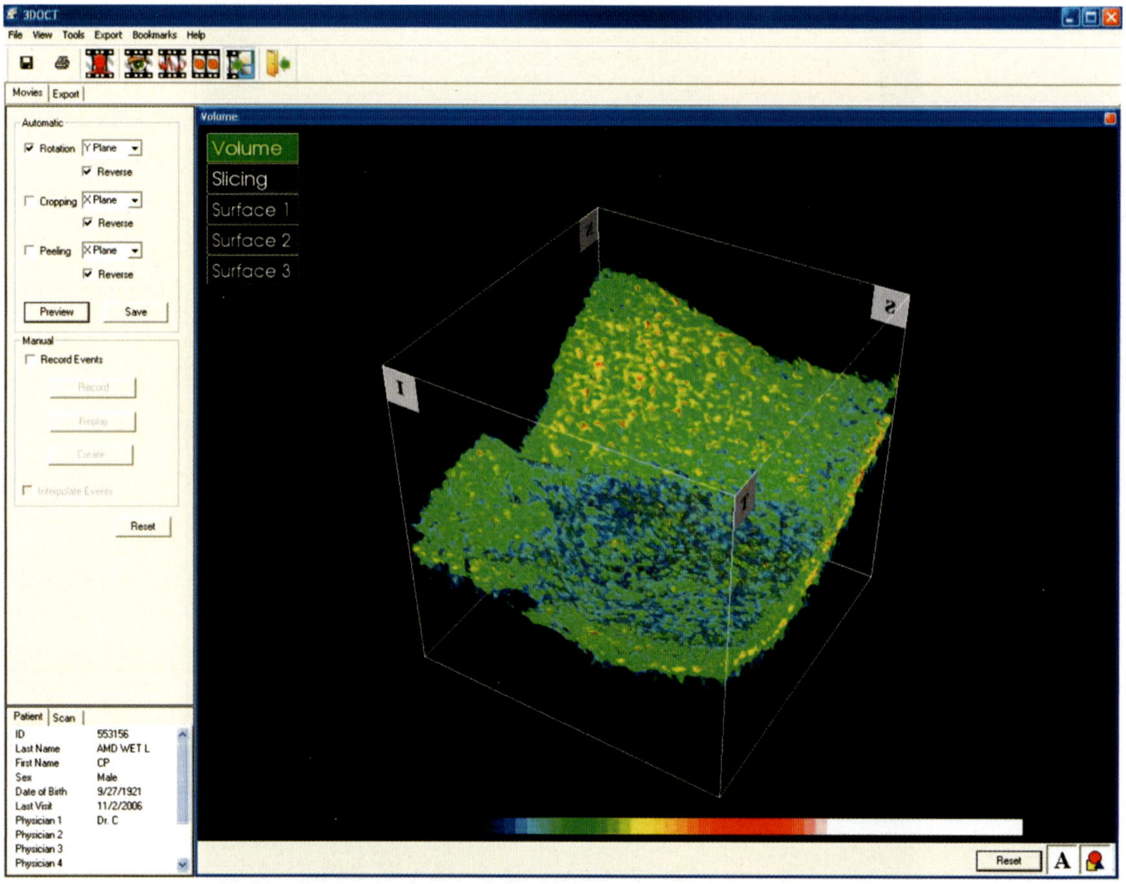

Figure 3.28: Movie window

Make Pre-arranged Movies—Automatic

a. Parameters (Figure 3.29):
   i. Rotation - (X-plane, Y-plane and Z-plane) and Reverse box.
   ii. Cropping - (X-plane, Y-plane, Z-plane, XZ-planes and XZY-planes) and Reverse box.
   iii. Peeling - RPE, (X-plane, Y-plane and Z-plane) and Reverse box.
b. Select among the above parameters to make an automatic movie.
c. Press Preview button.
d. (Optional) Press STOP in the process pop-up window to abort previewing procedure.
e. Repeat Steps (b) and (c) until desired affect is achieved.
   Press Reset button to restart the movie making process with the selected image.

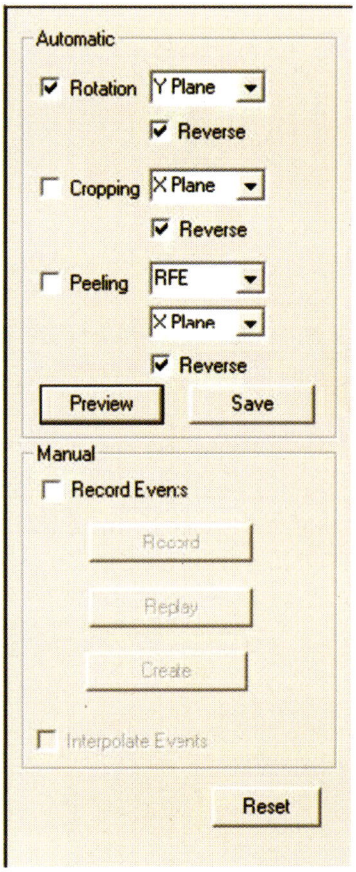

Figure 3.29: Movie option

Make sure that the Volume window is clear of any blocking images or other windows.

- Select Save button and in the pop-up Save-As window, enter the File name and press Save button.
- (Optional) Press STOP in the process pop-up window to abort saving procedure - Movie file will be saved up to that point.

Make Custom Movies—Manual

If you would like to make a movie where you control all the events, select this option. Your mouse movements will determine the final product.

- Check the Record Events checkbox to create a movie by recording your mouse movements.
- The manual parameters (Record, Replay and Create) are automatically enabled, while the Preview and Save buttons in the Automatic section are disabled.

Make sure that the Volume window is clear of any blocking images or other windows.

- Press the Record button.
- Using your mouse, apply manual movements such as cropping, peeling, rotation, slicing, zooming, or translating to the image in the Volume window.
- When done, press the Stop button.
- To preview, press Replay button.
- Repeat Steps (c) to (f) until desired effects are achieved. Press Reset button to restart the movie making process with the selected image.
- Note: If you would like to smooth out any jerky hand movements, check the Interpolate check box.
- Select Create button and in the pop-up Save As window, enter the File name and press the Save button.

SUGGESTED READING

1. User Manual 3D-Optical Coherence Tomography (3D-OCT)-1000.

4 3D OCT-2000

The Topcon 3D OCT-2000 is the first Spectral Domain OCT system to incorporate a high resolution fundus camera and a user-friendly color touch screen display in a compact space saving design. However, the resolution remains the same as the 3D OCT 1000 at 5 to 6 microns but the scanning speed has improved to 27,000A-scans/sec.The incorporation of a new software algorithm provides better color contrast of the B scan.

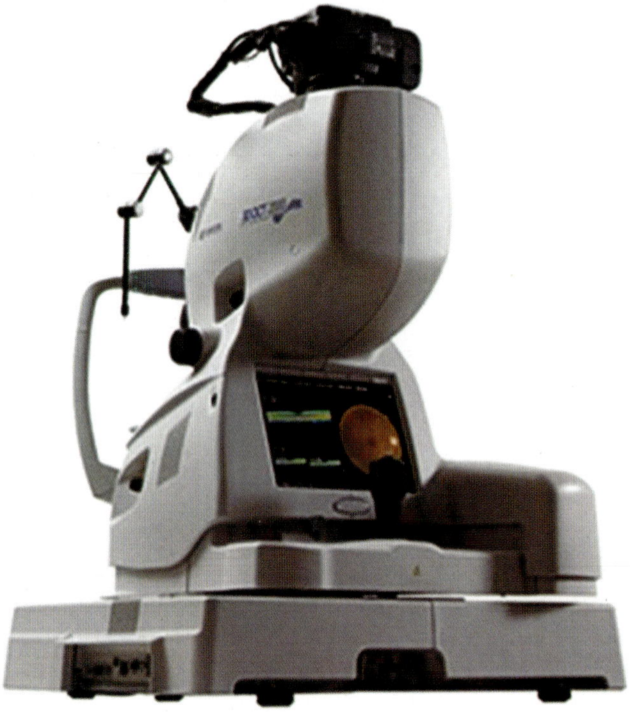

Figure 4.1: Topcon 3D OCT-2000

The 3D OCT-2000 is composed of the following three units:

- Main body unit
- Power supply unit
- Chin rest unit

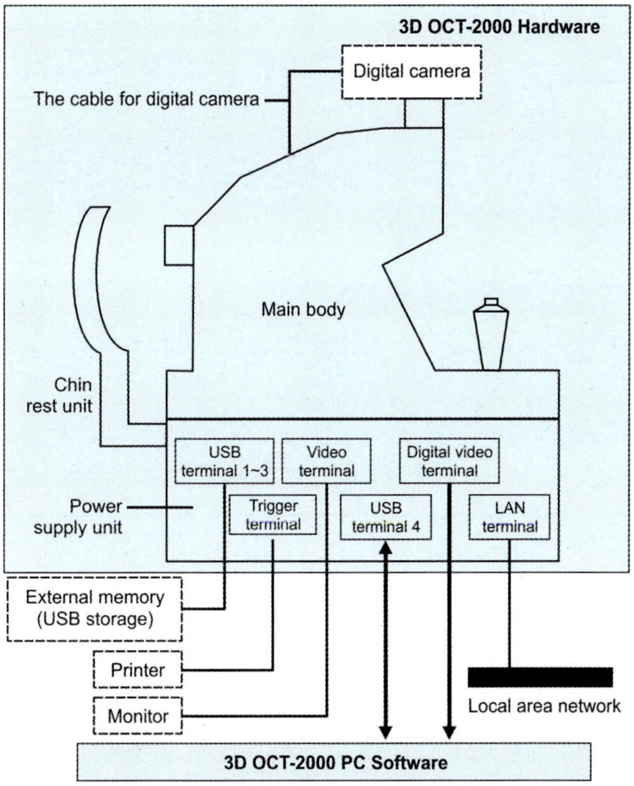

Figure 4.2: Diagrammatic cross-section of 3D OCT-2000 (*Courtesy:* Topcon 3D OCT-2000 Manual)

The 3D OCT-2000 has several advantages over the 3D OCT-1000.

1. **Display monitor:** It has a touch screen display monitor which enables quick and easy navigation (Figure 4.3).
2. **Scan size:** A larger scan size of 8.2 mm makes it possible to scan the optic disc and macula at one time (Figure 4.4).
3. **Anterior segment imaging** (Figures 4.5 to 4.15):
   - Cornea
     i. The epithelial layer, Bowman's membrane and endothelial layer can be demarcated (Figures 4.7 and 4.8)
     ii. It is possible to obtain central corneal thickness measurement, horizontal and vertical radius of curvature measurements and distribution of the corneal thickness (Figure 4.9).
     iii. Corneal abnormalities can be recognized (Figure 4.10)
   - Anterior chamber angle can be measured using the caliper tool (Figures 4.11 to 4.13).
   - Iris abnormalities can be visualized (Figures 4.14 and 4.15)
4. **Glaucoma**
   - Optic disc parameters can be obtained directly by scanning the disc in the 3D mode (Figure 4.16).
   - The autosearch function detects and tracks the optic disc position automatically thus enabling faster acquisition of the circle scan for RNFL analysis (Figure 4.17)
   - RNFL trend analysis is another new feature.
5. **Fundus photography:** An integrated high resolution (12.3MP) fundus camera makes it possible to capture even the periphery through an undilated pupil (Figure 4.18).

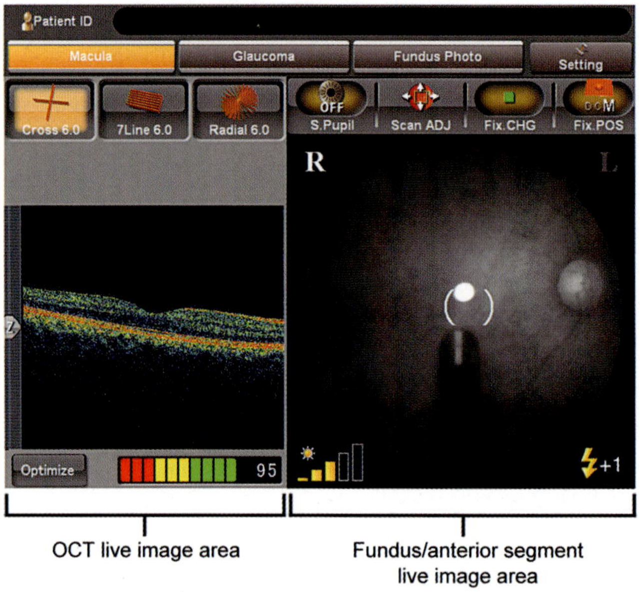

Figure 4.3: Touch screen (*Courtesy:* Topcon 3D OCT-2000 Manual)

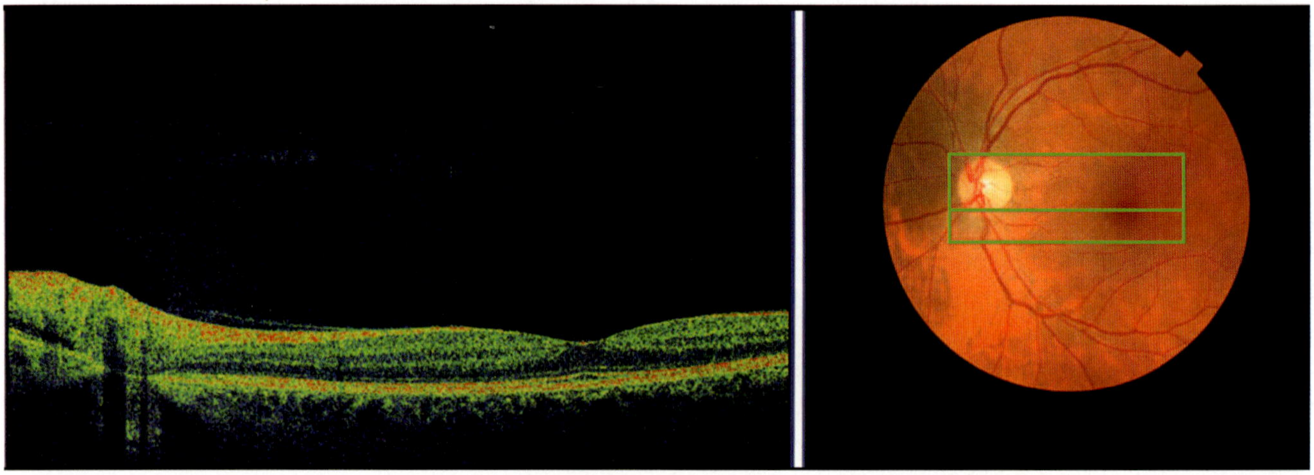

Figure 4.4: 8.2 x 3.0 mm scan showing disc and macula

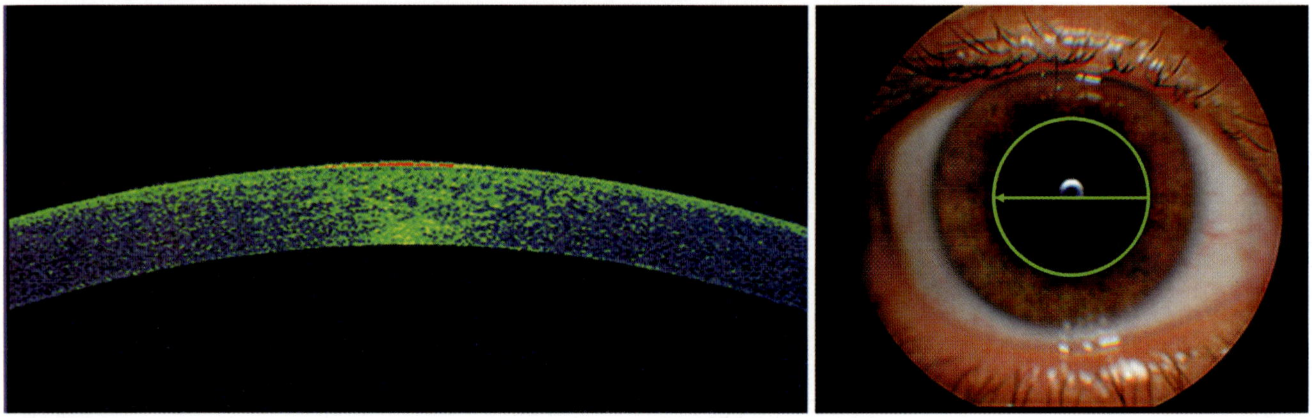

Figure 4.5: Normal cornea

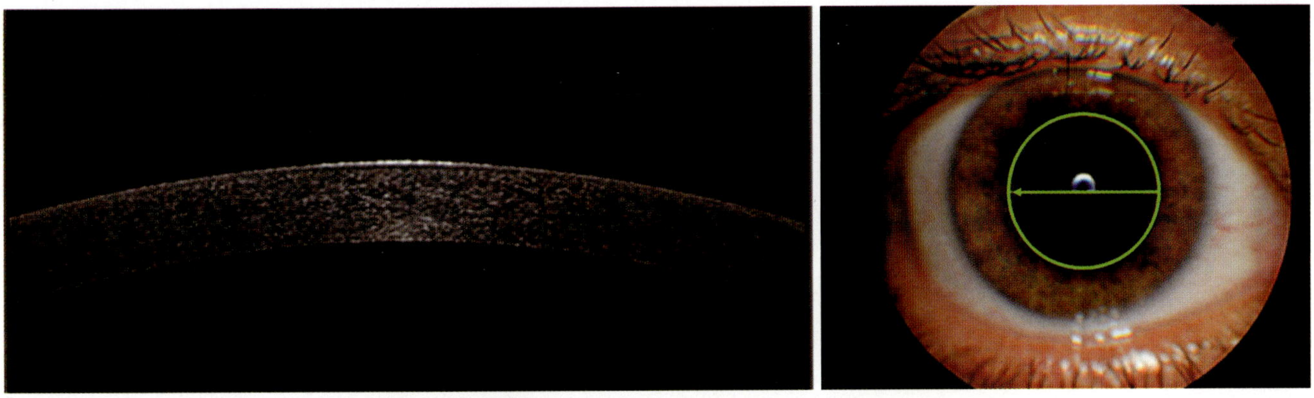

Figure 4.6: Normal cornea—Gray scale

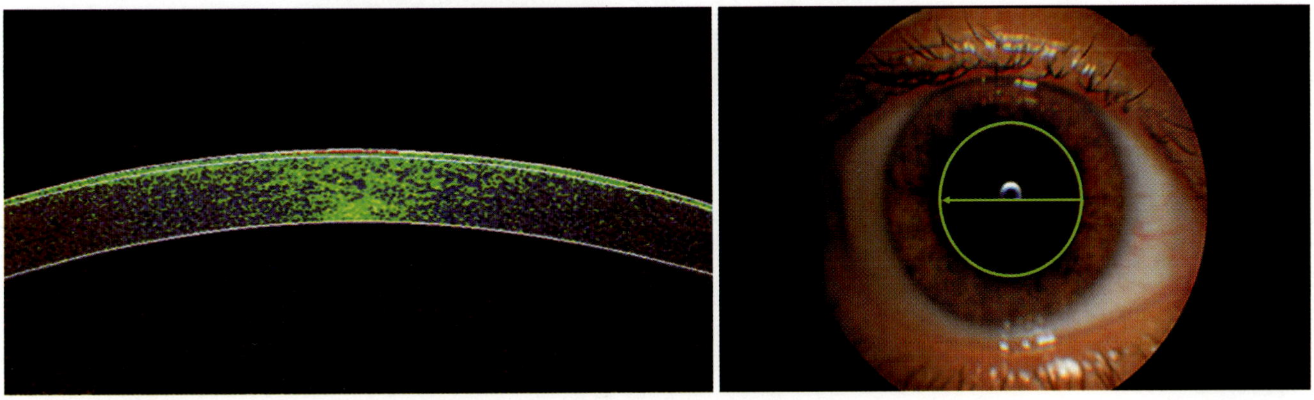

Figure 4.7: Normal cornea showing epithelial, Bowman's and endothelial layers

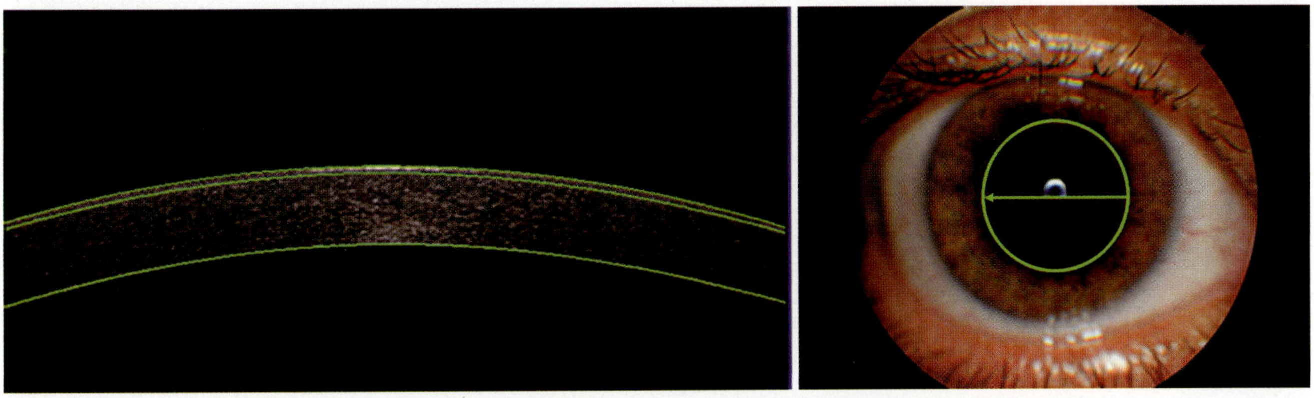

Figure 4.8: Normal cornea showing epithelial, Bowman's and endothelial layers—Gray scale

6. **3D Mosaic comparison feature** can be utilized to obtain the color fundus and the thickness map as a montage (Figures 4.19 and 4.20).
7. **Scan patterns:** 3D OCT 2000 enables scanning with three new scan patterns - 7 Line Raster, 7 Line Raster (V) and Radial scan (12 radial scans)(Figure 4.21).

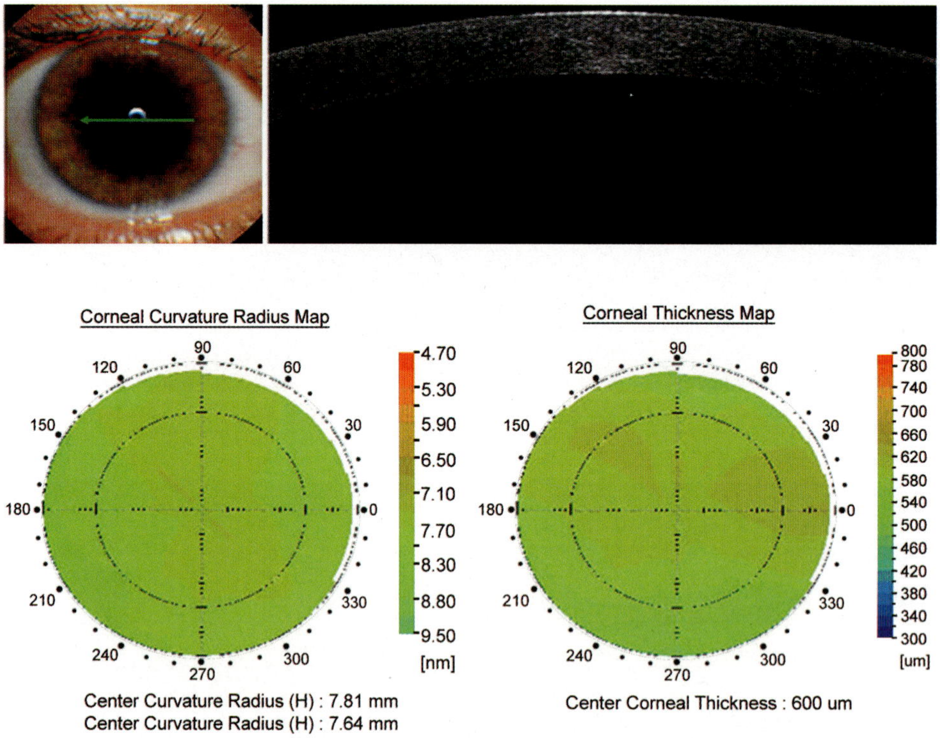

Figure 4.9: Report of a normal cornea

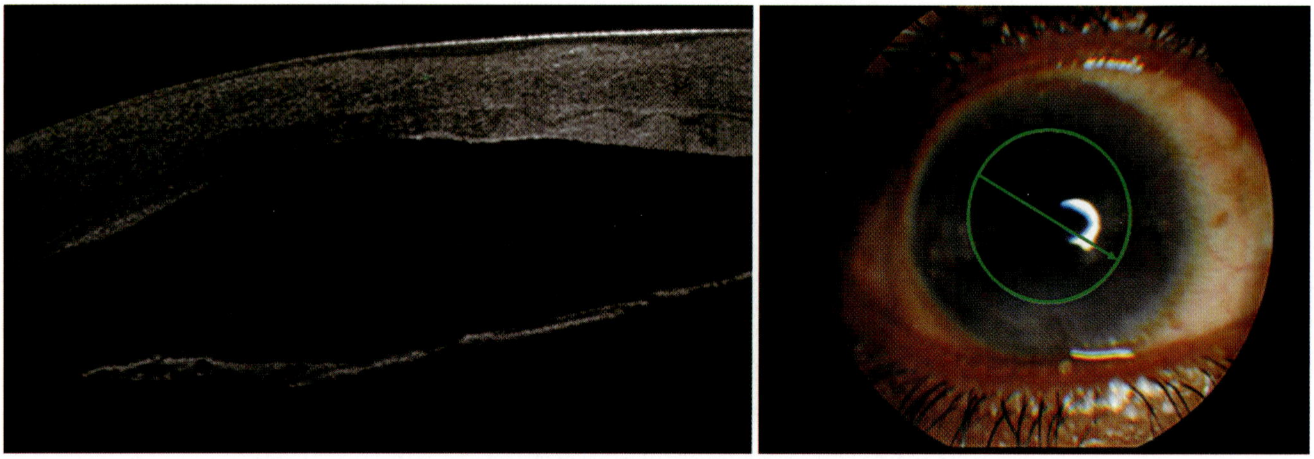

Figure 4.10: Descemet's folds

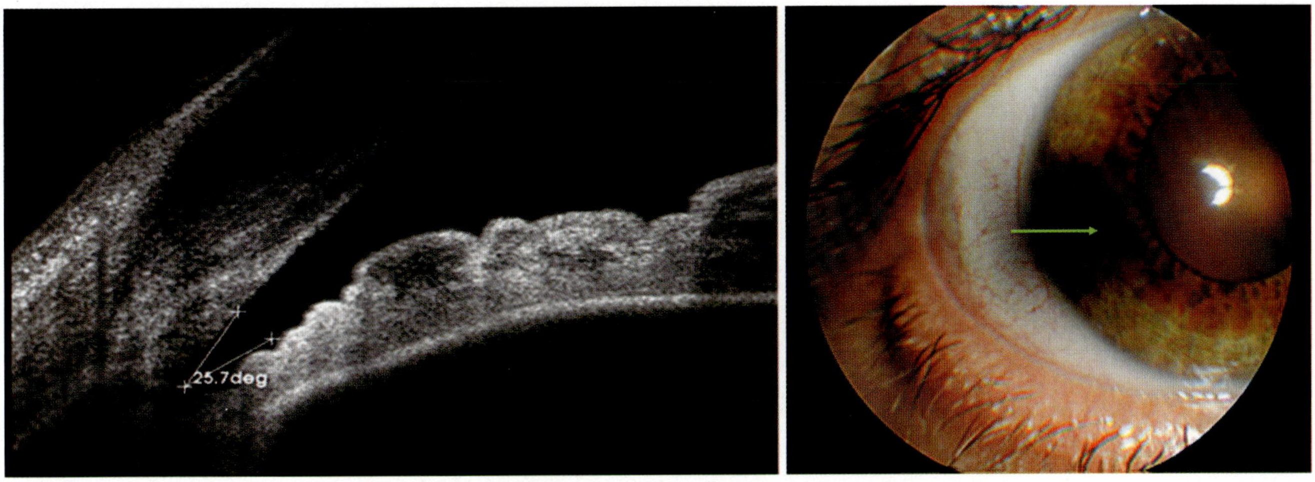

Figure 4.11: Angle in an emmetrope

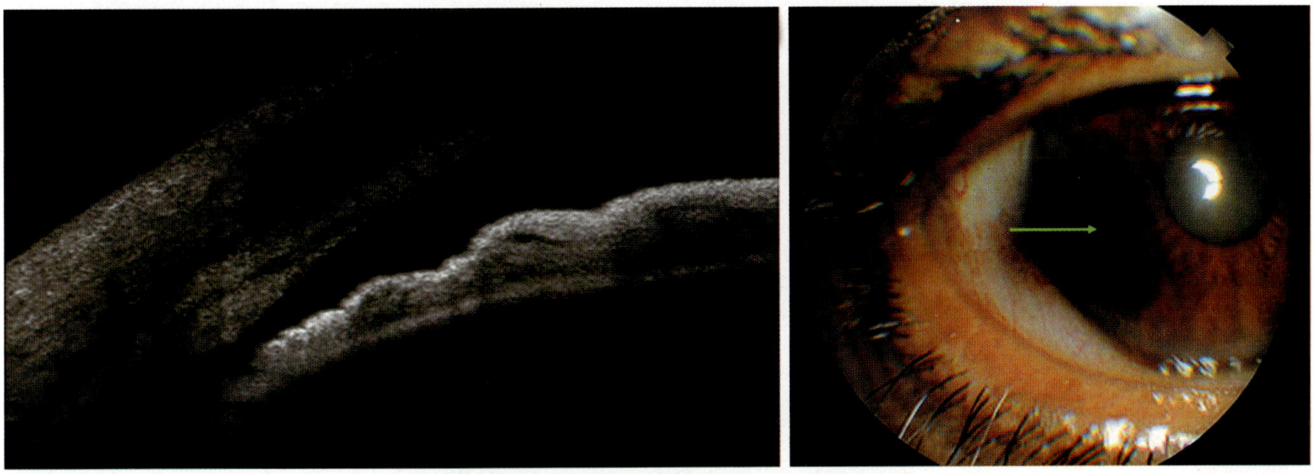

Figure 4.12: Narrow angle in a hypermetrope

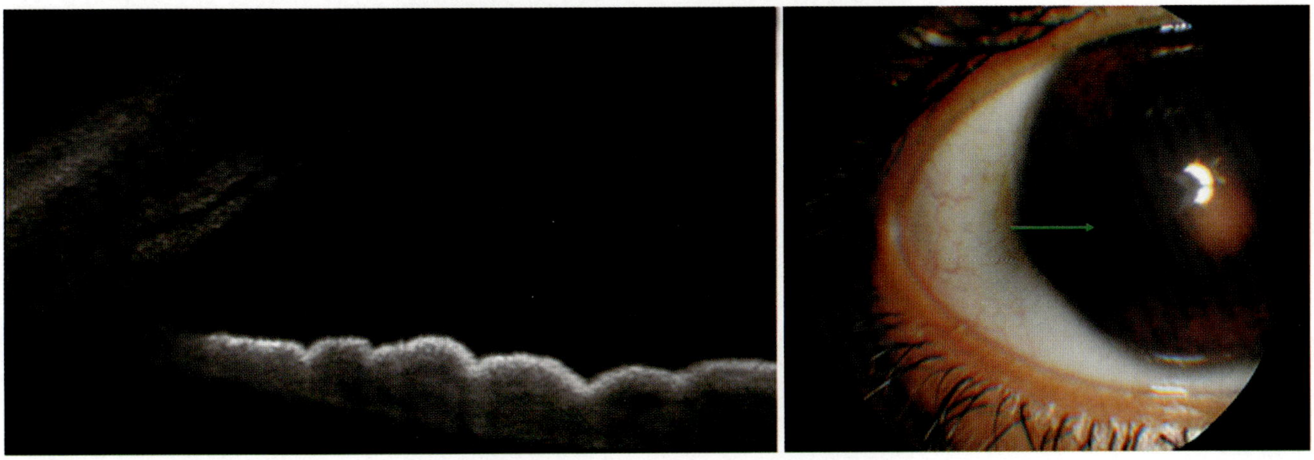

Figure 4.13: Wide angle in a myope

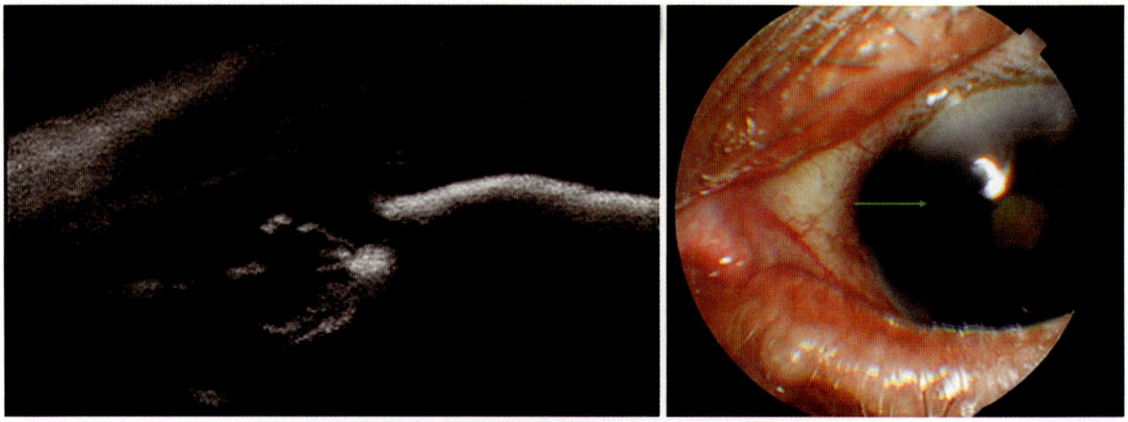

Figure 4.14: Incomplete YAG iridotomy

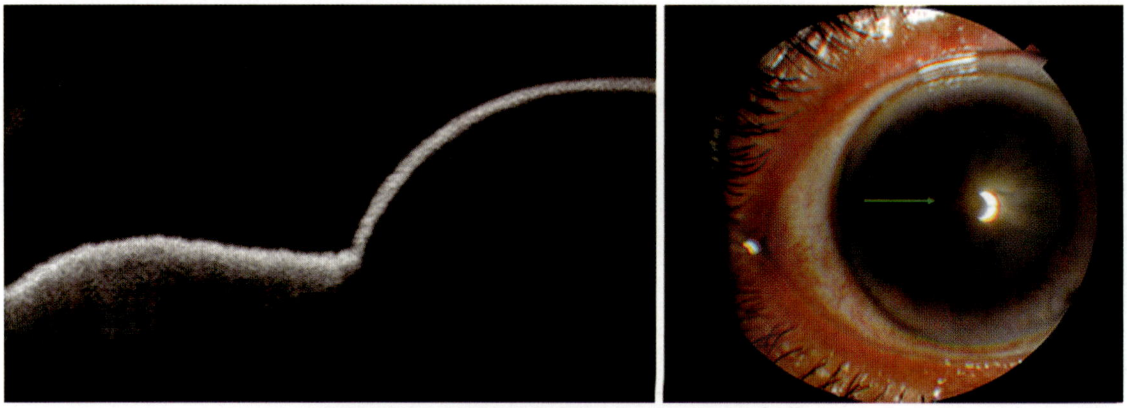

Figure 4.15: Iris cyst

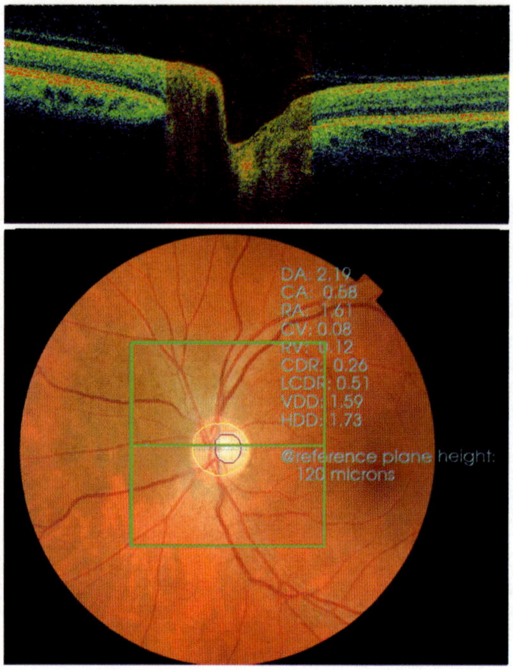

Figure 4.16: Optic disc parameters

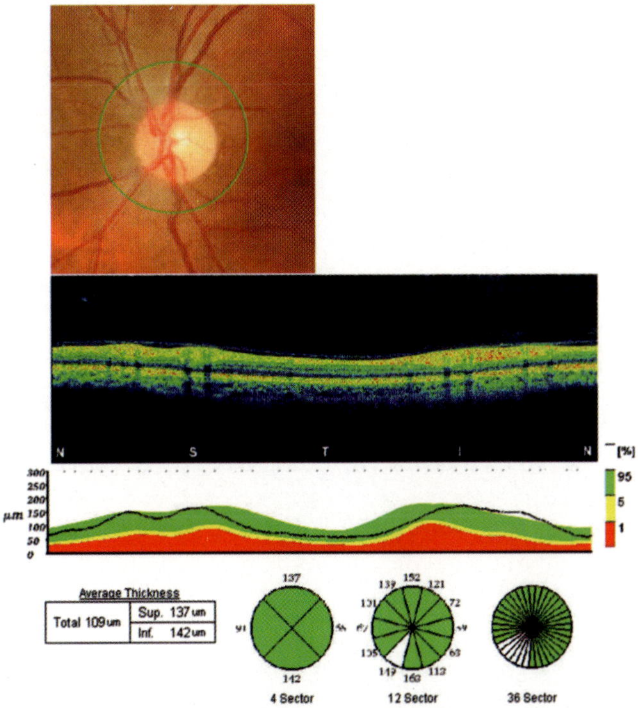

Figure 4.17: RNFL analysis report

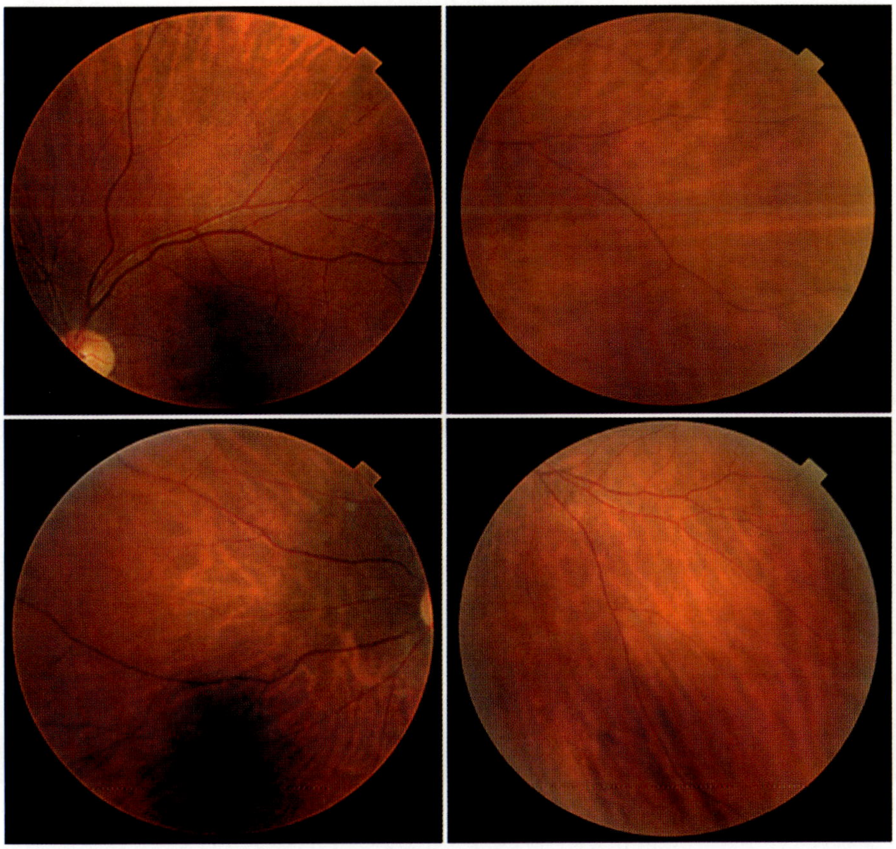

Figure 4.18: Fundus photographs through an undilated pupil

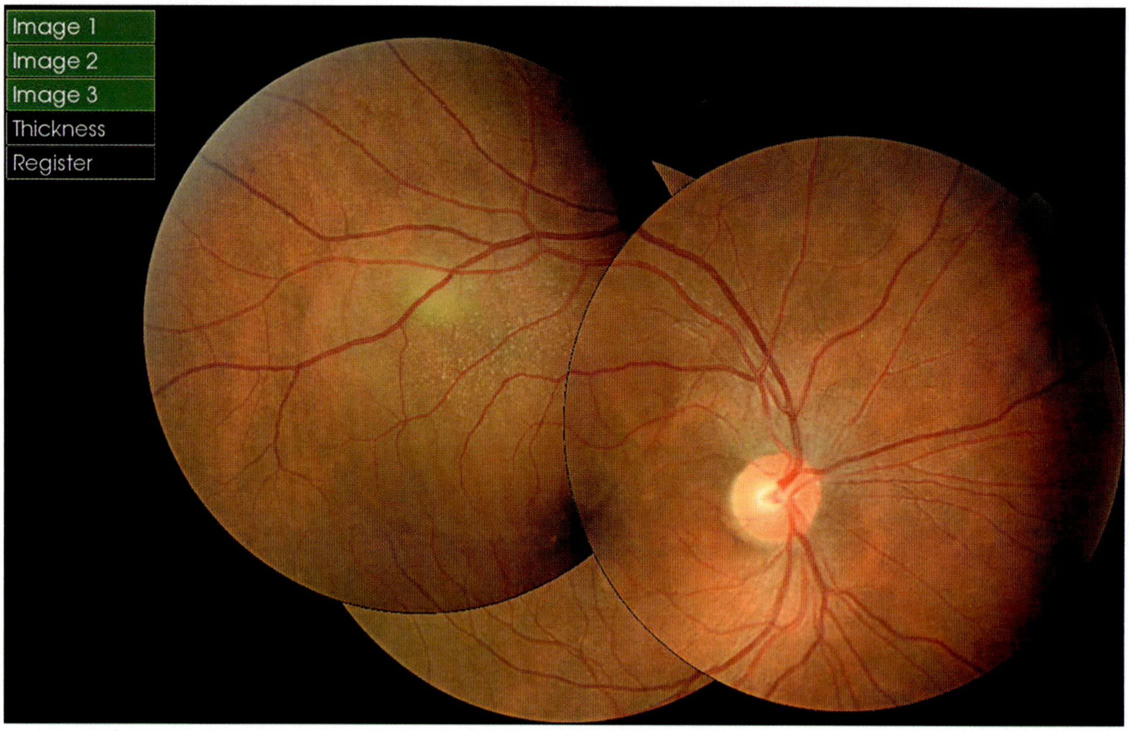

Figure 4.19: 3D Mosaic—Color fundus of a case of CSR

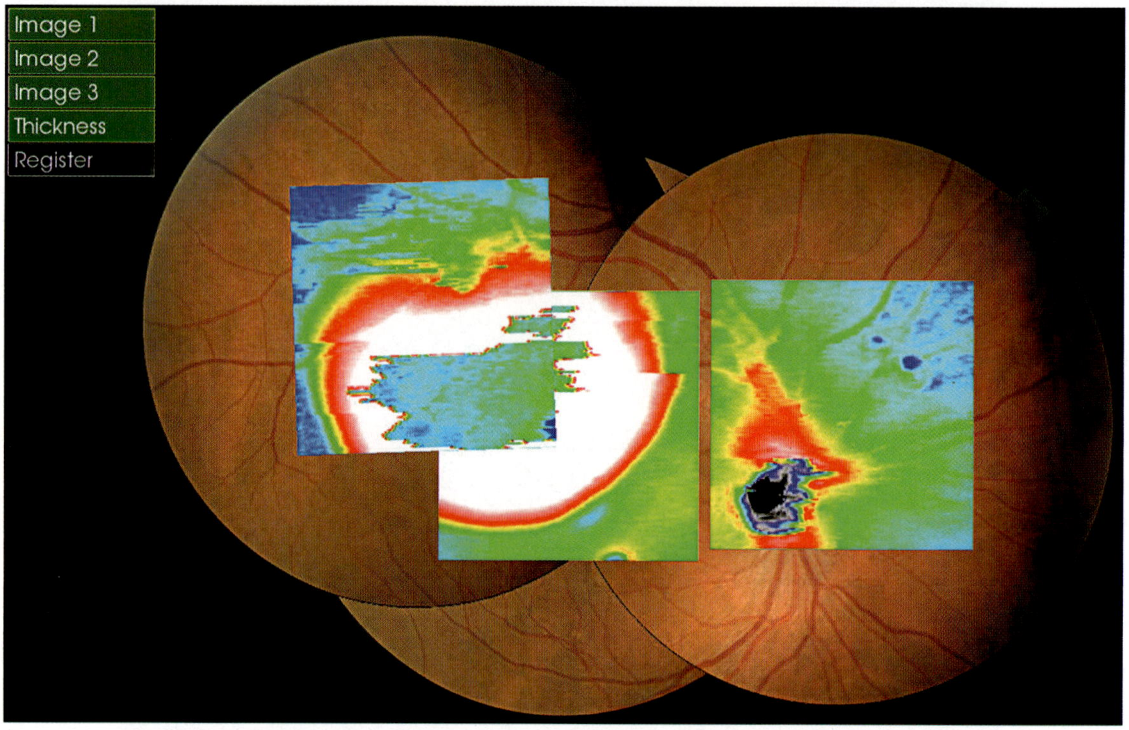

Figure 4.20: 3D Mosaic—Thickness map of a case of CSR

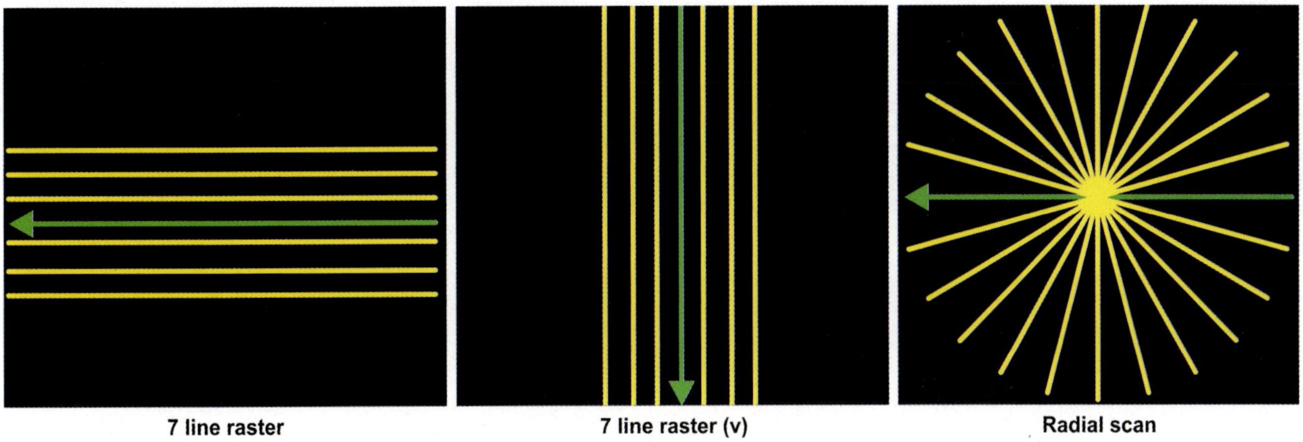

Figure 4.21: Scan patterns

SUGGESTED READING

1. User Manual 3D OCT-2000.

5 OCT Representation of the Normal Retina

OCT allows the retina to be studied in terms of cross-sections of the vitreous, and from the internal limiting membrane to the choriocapillaris and the superficial choroid layer (Figures 5.1 to 5.4).

The internal limiting membrane of the eye is clearly defined in OCT scans, due to the contrast between the non-reflective vitreous and the reflective retina. The posterior hyaloid is often visible as a very faint, fine and slightly reflective line. It may be in contact with the retina or detached. Immediately behind the vitreous lies the highly reflective retinal nerve fiber layer. The retinal nerve fiber is more visible on the nasal side of the fovea because of the density of the papillomacular bundle. The fovea, with its characteristic depression is easily recognizable in the retinal profile. The reflectivity of the inner and outer plexiform layers are greater than that of the inner and outer nuclear layers.

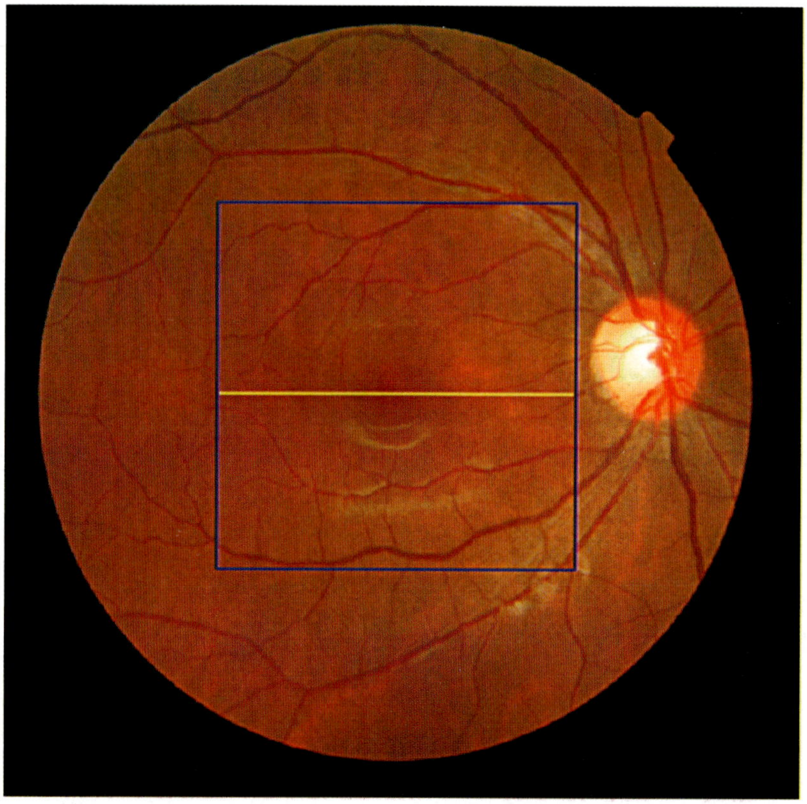

Figure 5.1A: Color photograph showing the line scan across the fovea

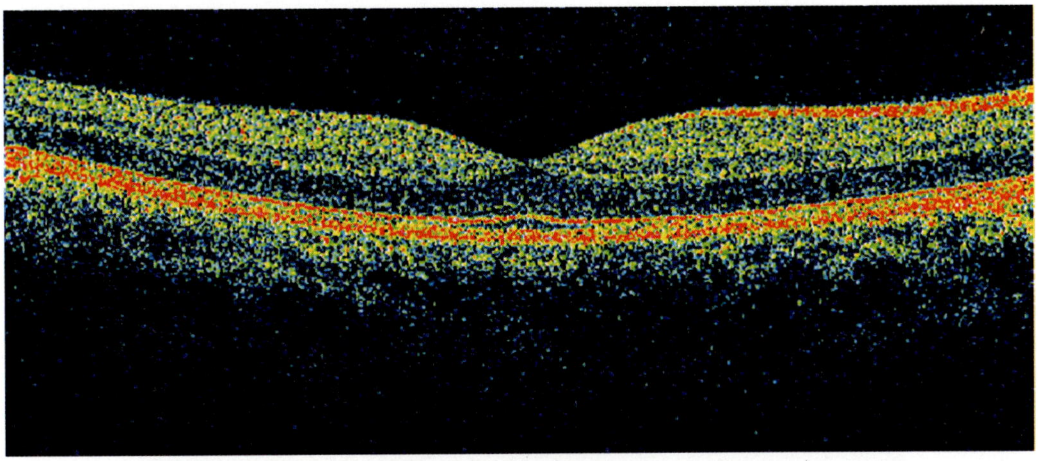

Figure 5.1B: Normal retina

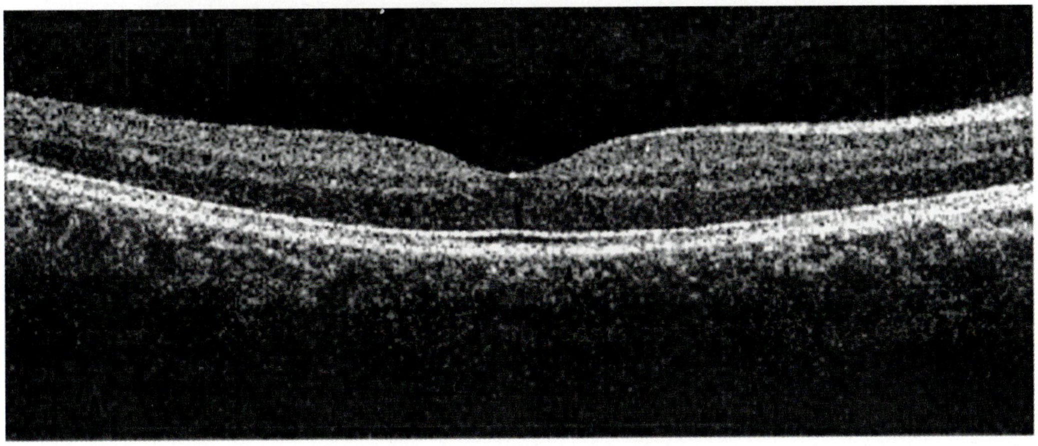

Figure 5.2: Normal retina—Gray scale variation

The external portion of the neural retina is bounded by a highly reflective band, while Bruch's membrane and the choriocapillaris appear as a single, less reflective structure in the optical scan. However, this band can be divided into three hyper-reflective structures: the first is the junction of inner and outer photoreceptor segments; the second is called Verhoeff's membrane and the third is the retinal pigment epithelium. There is a separation of the junction of the inner and outer photoreceptor segments from the Verhoeff's membrane in the foveola region due to the elongation of the outer segment of the cones (Figures 5.5A and B).

The external limiting membrane is seen as a faint line above the junction of inner and outer photoreceptor segments. The inner segment and outer segment of the photoreceptors is represented by the poorly reflective bands immediately in front and behind the junction of inner and outer photoreceptor segments. The poor reflectivity is due to the vertical orientation of the photoreceptors. The photoreceptor band is thicker in the area of the foveal depression.

Normal retinal vessels, which are located in the nerve fiber layer, cannot be clearly distinguished because of their blood content. However, they are easily located by the shadow cone that they form on the posterior layers (Figures 5.6A and B). The blood vessels are seen as dark lines in the C-scan (Figure 5.6C).

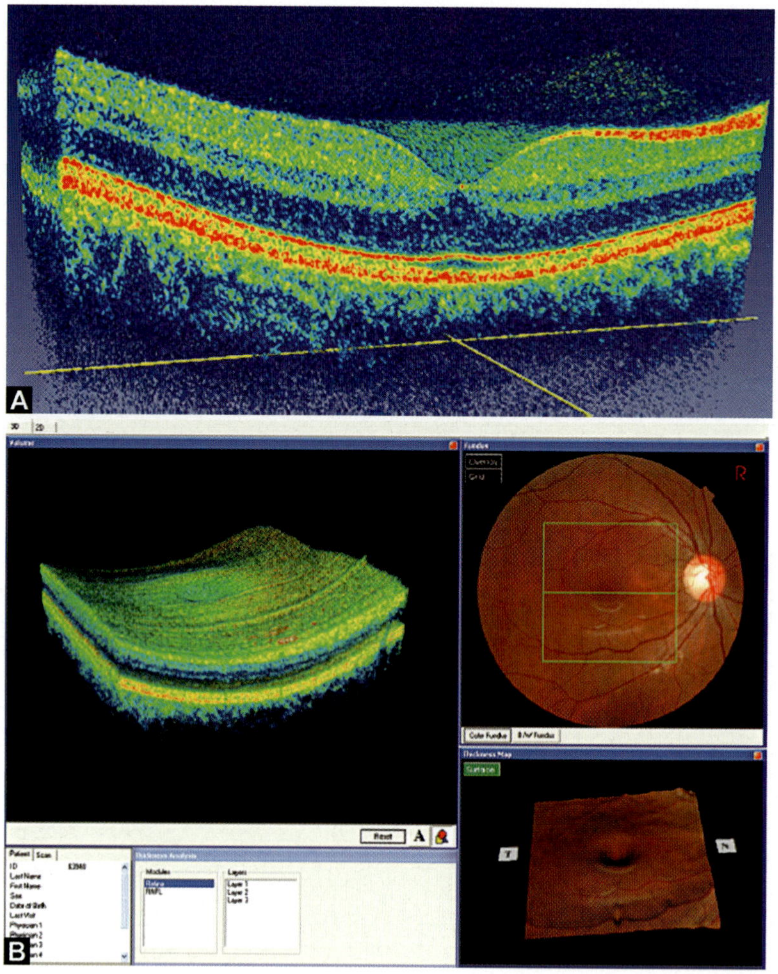

Figures 5.3A and B: Normal retina in three-dimension

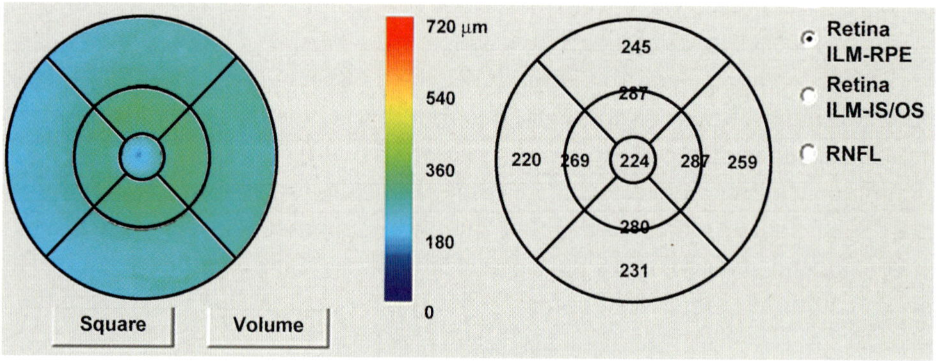

Figure 5.4: Normal retinal map

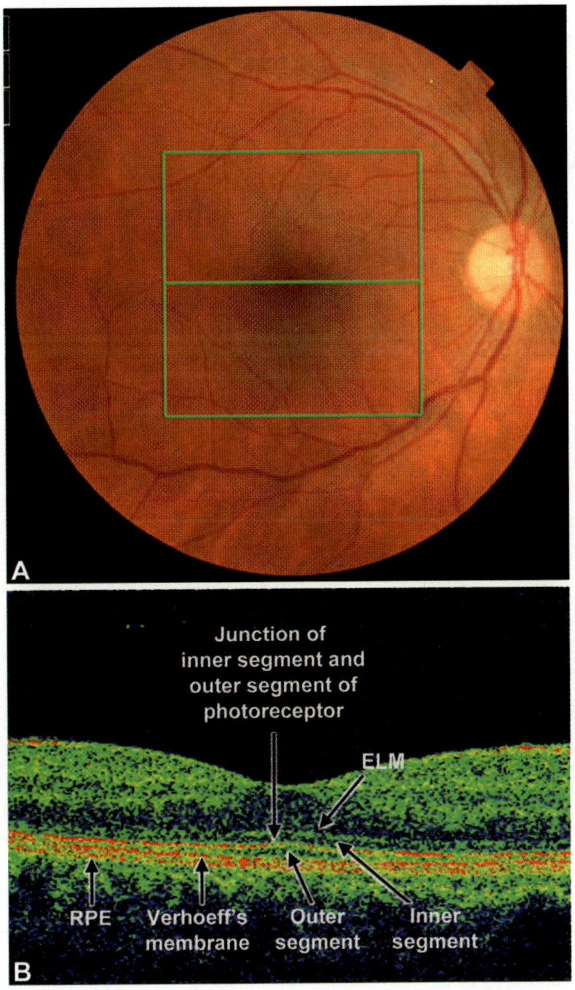

Figures 5.5A and B: Normal macula (Imaged with 3D OCT - 2000)

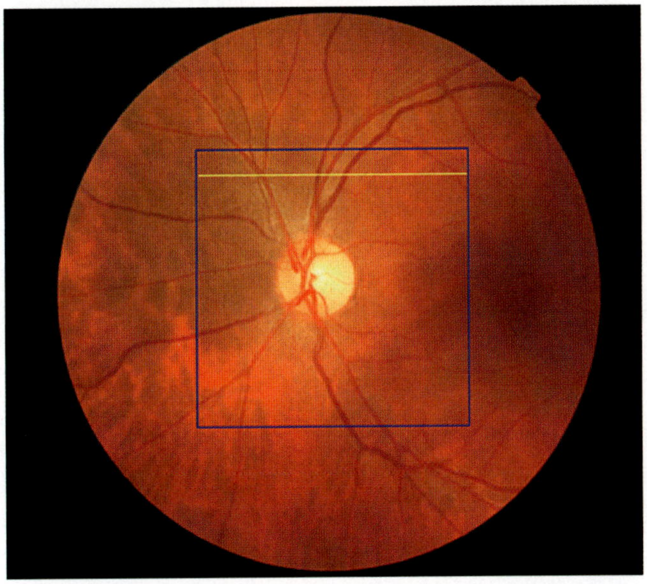

Figure 5.6A: Color photograph showing the line scan across the vessels

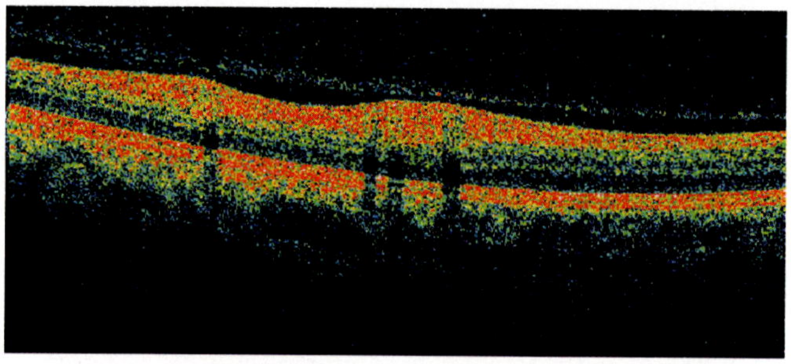

Figure 5.6B: Normal retinal vessels

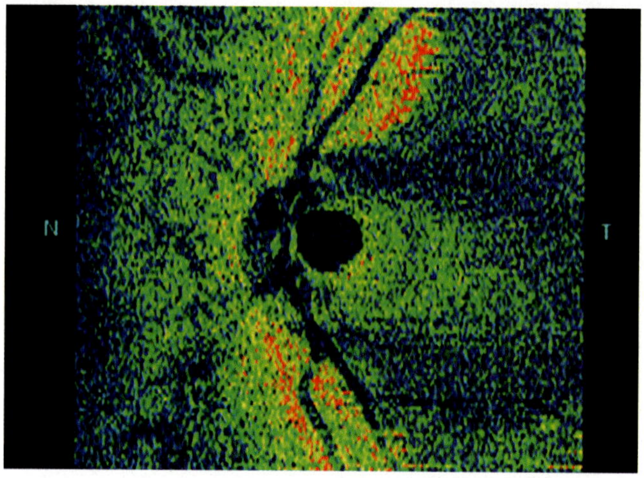

Figure 5.6C: C-scan showing blood vessels as dark lines (Image with 3D OCT 2000)

Table 5.1: Descriptive statistics of macular thickness measurements in normal Indian eyes (n = 76) with Topcon 3D OCT-1000 done in our institution

Variables (μm)	*Range (min-max)*	*Mean ± SD*	*95% confidence interval*
Foveal thickness	154 - 282	205.59 ± 30.60	198.55 - 212.63
Temporal inner macula	220 - 308	270.89 ± 17.89	266.78 - 275.01
Superior inner macula	248 - 325	288.72 ± 17.54	284.69 - 292.76
Nasal inner macula	231 - 322	286.28 ± 21.50	281.33 - 291.23
Inferior inner macula	210 - 311	272.77 ± 21.91	267.73 - 277.82
Temporal outer macula	210 - 276	237.49 ± 16.33	233.74 - 241.25
Superior outer macula	217 - 283	248.88 ± 13.86	245.69 - 252.07
Nasal outer macula	217 - 311	272.71 ± 16.68	268.87 - 276.55
Inferior outer macula	224 - 311	255.76 ± 19.02	251.38 - 260.14

OCT REPRESENTATION OF THE OPTIC DISC (FIGURES 5.7A TO C)

A horizontal OCT scan reveals the physiological cup into which the highly reflective nerve fibers penetrate. The retina is interrupted at the limits of the optic disc. The retinal pigment epithelium and the choriocapillaris are sharply truncated, while the superficial nerve fibers display continuity with the fibers of the optic nerve. The scleral ring can be seen.

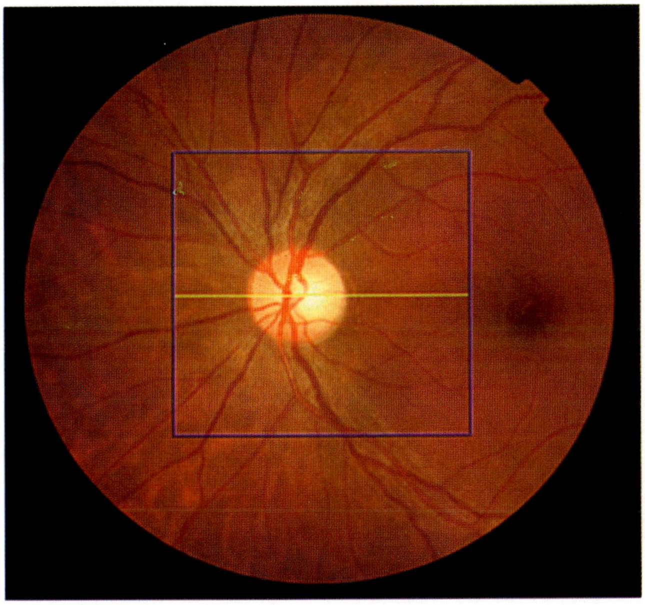

Figure 5.7A: Color photograph showing the line scan passing through the center of the disc

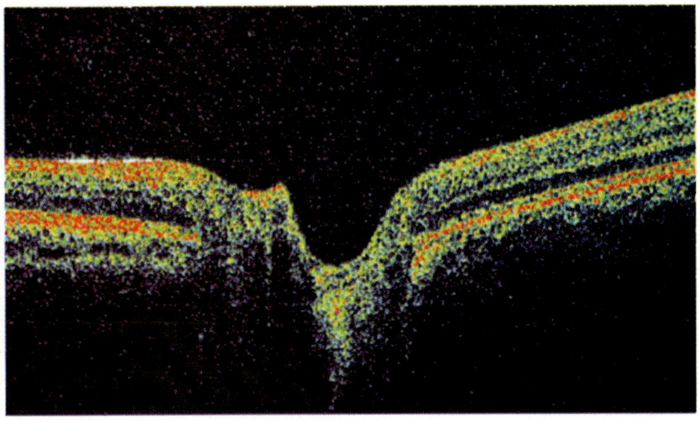

Figure 5.7B: Normal optic disc

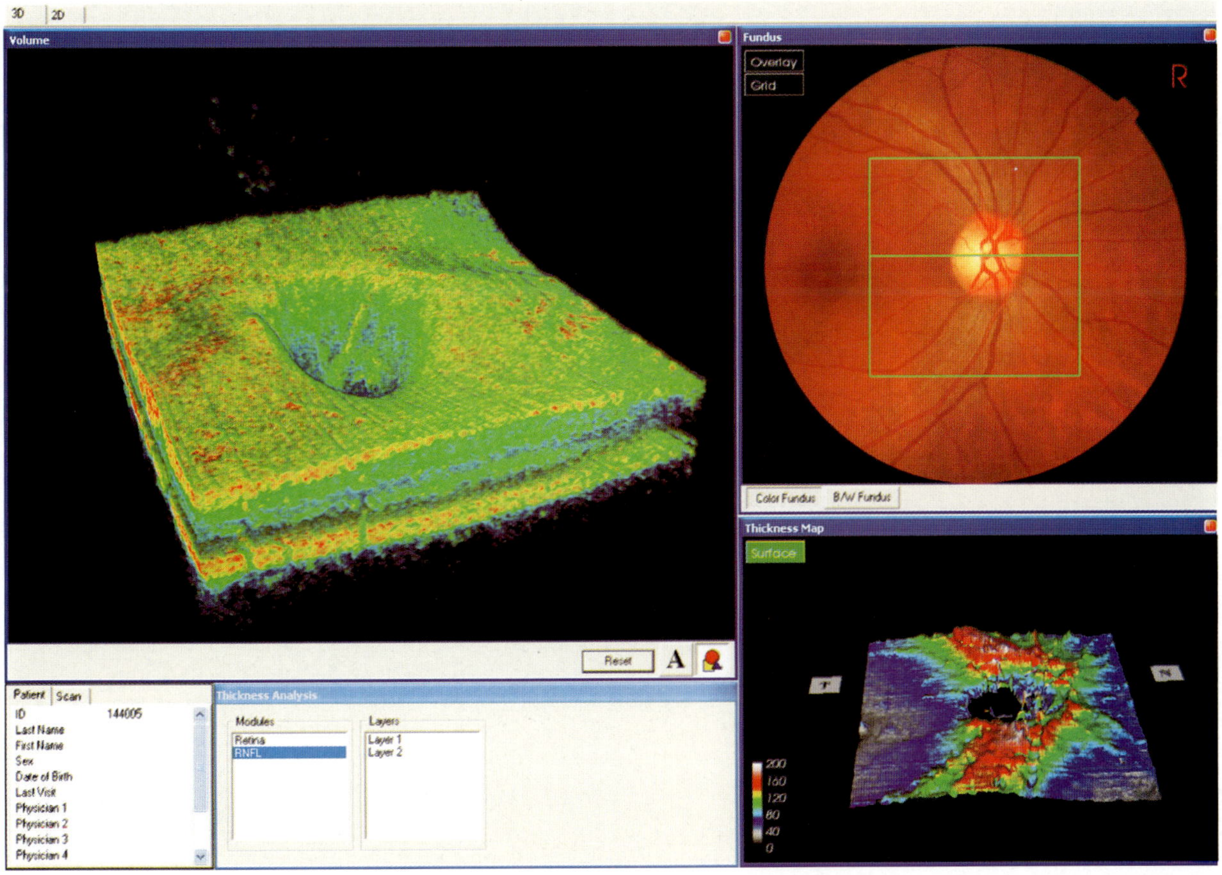

Figure 5.7C: Normal optic disc in three-dimension

CONCLUSION

3D OCT- 2000 allows improved visualization of the ELM, inner segment, outer segment and Verhoeff's membrane.

SUGGESTED READING

1. Hee MR, Izatt JA, Swanson EA, et al. Optical coherence tomography of the human retina. Arch Ophthalmol 1995;113:325-32.
2. Schuman JS, Puliafito CA, Fujimoto JG. Optical Coherence Tomography of Ocular Diseases. 2nd ed. Slack Incorporated 2004.

Section

2

OCT Patterns in Various Diseases

6 Central Serous Chorioretinopathy

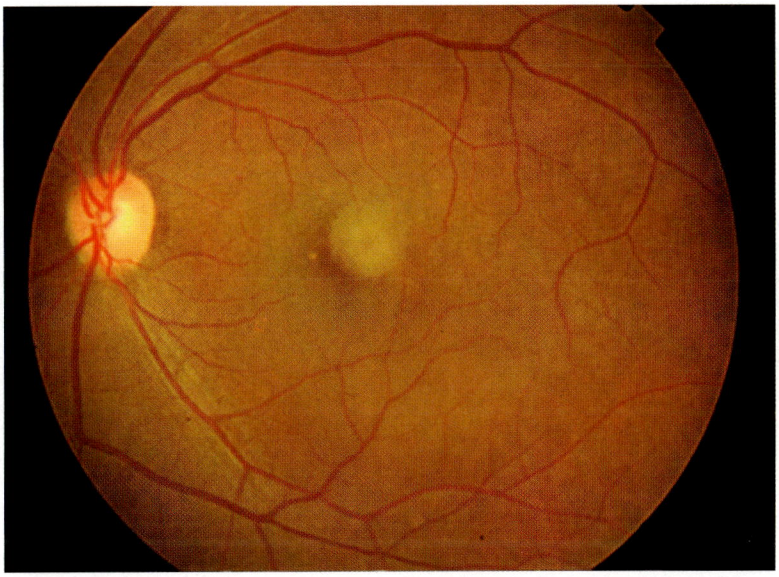

Idiopathic central serous chorioretinopathy is a disease in which a serous detachment of the neurosensory retina occurs over an area of leakage from the choriocapillaris through the retinal pigment epithelium (RPE). It is a self limiting disease, however, recurrences can occur.

Classically, ICSC is most common in male patients aged 20-55 years with type A personality. This condition affects men 6-10 times more often than it affects women. Patients diagnosed at 50 years or older are found to have bilateral disease and show more diffuse RPE changes.

Optical coherence tomography (OCT) reveals many aspects of the pathophysiology of ICSC, ranging from subretinal fluid, pigment epithelial detachments, and retinal atrophy following chronic disease. OCT is especially helpful in identifying subtle, even subclinical, neurosensory macular detachments.

ICSC may be divided into two distinct clinical presentations. FA of classic ICSC shows one or more focal leaks at the level of the RPE. The classic "smokestack" appearance of the fluorescein leak is seen only in 10-15% of cases. FA of diffuse retinal pigment epitheliopathy demonstrates focal granular hyperfluorescence corresponding to window defects and blockage caused by RPE atrophy and clumping with one or more areas of subtle continued leakage.

ICG angiography shows hypofluorescent areas early in the angiogram followed by late hyperfluorescence and leakage in choroidal vasculature. Often, multiple areas of leakage are seen on ICG angiography that are not evident clinically or on FA.

CASE 6.1: ICSC WITH SEROUS RETINAL DETACHMENT

Case Summary

A 45-year-old male was seen with complaints of diminished vision in the left eye of one day duration. His best-corrected vision in this eye was 6/9. Fluorescein angiography showed a smoke stack appearance, confirming the diagnosis of ICSC (Figures 6.1.1 and 6.1.2).

Optical Coherence Tomography

A horizontal line scan through the fovea showed elevation of the neurosensory retina with an optically clear space underneath corresponding to the presence of serous fluid under the fovea The retinal map showed a foveal thickness of 519 microns (Figures 6.1.3A to D).

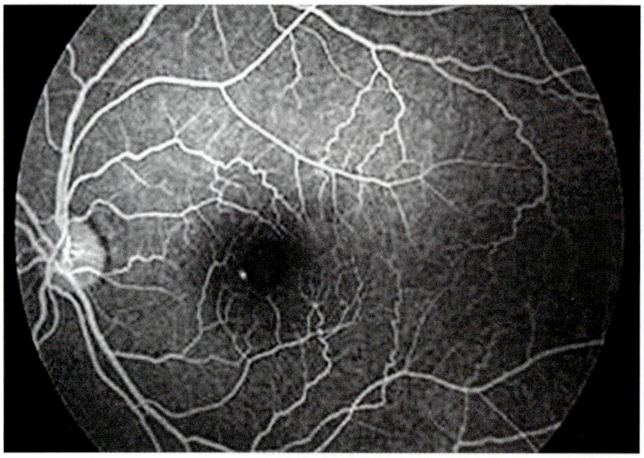

Figure 6.1.1: Early phase fluorescein angiogram shows a single pinpoint leak

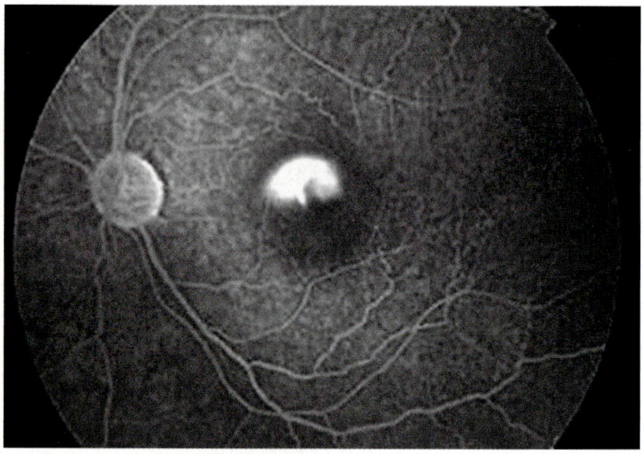

Figure 6.1.2: Late phase fluorescein angiogram shows the typical smokestack appearance

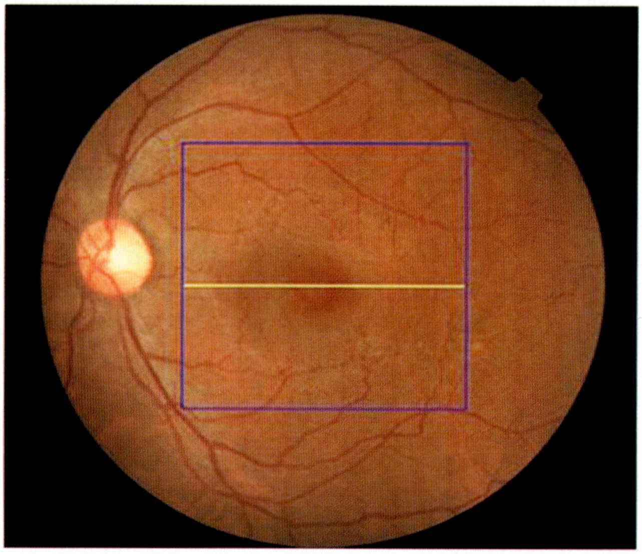

Figure 6.1.3A: Color fundus photograph showing the horizontal line scan through the fovea

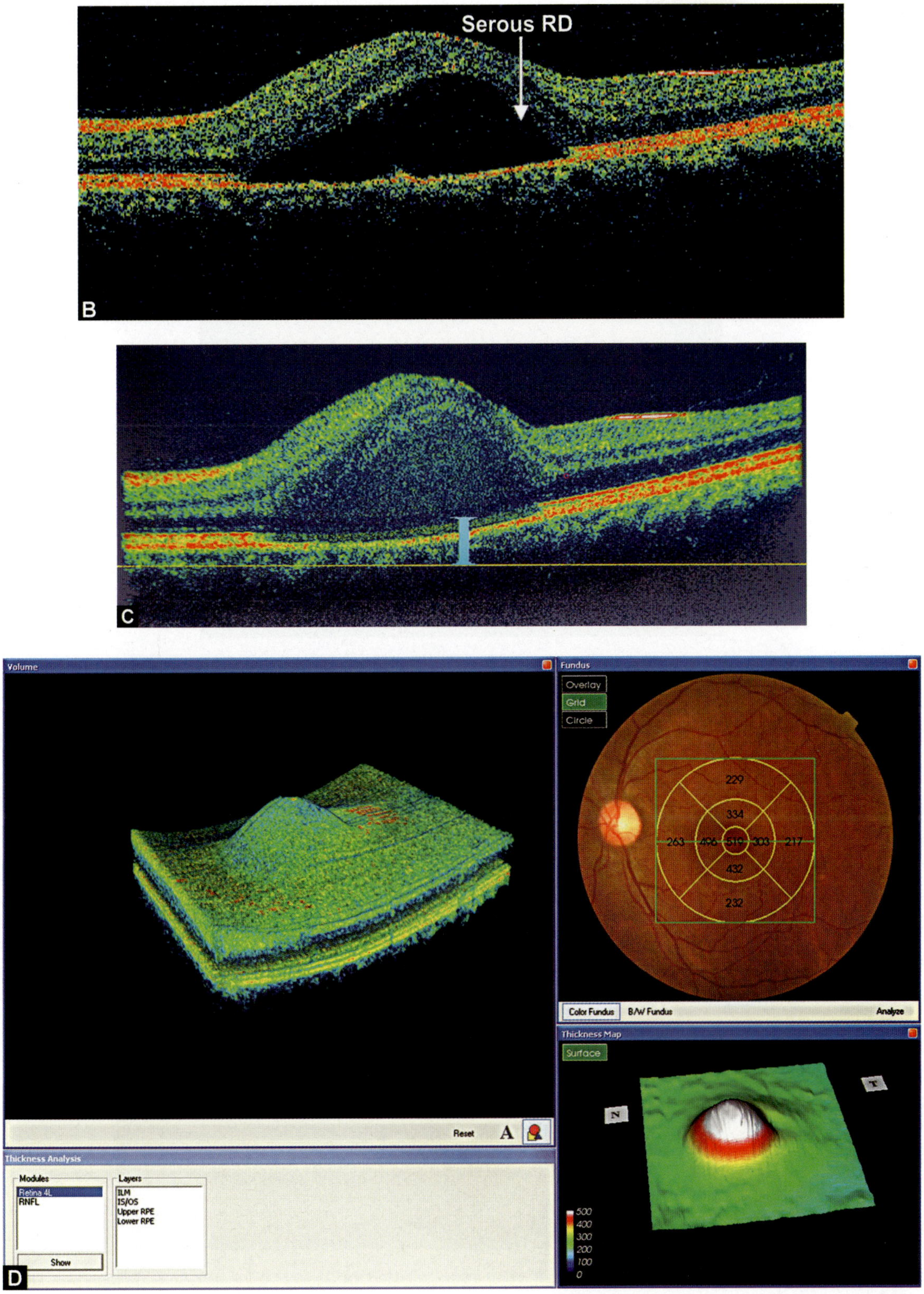

Figures 6.1.3B to D: (B) Horizontal line scan 2D image showing serous retinal detachment; (C) Cropped 3D image showing serous retinal detachment; (D) 3D image of case 6.1. Retinal map showing foveal thickness of 519 µm.Color surface thickness map

Follow-up

Patient was managed conservatively and when followed up at 3 months, the visual acuity had improved to 6/6. Repeat OCT showed return of the foveal contour with reduction in the serous retinal detachment and foveal thickness now measured 280 microns (Figures 6.1.3E to H).

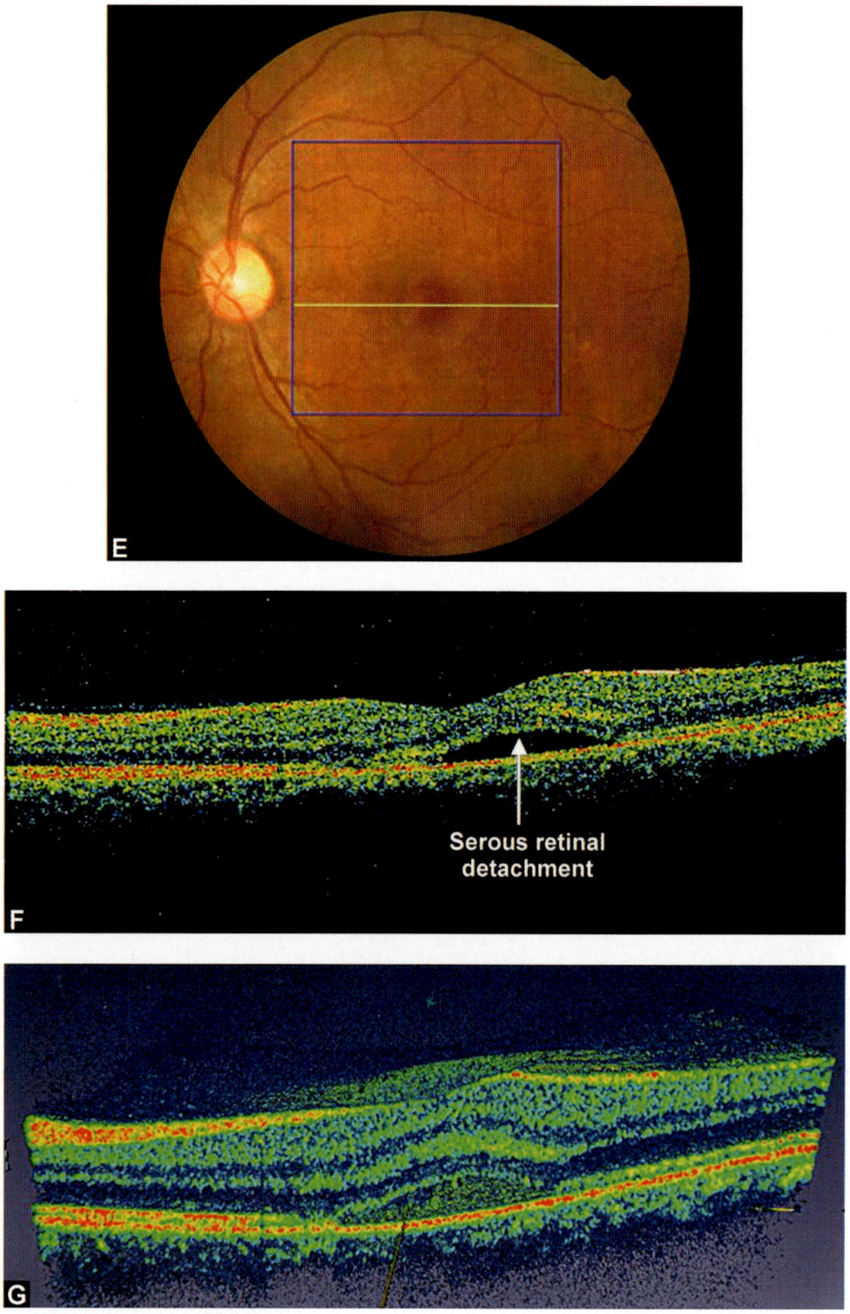

Figures 6.1.3E to G: (E) Repeat Color fundus photograph 3 months later showing the horizontal line scan through the fovea. (F) Horizontal line scan 2D image showing reduction of serous retinal detachment. (G) Cropped 3D image showing reduction of serous retinal detachment

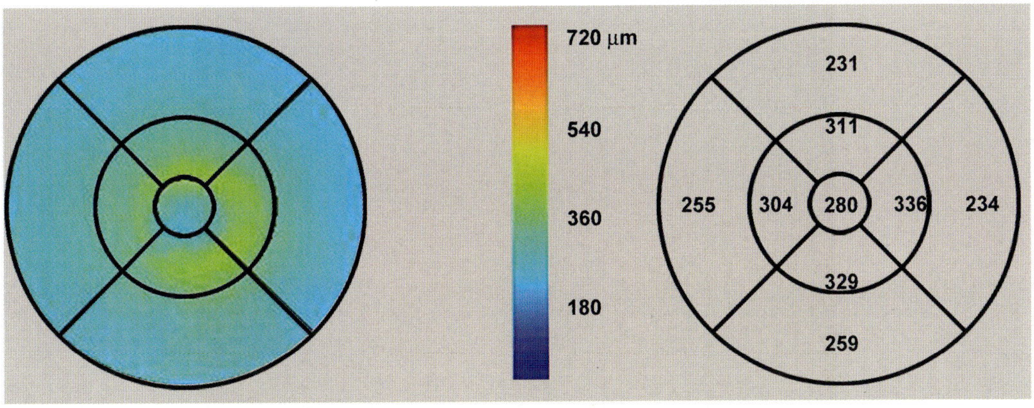

Figure 6.1.3H: Retinal map showing reduction in foveal thickness measuring 280 µm

CASE 6.2: ICSC WITH SEROUS RETINAL DETACHMENT AND PIGMENT EPITHELIAL DETACHMENT IN ONE EYE AND MULTIPLE PEDS IN THE OTHER EYE

Case Summary

A 37-year-old male was seen with complaints of diminished vision in the right eye of 2 months duration. His best-corrected vision in this eye was 6/9. Fluorescein angiography showed a smoke stack appearance with serous retinal elevation, confirming the diagnosis of ICSC (Figures 6.2.1and 6.2.2).

Optical Coherence Tomography–1

A horizontal line scan through the foveal center showed the presence of a hyporeflective area under the fovea suggestive of serous fluid accumulation with a small PED within it (Figures 6.2.3A to D)

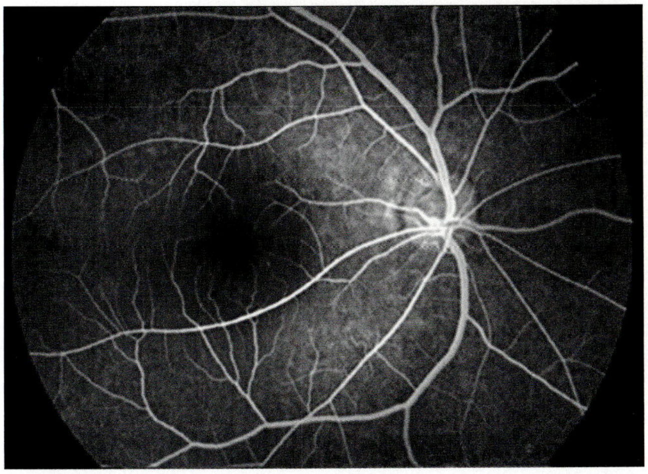

Figure 6.2.1: Early phase fluorescein angiogram shows a single pinpoint leak

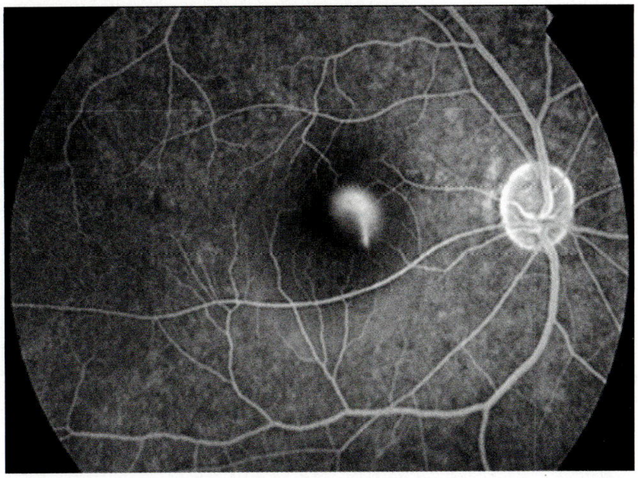

Figure 6.2.2: Late phase fluorescein angiogram shows the typical smokestack appearance

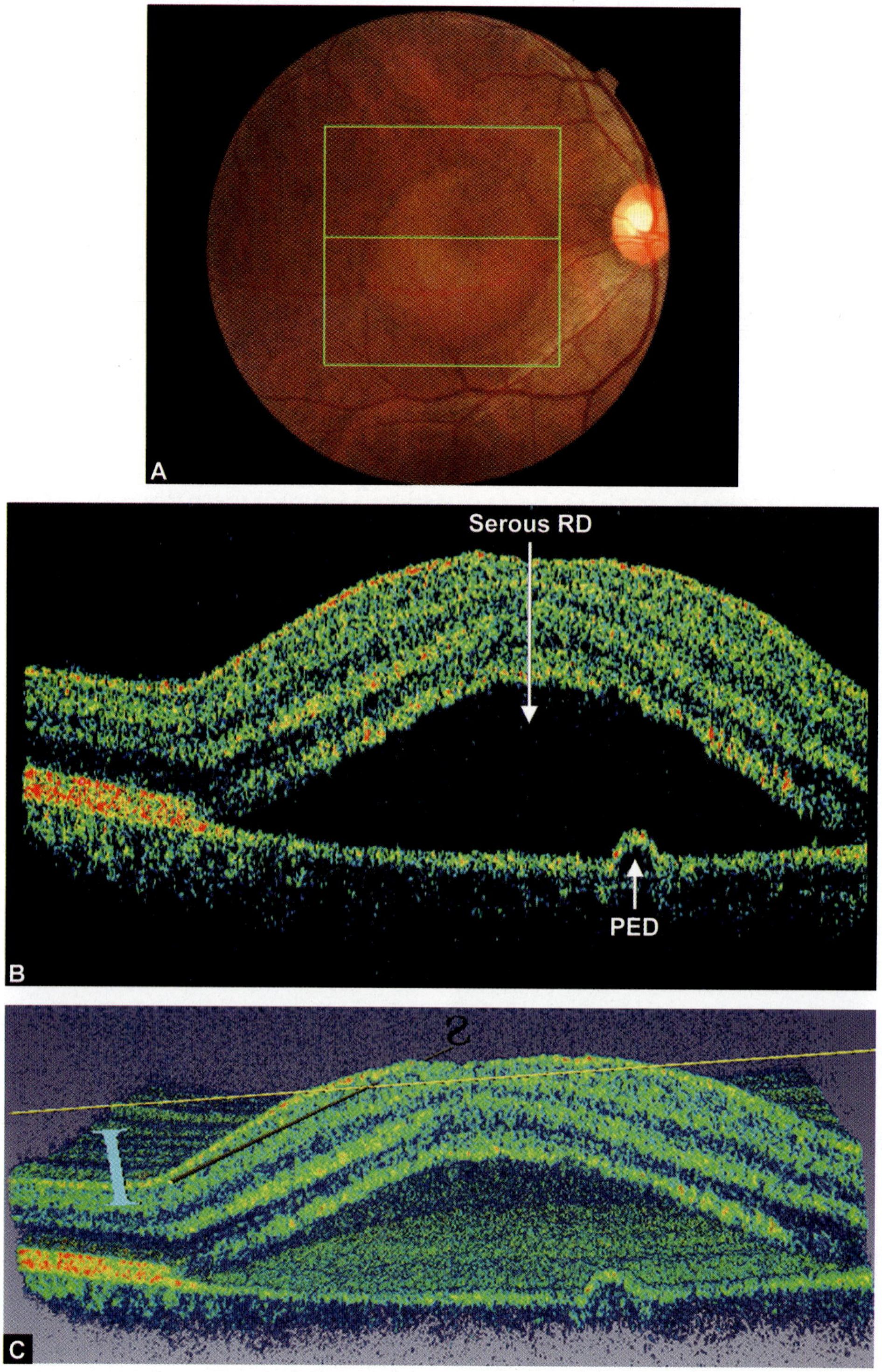

Figures 6.2.3A to C: (A) Color fundus photograph of right eye showing the horizontal line scan through the fovea. (B) Horizontal line scan 2D image showing serous retinal detachment with a PED within it. (C) Cropped 3D image showing serous retinal detachment with a PED within it

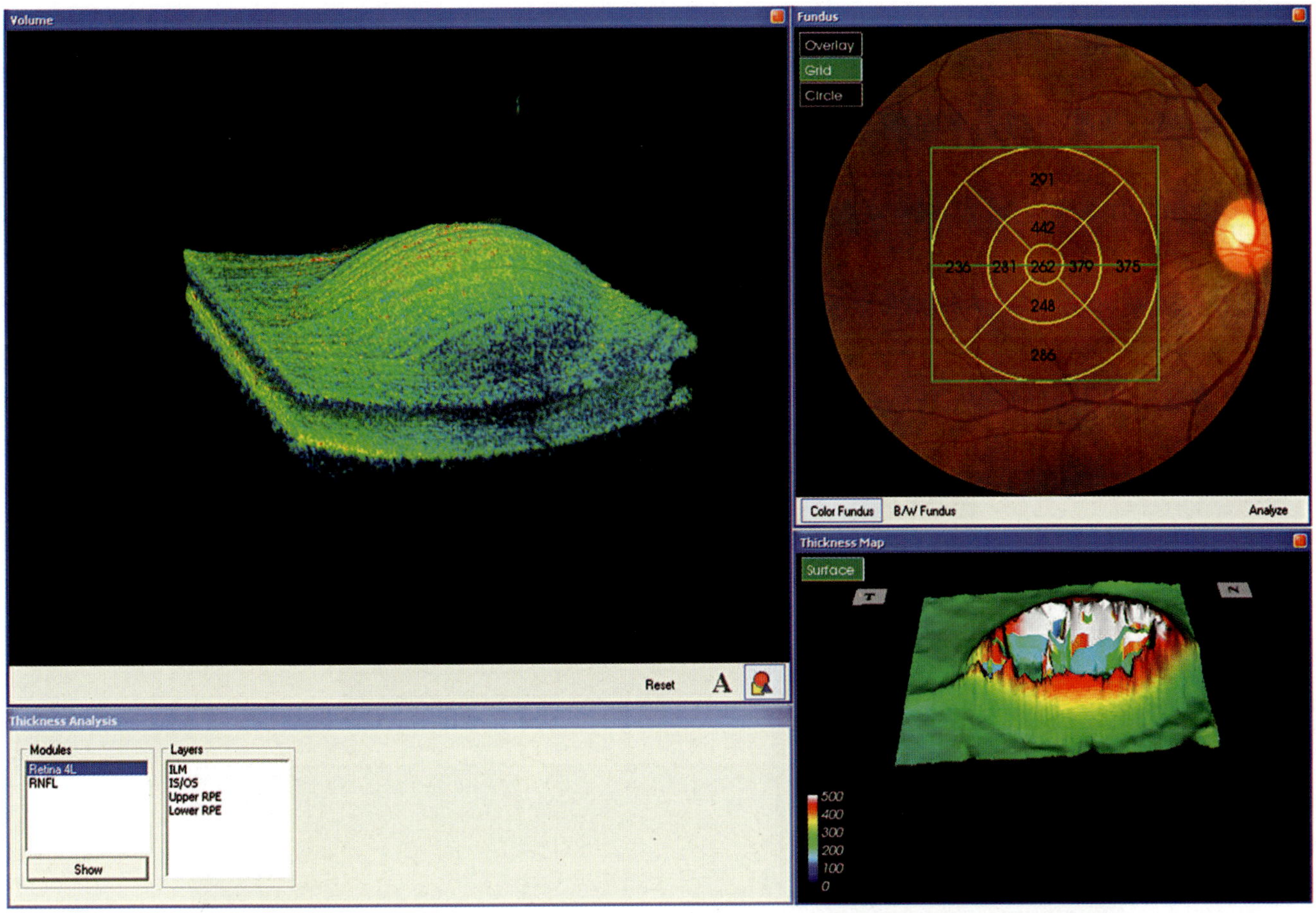

Figure 6.2.3D: 3D image of the right eye of Case 6.2. Retinal map showing foveal thickness of 262 μm. Color surface thickness map

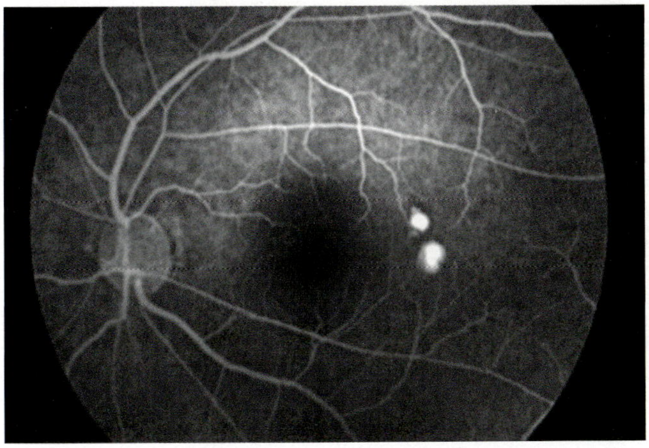

Figure 6.2.4: Early phase fluorescein angiogram shows multiple PED

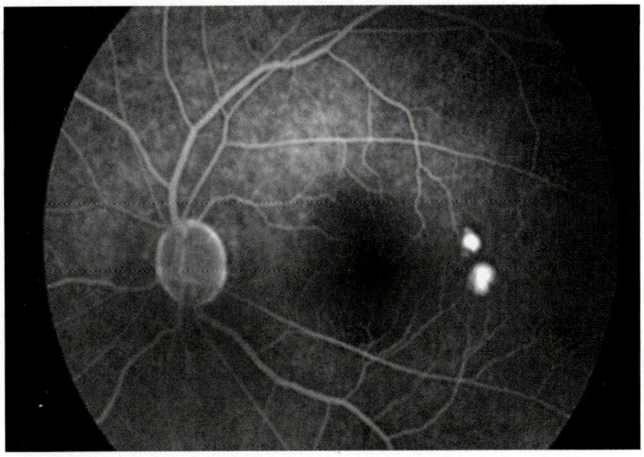

Figure 6.2.5: Late phase fluorescein angiogram shows multiple PED

The best-corrected visual acuity in the left eye of the patient was 6/6. Fluorescein angiography showed hyperfluorescent spots suggestive of pigment epithelial detachments (Figures 6.2.4 and 6.2.5).

Optical Coherence Tomography–2

Horizontal line scans at different levels showed dome-shaped hyporeflective spaces temporal to the fovea consistent with pigment epithelial detachments (Figures 6.2.6A to G).

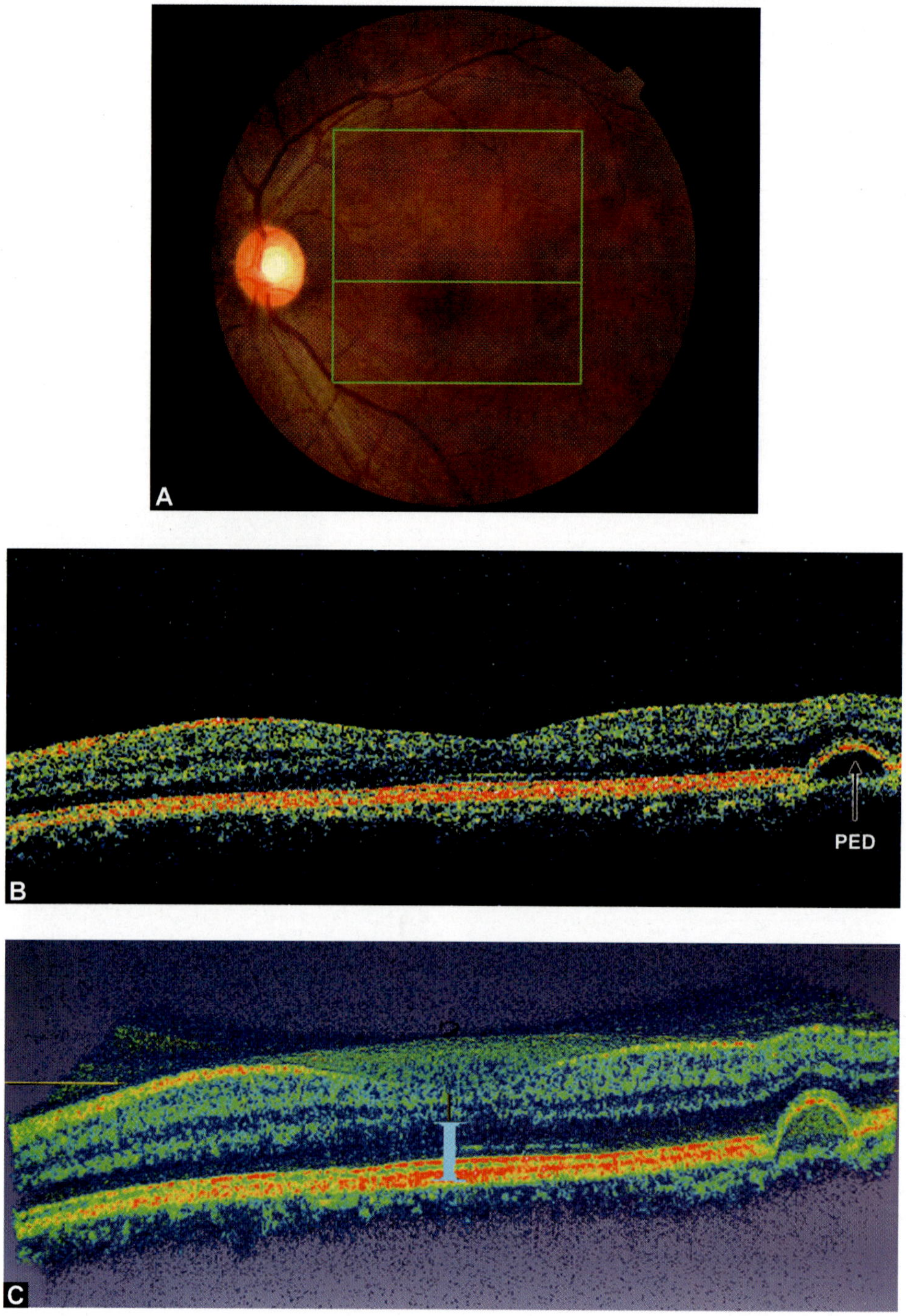

Figures 6.2.6A to C: (A) Color fundus photograph of the left eye showing the horizontal line scan through the upper PED. (B) Horizontal line scan 2D image showing PED temporal to the fovea. (C) Cropped 3D image showing PED temporal to the fovea

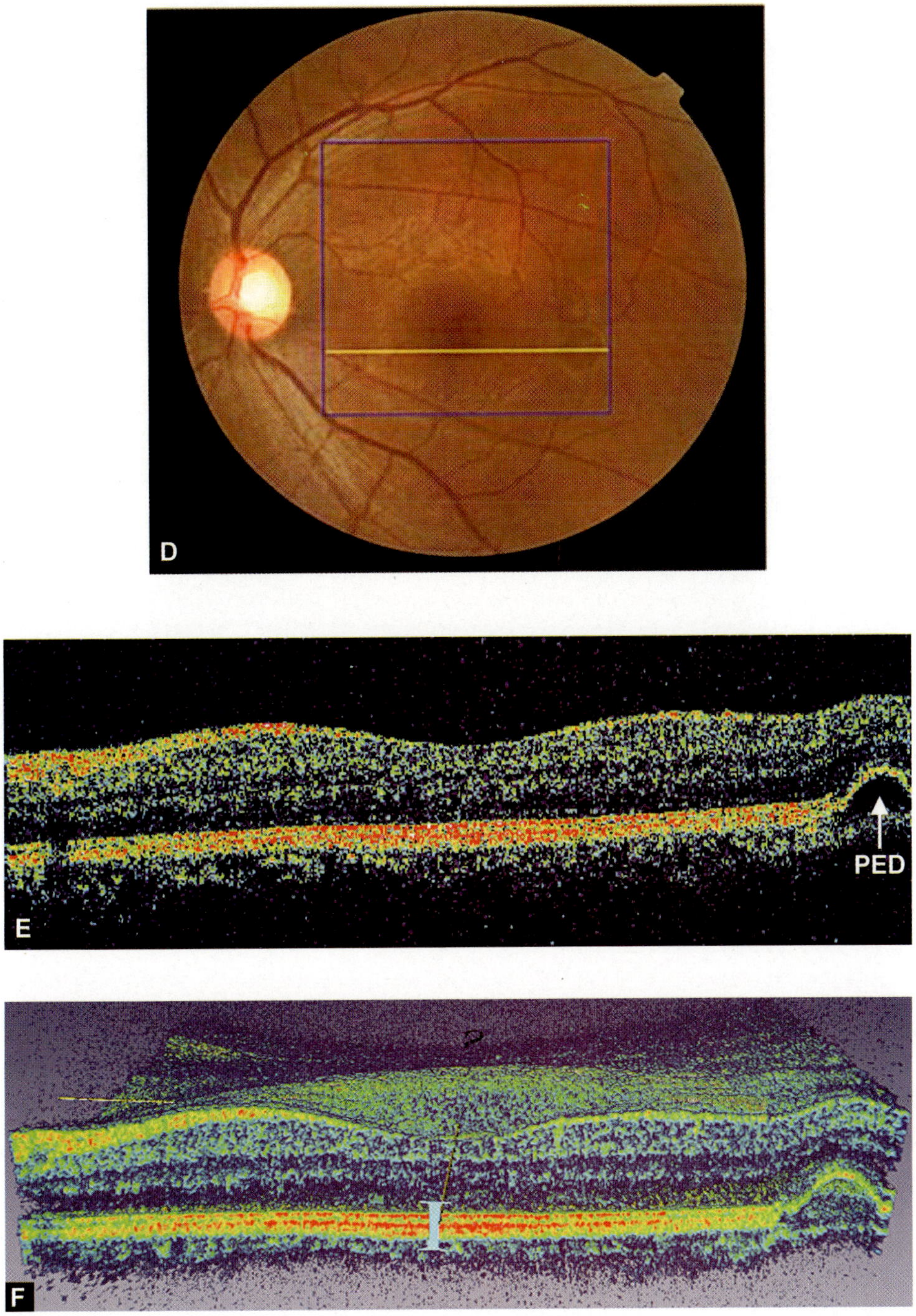

Figures 6.2.6D to F: (D) Color fundus photograph of the left eye showing the horizontal line scan through the lower PED. (E) Horizontal line scan 2D image showing PED temporal to the fovea. (F) Cropped 3D image showing PED temporal to the fovea

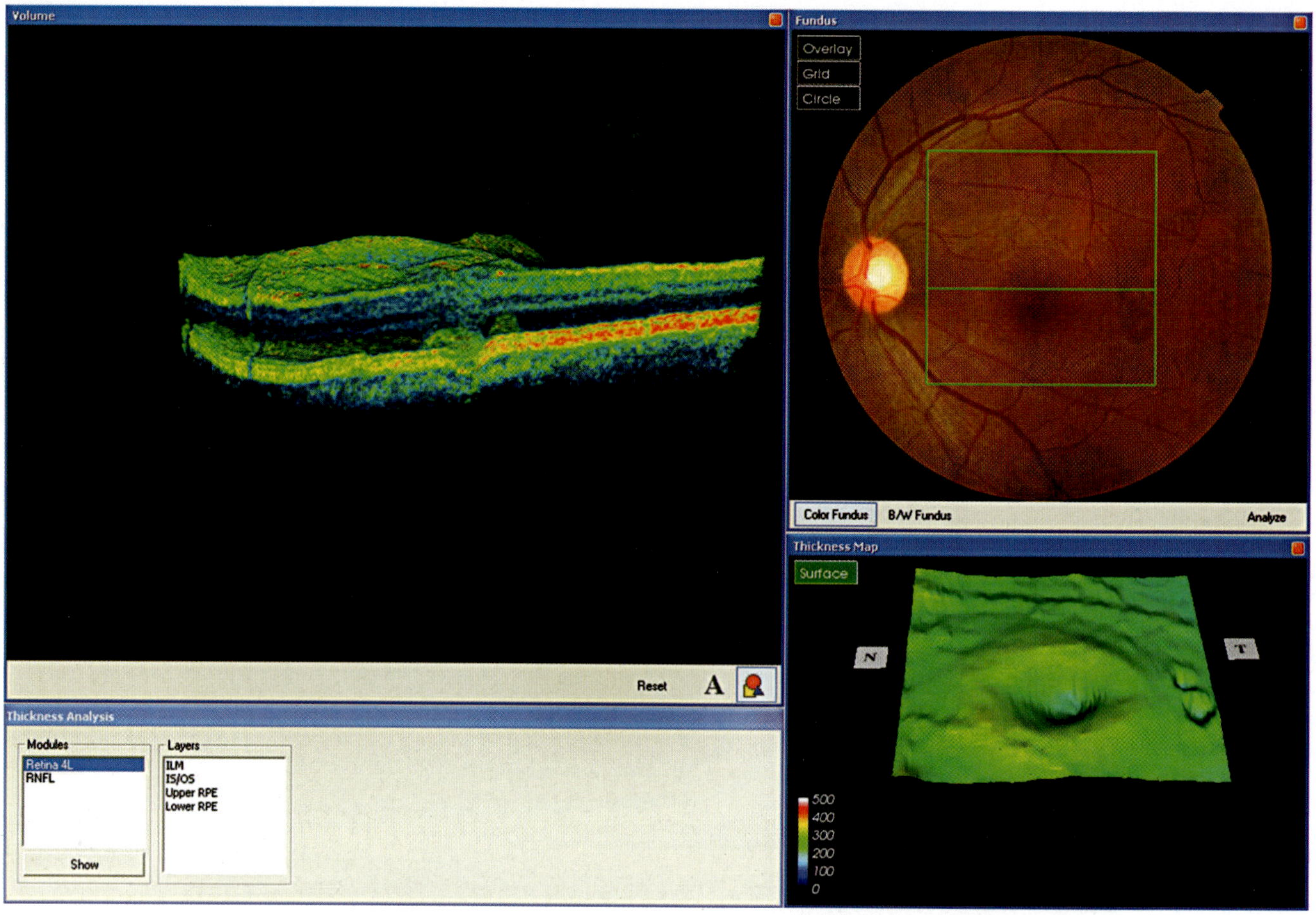

Figure 6.2.6G: 3D image of the left eye of Case 6.2

CASE 6.3: ICSC WITH SEROUS RETINAL DETACHMENT AND PIGMENT EPITHELIAL DETACHMENT

Case Summary

A 36-year-old male presented with diminished vision in the left eye of one month duration. His best- corrected visual acuity in this eye was 6/24.

Optical Coherence Tomography

Horizontal line scan through the fovea showed a hyporeflective space consistent with serous retinal detachment (Figures 6.3.1A and B).

Horizontal line scan passing temporal to the fovea showed serous retinal detachment and pigment epithelial detachment (Figures 6.3.1C to F).

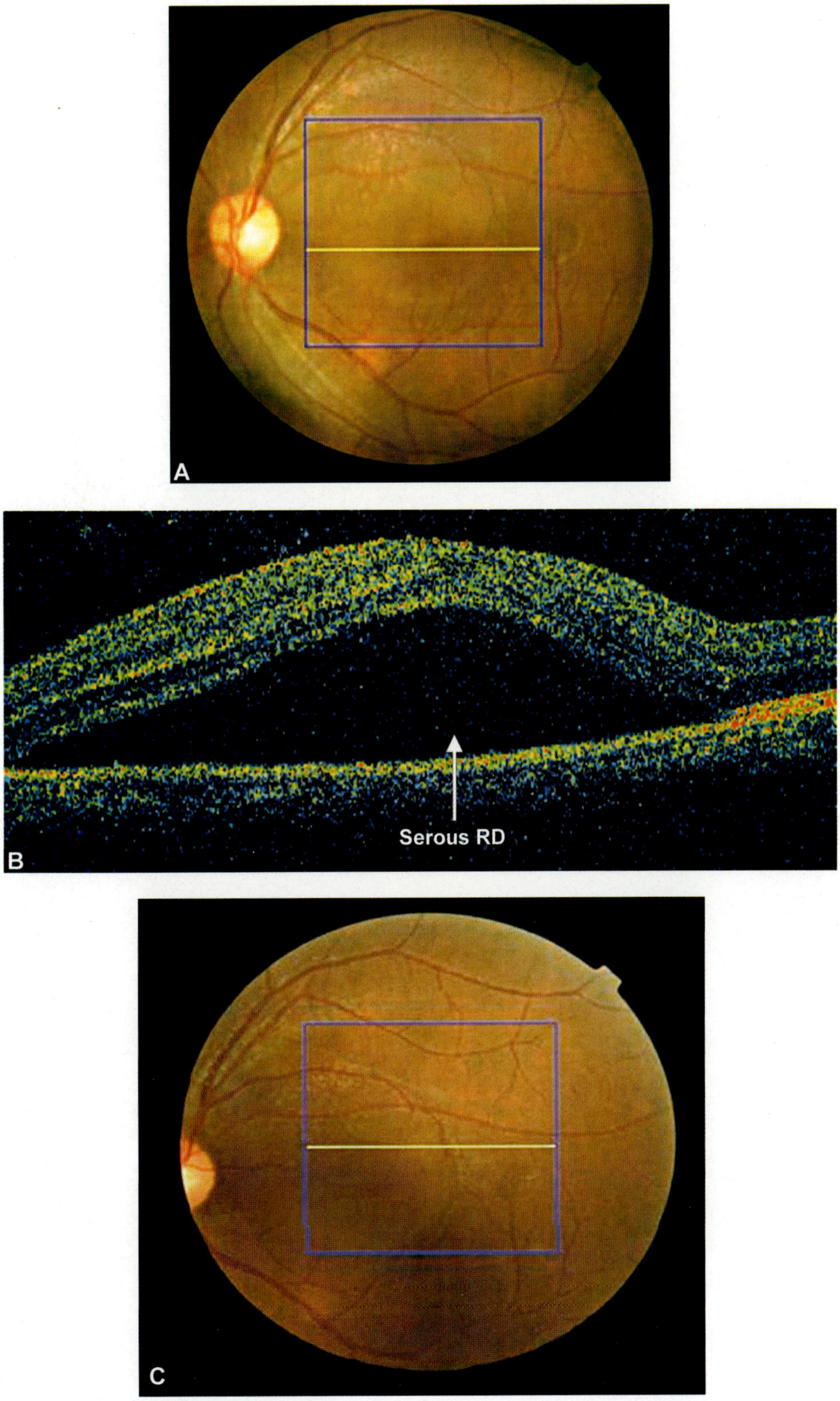

Figures 6.3.1A to C: (A) Color fundus photograph of the left eye showing the horizontal line scan through the fovea. (B) Horizontal line scan 2D image showing serous retinal detachment. (C) Color fundus photograph showing the horizontal line scan temporal to the fovea

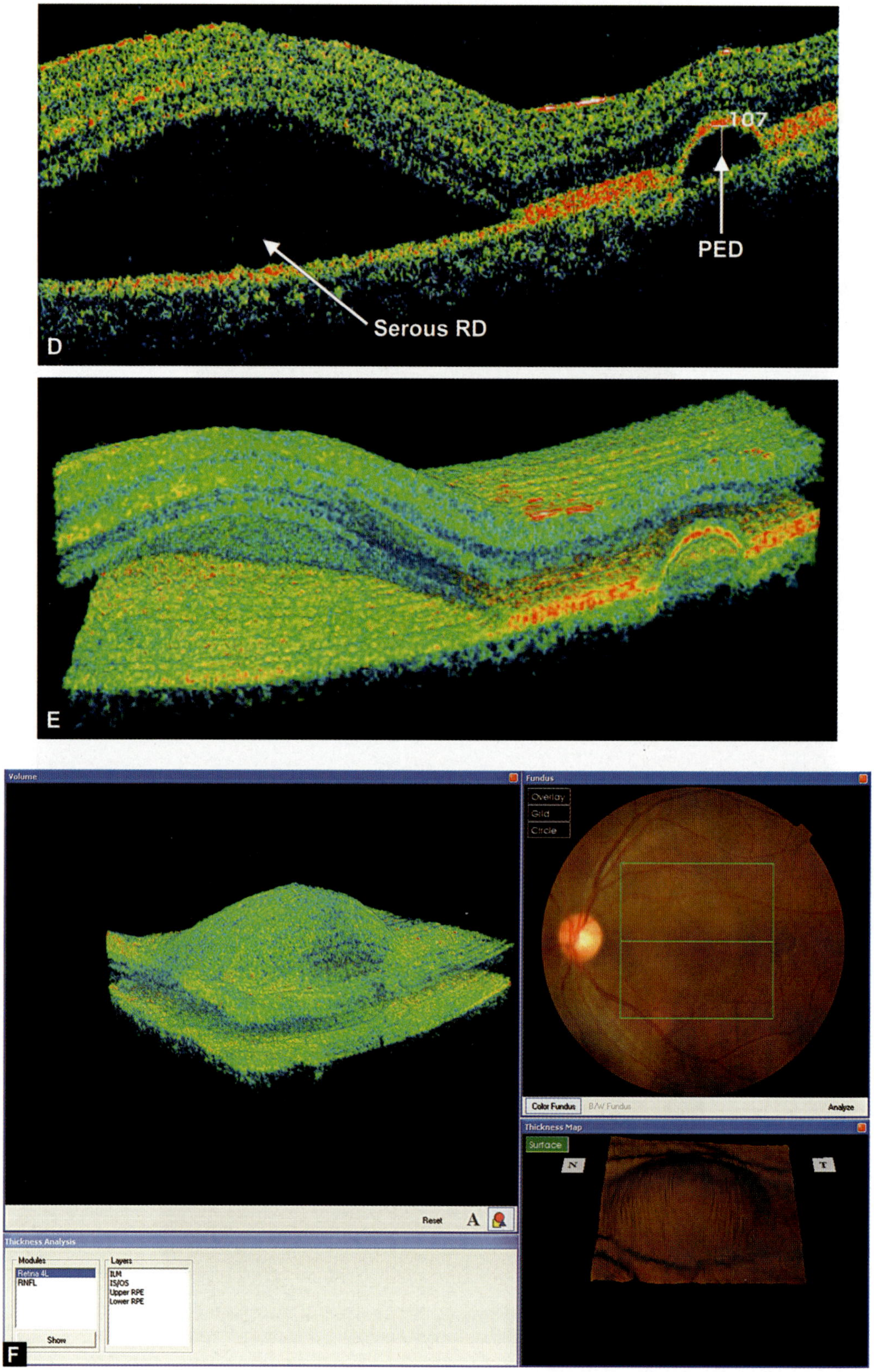

Figures 6.3.1D to F: (D) Horizontal line scan 2D image showing serous retinal detachment and PED. (E) Cropped 3D image showing serous retinal detachment and PED. (F) 3D image of Case 6.3

CASE 4: ICSC WITH SEROUS RETINAL DETACHMENT AND MULTIPLE PIGMENT EPITHELIAL DETACHMENTS

Case Summary

A 39-year-old male presented with diminished vision in the right eye of one month duration. His best corrected visual acuity in this eye was 6/60. Fluorescein angiography showed inkblot appearance with serous retinal elevation, confirming the diagnosis of ICSC (Figures 6.4.1 and 6.4.2).

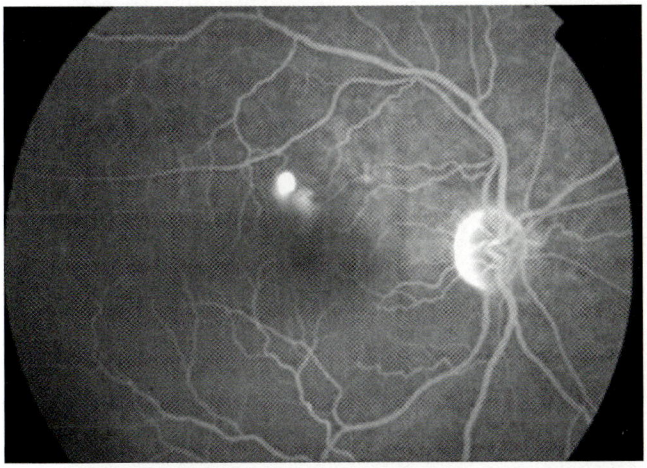

Figure 6.4.1: Early phase fluorescein angiogram shows two hyperfluorescent areas

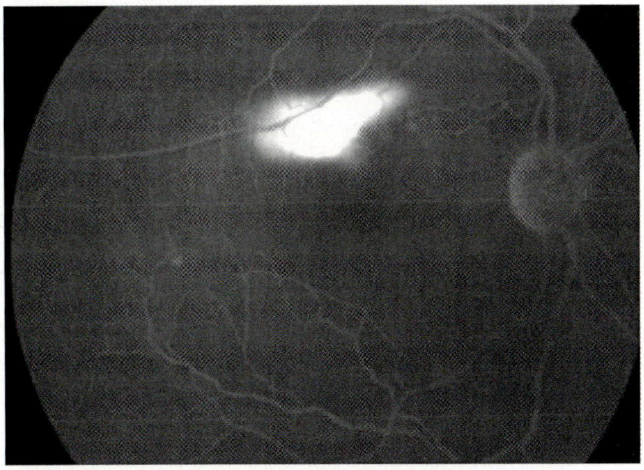

Figure 6.4.2: Late phase fluorescein angiogram shows inkblot appearance and serous retinal elevation

Optical Coherence Tomography

Horizontal line scans at different levels showed the presence of serous retinal detachment with multiple pigment epithelial detachments (Figures 6.4.3A to G).

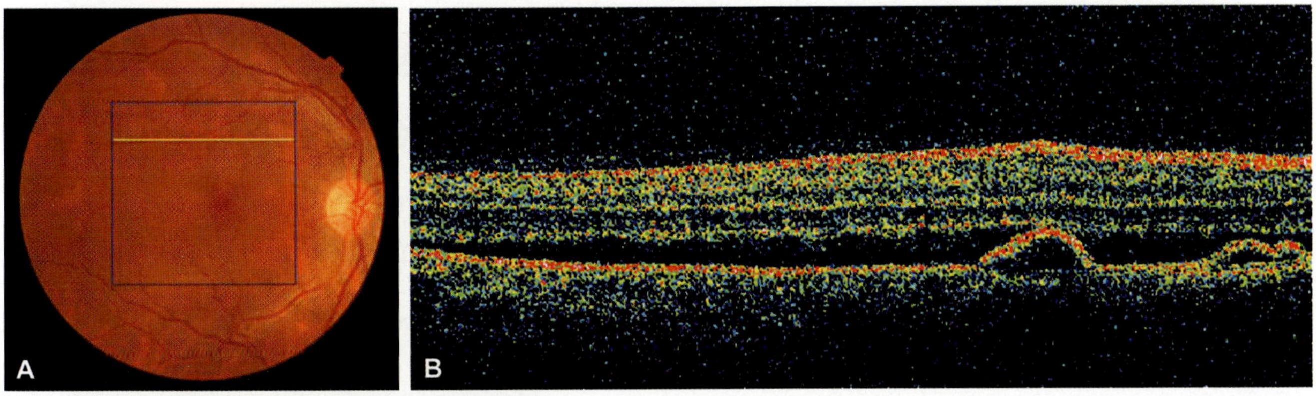

Figures 6.4.3A and B: (A) Color fundus photograph of the right eye showing the horizontal line scan above the fovea. (B) Horizontal line scan 2D image showing multiple PED within the serous retinal detachment

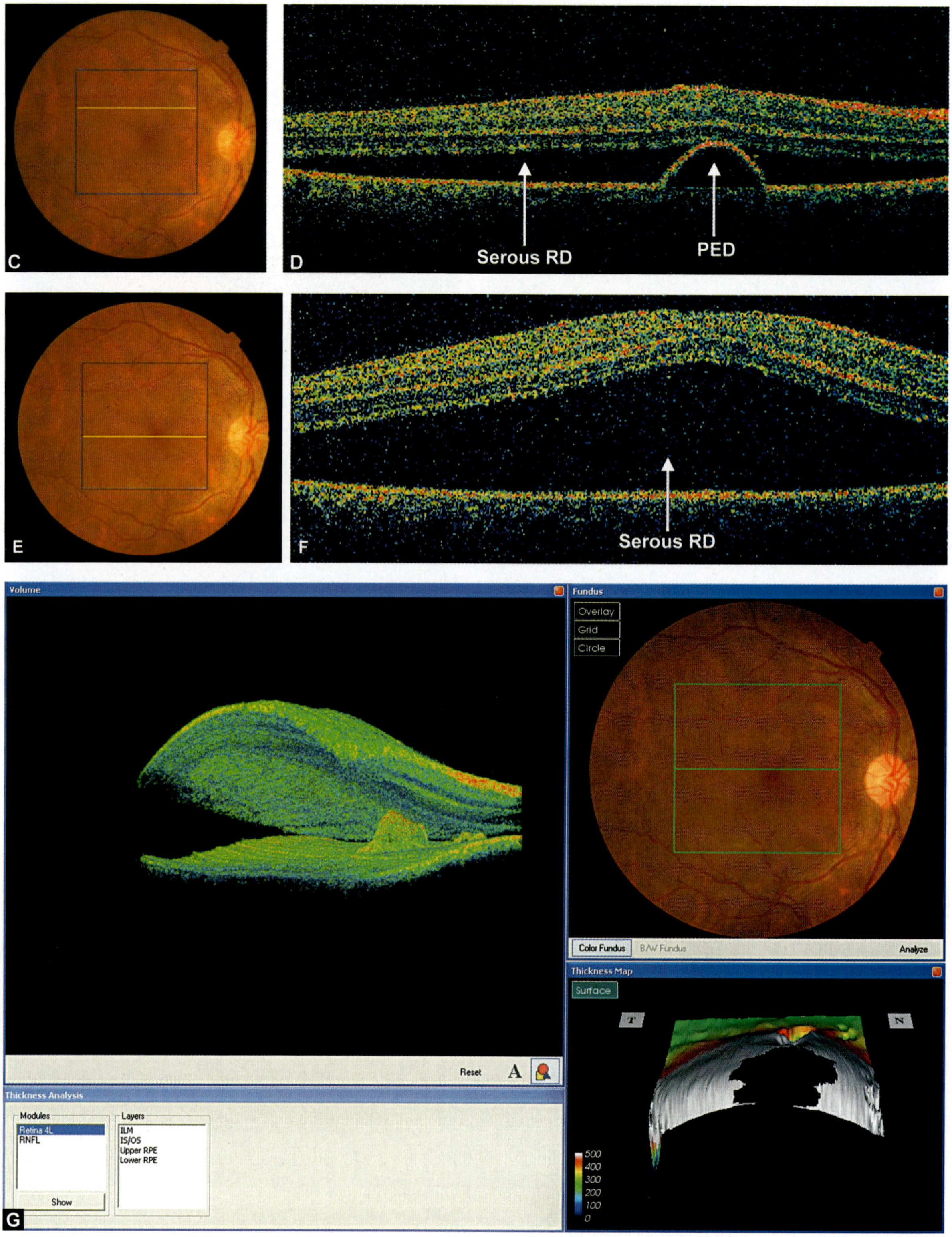

Figures 6.4.3C to G: (C) Color fundus photograph showing the horizontal line scan above the fovea. (D) Horizontal line scan 2D image showing PED within the serous retinal detachment. (E) Color fundus photograph showing the horizontal line scan through the fovea; (F) Horizontal line scan 2D image showing serous retinal detachment. (G) 3D image of Case 6.4 showing multiple PED within the serous retinal detachment

CASE 6.5: MULTIFOCAL ICSC

Case Summary

A 48-year-old man was seen with history of decreased vision in the left eye of two weeks duration. His best-corrected visual acuity was 6/12 in the left eye. Fluorescein angiography showed multifocal central serous chorioretinopathy with serous retinal elevation (Figures 6.5.1 and 6.5.2).

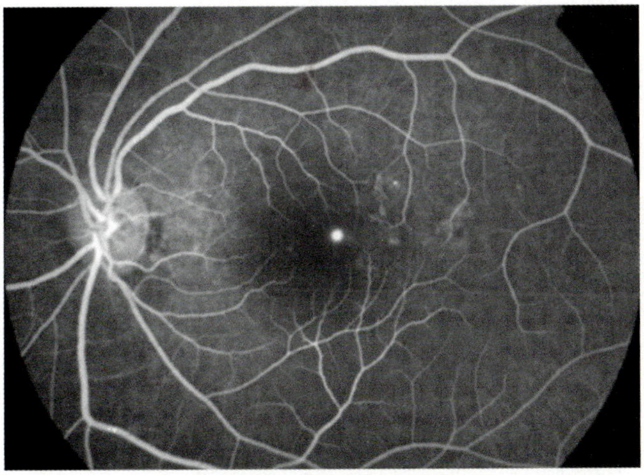

Figure 6.5.1: Early phase fluorescein angiogram shows two hyperfluorescent areas

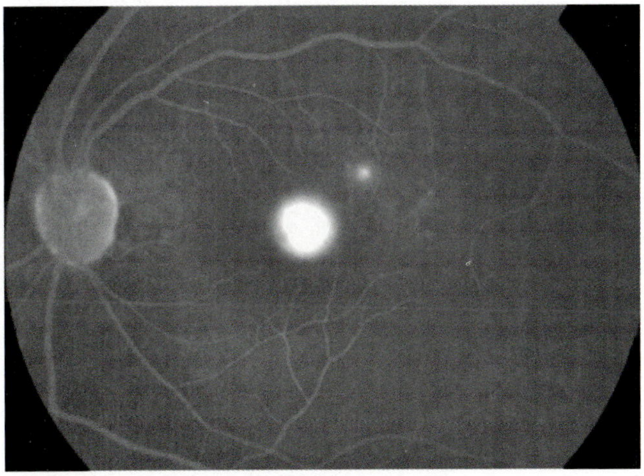

Figure 6.5.2: Late phase fluorescein angiogram shows inkblot appearance and serous retinal elevation

Optical Coherence Tomography

Horizontal line scan through the fovea showed fibrinous exudation within the serous retinal detachment. The hyporeflective area within the exudation is due to clearing of the exudation. A significant degree of hyper-reflectivity is seen in the foveal area in the vicinity of the elevated photoreceptors. A small protrusion from the RPE is seen nasal to the fovea (Figures 6.5.3A to D).

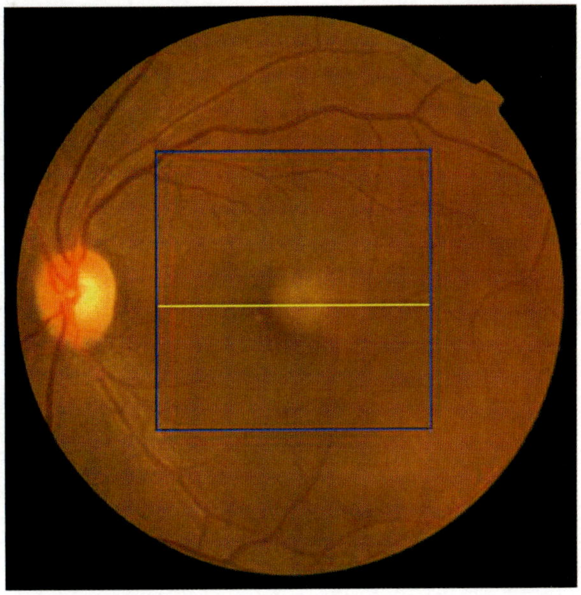

Figure 6.5.3A: Color fundus photograph of the left eye showing the horizontal line scan through the fovea

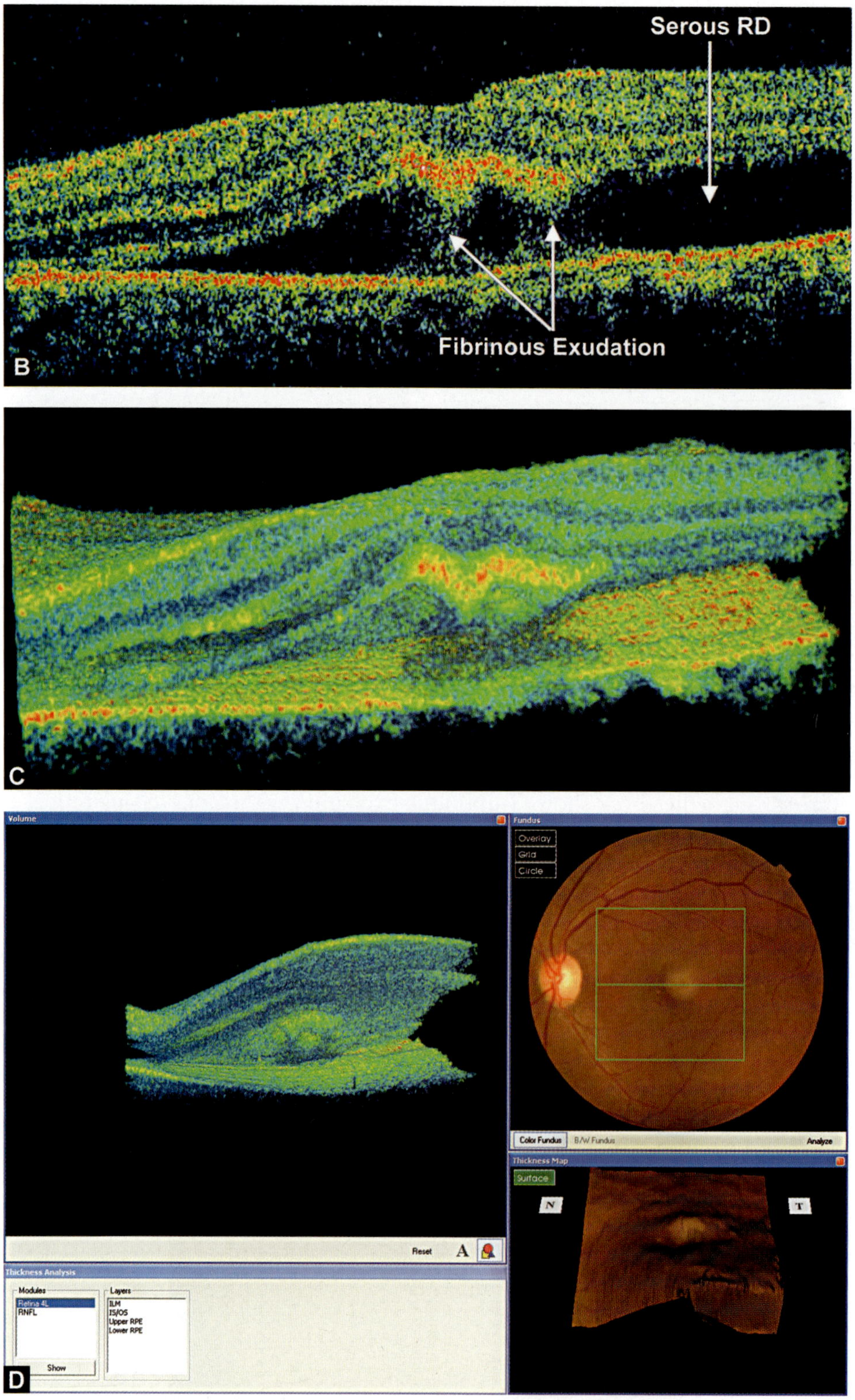

Figures 6.5.3B to D: (B) Horizontal line scan 2D image showing fibrinous exudation within the serous retinal detachment. (C) Cropped 3D image showing fibrinous exudation within the serous retinal detachment. (D) 3D image of Case 6.5 showing fibrinous exudation within the serous retinal detachment

CASE 6.6: ICSC WITH SEROUS RETINAL DETACHMENT AND MULTIPLE PIGMENT EPITHELIAL DETACHMENTS

Case Summary

A 38-year-old man presented with complaints of seeing a black patch in the right eye of two days duration. His best-corrected vision in this eye was 6/24. Fluorescein angiography showed pigment epithelial detachments, inkblot appearance, RPE degeneration and serous retinal elevation (Figures 6.6.1 and 6.6.2).

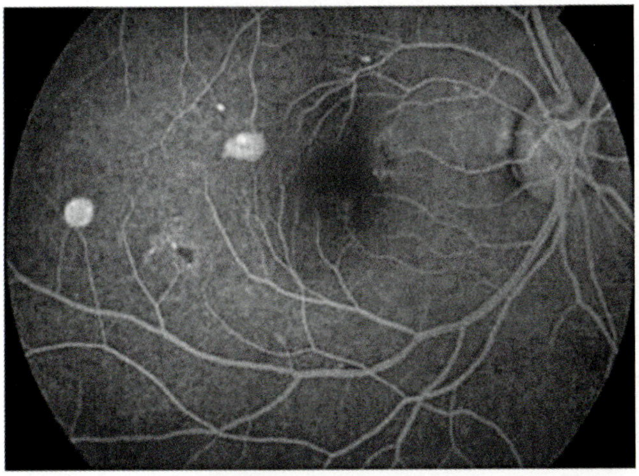

Figure 6.6.1: Early phase fluorescein angiogram shows multiple PED

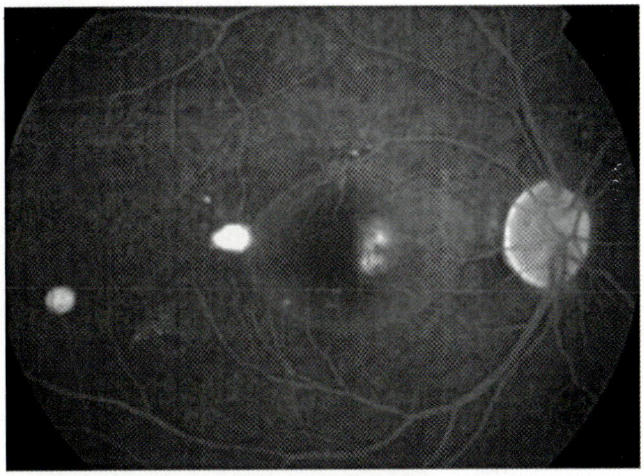

Figure 6.6.2: Late phase fluorescein angiogram shows PED, inkblot appearance and serous retinal elevation

Optical Coherence Tomography

Horizontal line scan showed the presence of serous retinal detachments and two pigment epithelial detachments (Figures 6.6.3A to C). The two PEDs are seen as hyporeflective areas in the C-scan in Figure 6.6.3D.

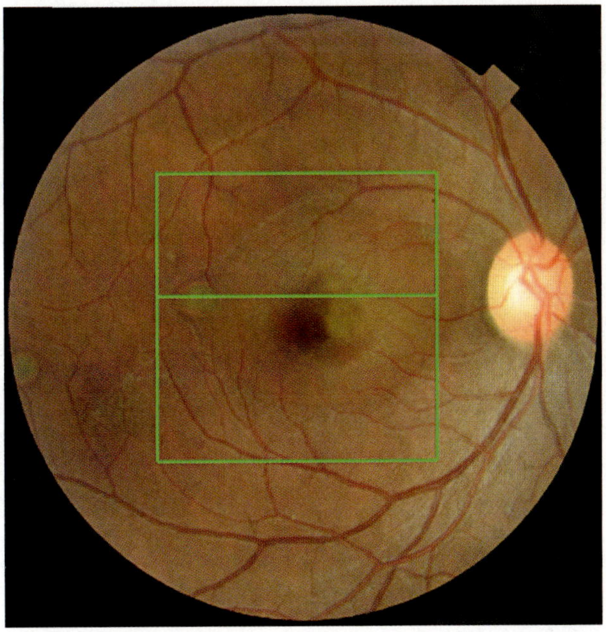

Figure 6.6.3A: Color fundus photograph of the right eye showing the horizontal line scan

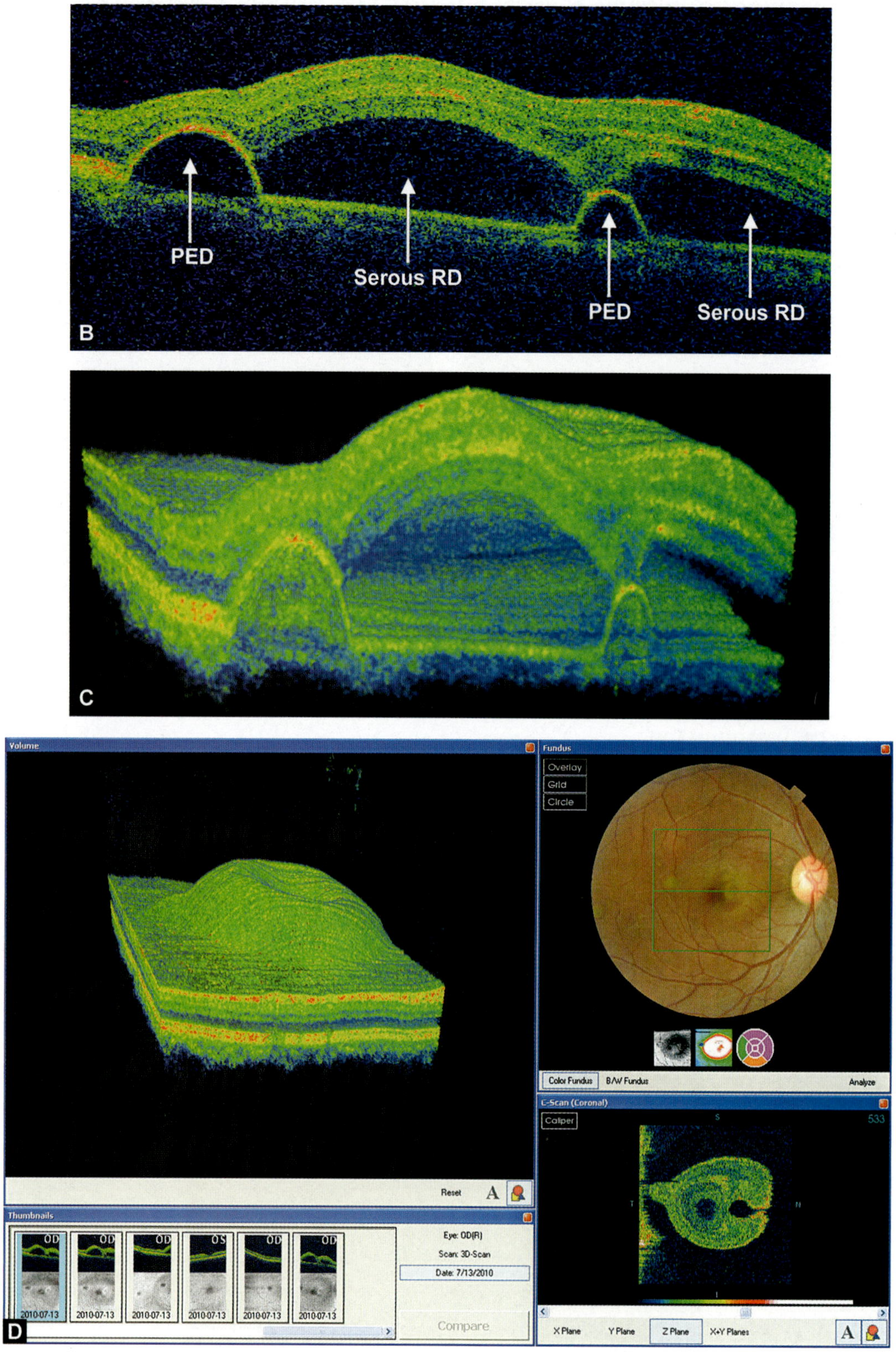

Figures 6.6.3B to D: (B) Horizontal line scan 2D image showing multiple PED within the serous retinal detachment. (C) Cropped 3D image showing multiple PED within the serous retinal detachment. (D) 3D image of Case 6.6. The PED are seen as hyporeflective areas in the C scan **(Images with Topcon 3D OCT-2000)**

CASE 6.7: FOCAL RETINAL PIGMENT EPITHELIAL BREAK IN ICSC (IMAGING WITH TOPCON 3D OCT-2000)

Case Summary

A 50-year-old male patient presented with diminished vision in the left eye of 2 months duration. His best-corrected visual acuity in this eye was 6/60. Fluorescein angiography showed inkblot appearance, multiple pigment epithelial detachments and a large area of serous retinal elevation (Figures 6.7.1 and 6.7.2).

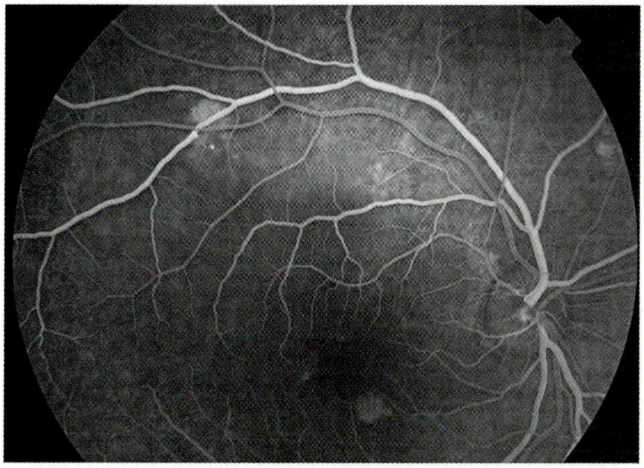

Figure 6.7.1: Early phase fluorescein angiogram shows multiple hyperfluorescent areas

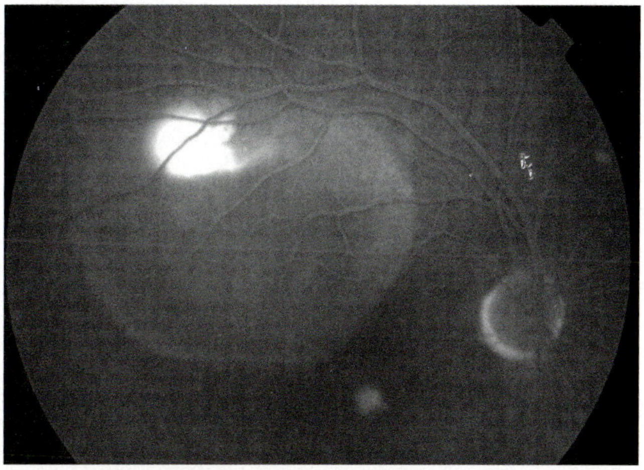

Figure 6.7.2: Late phase fluorescein angiogram shows PED, inkblot appearance and serous retinal elevation

Optical Coherence Tomography

Horizontal line scan passing through the focal leak showed the RPE disruption (pink arrow) within a RPE detachment. Subretinal exudation is visible within the neurosensory detachment. (Figures 6.7.3A and B; 6.7.5 and 6.7.6).

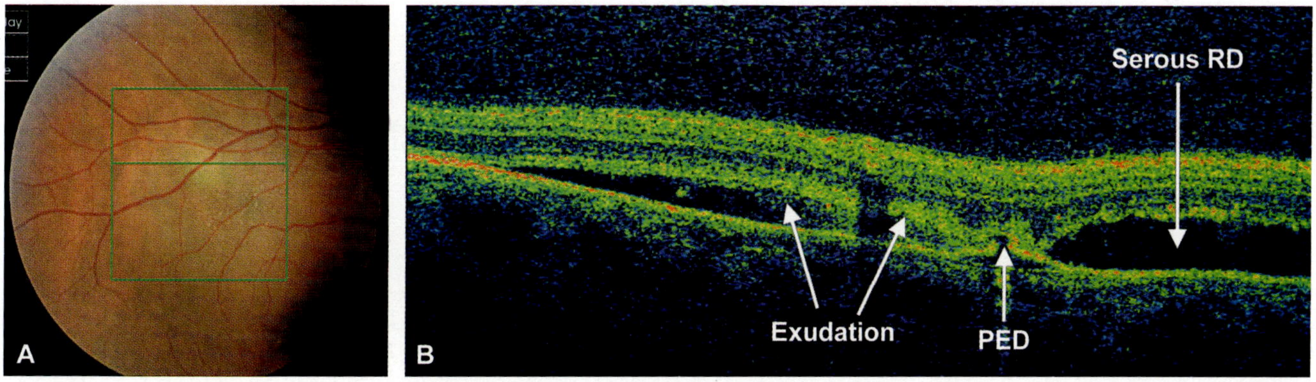

Figures 6.7.3A and B: (A) Color fundus photograph of the right eye showing the horizontal line scan through the area corresponding to the inkblot appearance in the angiogram. (B) Horizontal line scan 2D image showing serous retinal detachment with fibrinous exudation and PED. A focal retinal pigment epithelial break is also evident

Hyper-reflective areas (short arrows) can be seen on the posterior surface of the detached neurosensory retina which correspond to the precipitates seen clinically (Figures 6.7.3C and D).

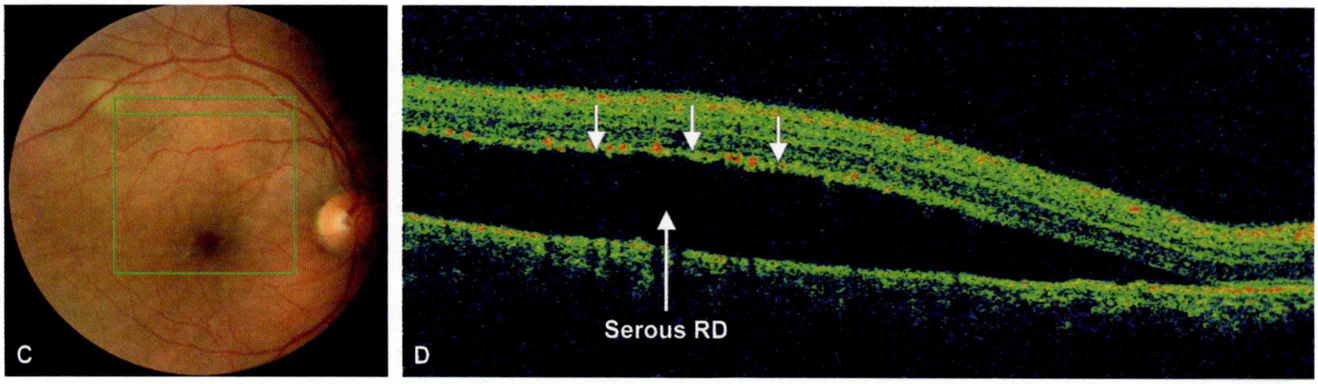

Figures 6.7.3C and D: (C) Color fundus photograph of the right eye showing the horizontal line scan above the fovea. (D) Horizontal line scan 2D image showing hyper-reflective areas on the posterior surface of the detached neurosensory retina

Horizontal line scan passing above the fovea showed the extent of the neurosensory detachment (Figures 6.7.3E and F)

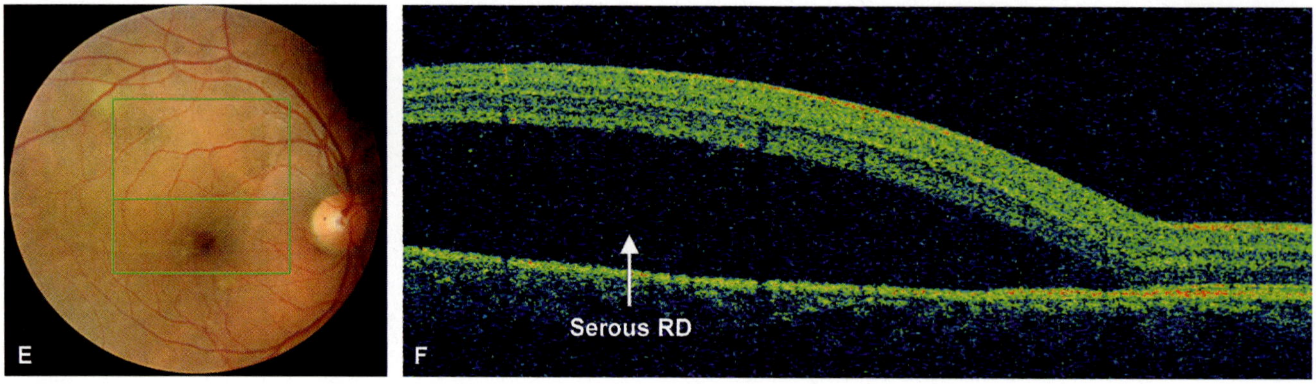

Figures 6.7.3E and F: (E) Color fundus photograph of the right eye showing the horizontal line scan above the fovea. (F) Horizontal line scan 2D image showing serous retinal detachment

Horizontal line scan passing below the fovea showed a pigment epithelial detachment (Figures 6.7.3G and H).

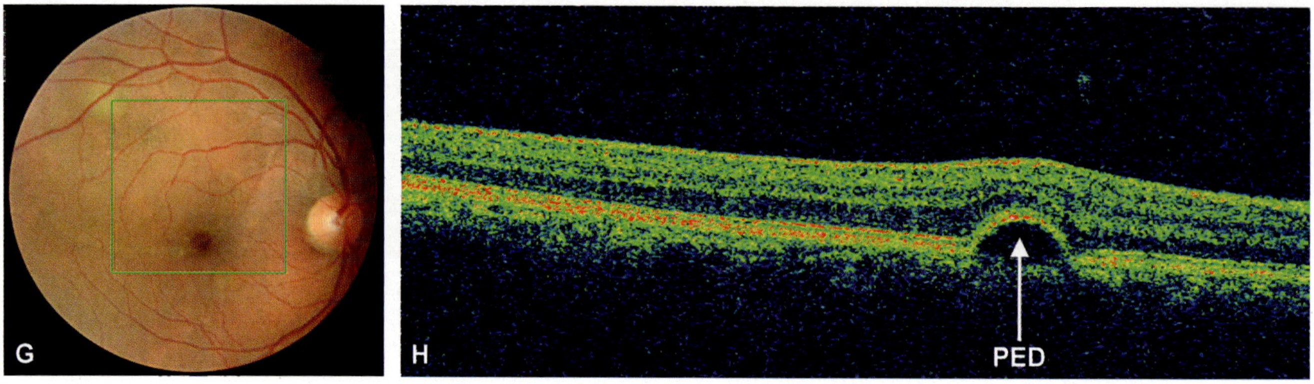

Figures 6.7.3G and H: (G) Color fundus photograph of the right eye showing the horizontal line scan below the fovea. (H) Horizontal line scan 2D image showing PED

Horizontal line scans at different levels showed the presence of pigment epithelial detachments (Figures 6.7.4A to D).

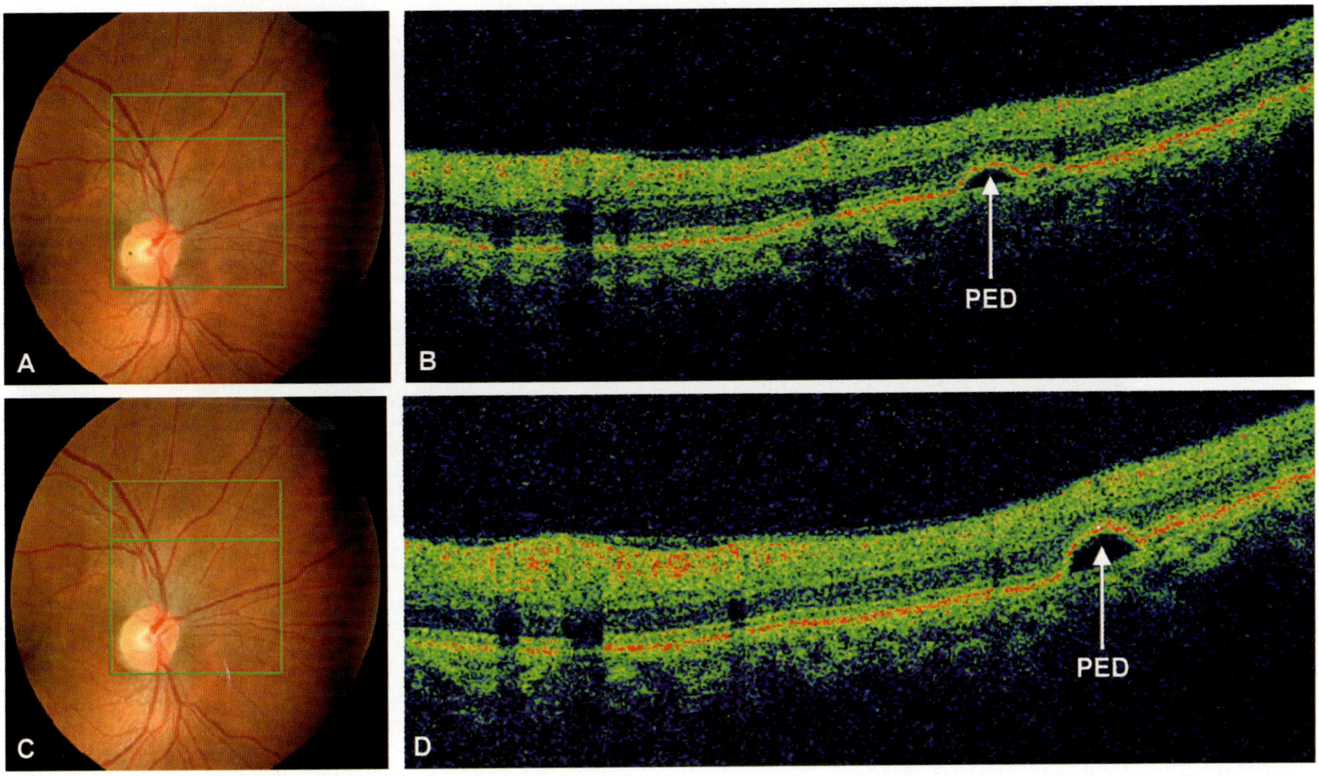

Figures 6.7.4A to D: (A) Color fundus photograph of the right eye showing the horizontal line scan above the disc. (B) Horizontal line scan 2D image showing PED. (C) Color fundus photograph of the right eye showing the horizontal line scan above the disc. (D) Horizontal line scan 2D image showing PED

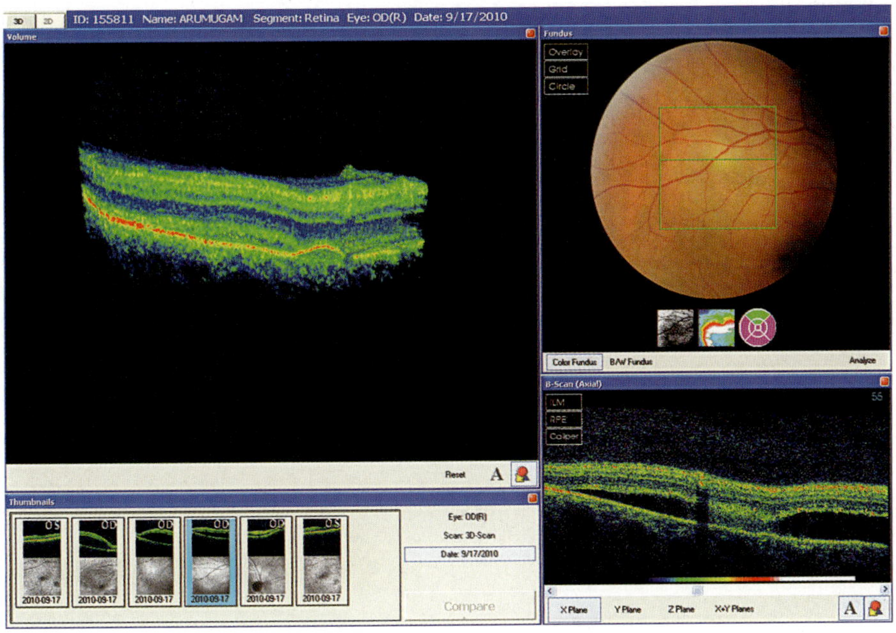

Figure 6.7.5: Cropped 3D image of Case 6.7

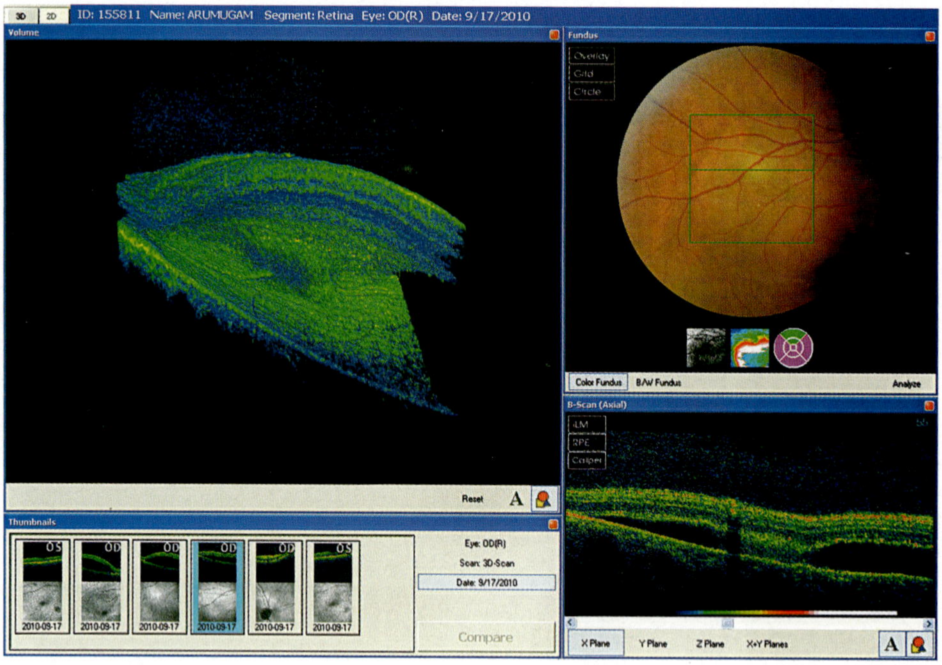

Figure 6.7.6: 3D image of Case 6.7

SUGGESTED READING

1. Iida T, Hagimura N, Sato T, Kishi S. Evaluation of central serous chorioretinopathy with optical coherence tomography. Am J Ophthalmol.2000 Jan;129(1):16-20.
2. Montero JA, Ruiz – Moreno JM. Optical coherence tomography characterization of idiopathic central serous chorioretinopathy. Br J Ophthalmol. 2005;89(5):562-4.
3. Ober MD, Eandi CM, Jampol LM, et al. Focal retinal pigment epithelial breaks in central serous chorioretinopathy. Retinal Cases and Brief Reports 2007;1:271-273.
4. Rezai KA, Eliott D. Optical coherence tomographic findings in pregnancy associated central serous chorioretinopathy.Graefes Arch Clin Exp Ophthalomol.2004;242(12):1014-6.
5. Saito M, Iida T, Kishi S. Ring shaped subretinal fibrinous exudates in central serous chorioretinopathy. Jpn J Ophthalmol 2005;49(6):516-9.

7 Choroidal Disorders

Choroidal coloboma is a congenital defect caused by defective closure of embryonal fissure. Closure of the fissure normally takes place during the 6th week of gestation. Genetic as well as environmental factors have been proposed to cause an intrauterine insult that can lead to defective closure of the embryonal fissure leading to coloboma of the fundus. The spectrum of this anomaly can vary from small colobomas located in the equatorial region that do not interfere with vision, to large colobomas involving the disc and macula with severe impairment of vision. Retinal detachment occurs in 40 percent of eyes with choroidal coloboma. Histologically, the colobomatous area is deficient in normal choroid, retinal pigment epithelium and the retina. The neurosensory retina continues as the intercalary membrane (ICM) in the area of coloboma.

ROLE OF OPTICAL COHERENCE TOMOGRAPHY

The margin of the choroidal coloboma holds important information because it is the transition zone between the normal and the abnormal part of the fundus and the site of communication between the subintercalary membrane space and subretinal space.

OCT is useful in evaluating the margins of choroidal colobomas. It helps in the detection of subclinical retinal detachment along the margin and identification of the location of communications between sub-ICM space and subretinal space which may be important in planning the management of these eyes.

CASE 7.1: CHOROIDAL COLOBOMA

Case Summary

A 23-year-old male was seen for routine eye check-up. His best-corrected visual acuity in the right eye was 6/60. Anterior segment showed an iris coloboma.

Optical Coherence Tomography

Horizontal line scan passing through the margin of the coloboma showed normal retina with a total defect (absence of retina, retinal pigment epithelium and choroid) in the region of the coloboma (Figures 7.1.1A to D).

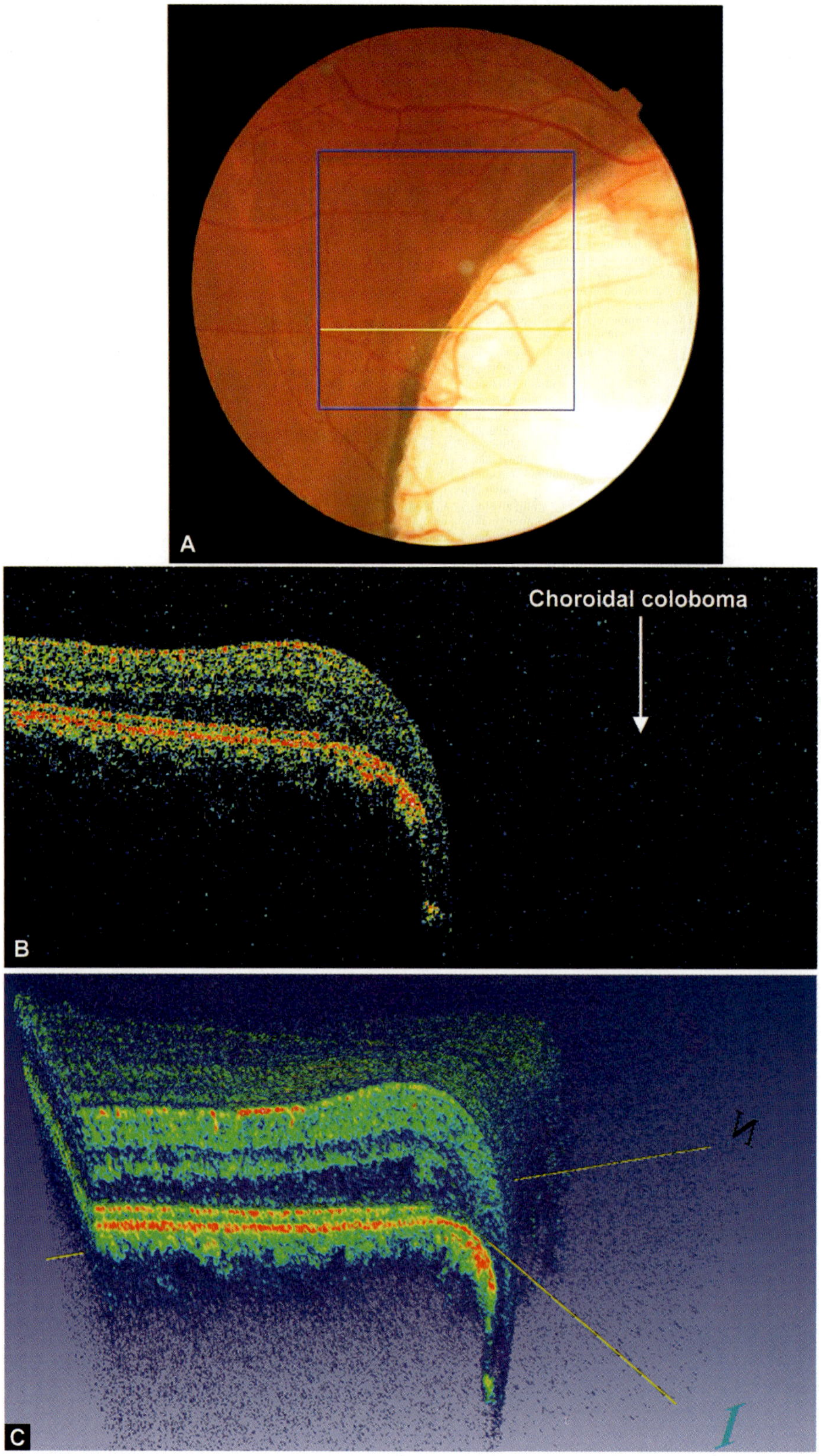

Figures 7.1.1A to C: (A) Color fundus photograph showing the horizontal line scan through the margin of the coloboma. (B) Horizontal line scan through the margin of the coloboma, 2D image showing normal retina with total defect in the region of the coloboma. (C) Cropped 3D image showing normal retina with total defect in the region of the coloboma

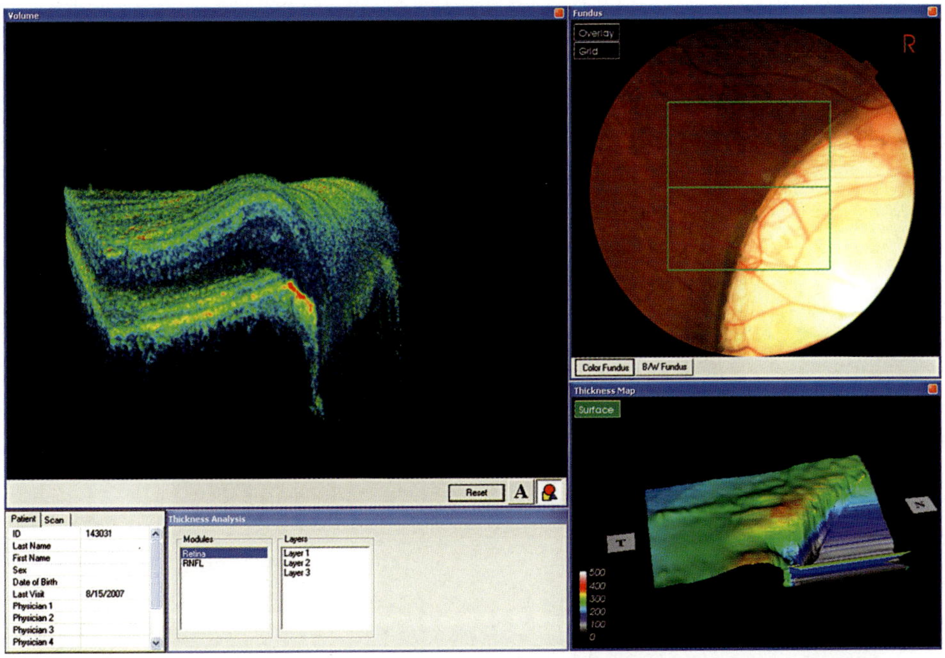

Figure 7.1.1D: 3D image of Case 7.1

CHOROIDAL FOLDS

Choroidal folds are undulations involving the inner layers of the choroid, Bruch's membrane and the retinal pigment epithelium. They appear as alternate yellow and dark streaks—yellow corresponding to the crest of the folds. The folds may be horizontal, vertical or oblique and are parallel to each other. They can be either idiopathic or secondary to hypotony, posterior scleritis, orbital tumors etc.

Fluorescein angiography shows alternating dark and light bands. The crest of the fold appears hyperfluorescent while the trough appears hypofluorescent.

Role of Optical Coherence Tomography

OCT helps to differentiate between chorioretinal and choroidal folds. Chorioretinal folds are indicated by undulating retinal and RPE lines of normal thickness while choroidal folds are evidenced by a wavy appearance of the RPE and a flat retinal surface.

CASE 7.2: IDIOPATHIC CHOROIDAL FOLDS

Case Summary

A 48-year-old female was seen for routine eye check-up. Her best-corrected visual acuity was 6/6 in both eyes.

Optical Coherence Tomography

Horizontal line scan passing through the area of folds showed wavy appearance of the retinal pigment epithelium (Figures 7.2.1A and B). The retinal layers from the ILM to the photoreceptor layers have been peeled in Figure 7.2.1C to show the folds on the RPE layer.

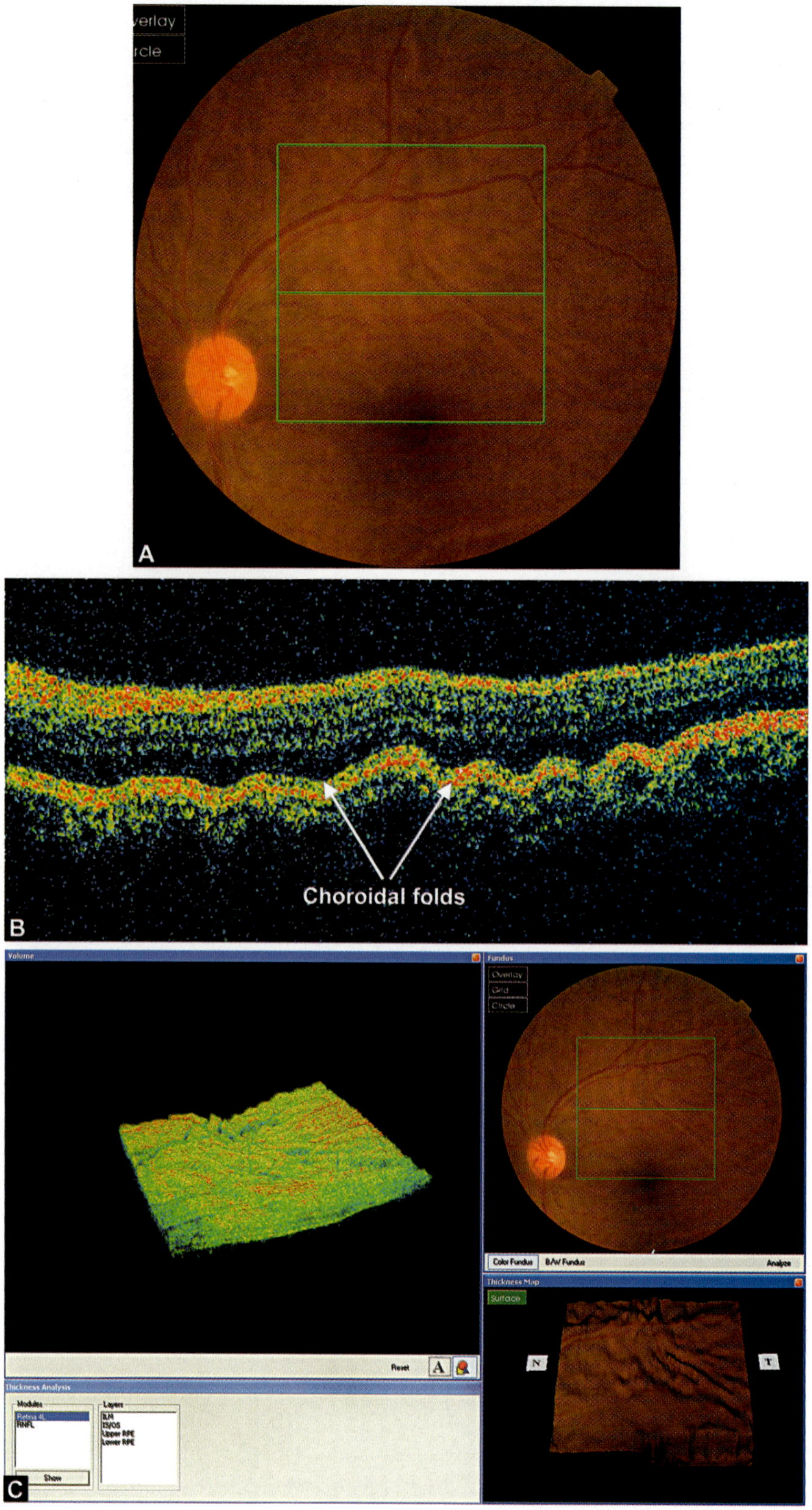

Figures 7.2.1A to C: (A) Color fundus photograph showing the horizontal line scan through the choroidal folds. (B) Horizontal line scan, 2D image showing wavy appearance of the RPE corresponding to the choroidal folds. (C) Retinal layers have been peeled to show the folds on the RPE layer corresponding to the choroidal folds

CONCLUSION

OCT is helpful in differentiating chorioretinal folds from choroidal folds and can reveal the relationship between the folds and the posterior vitreous surface.

CHOROIDAL METASTASIS

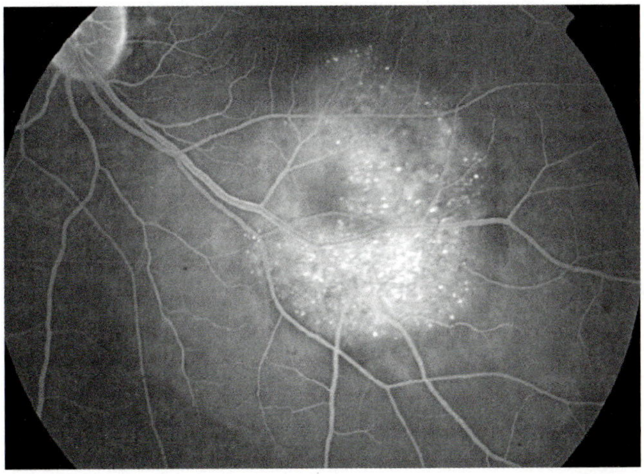

Metastatic carcinoma to the choroid is now recognized as the most common intraocular neoplasm. Eighty percent of cases are unilateral and unifocal whereas 20 percent have multiple or bilateral tumors. The typical metastatic carcinoma to the choroid from breast, lung or gastrointestinal tract appears as a golden yellow to yellowish white, round to oval lesion. Tumors of the kidney and prostate are also known to metastasize to the choroid.

Fluorescein angiography of metastatic carcinoma to the choroid shows few or no large caliber intralesional vessels, relative hypofluorescence of the lesion in the early phase and diffuse hyperfluorescence in the late phase. In some cases, multiple hyperfluorescent dots are evident on the surface of the lesion in the venous and late phase.

Optical Coherence Tomography

Schaudig et al have shown that the OCT beam is strongly reflected by the RPE and reflections from the tumor mass are weak, therefore, OCT is not useful for *in vivo* histological typing of choroidal tumors. However, OCT can demonstrate the secondary changes in the overlying retina and retinal pigment epithelium known to be associated with metastatic carcinoma to the choroid. The OCT features of choroidal metastasis include serous retinal detachment, highly reflective lesions overlying the RPE-choriocapillaris complex, thickened retinal RPE-choriocapillaris complex, highly reflective points inside the neurosensory retina and in the subretinal space and intraretinal splitting.

CASE 7.3: CHOROIDAL METASTASIS SECONDARY TO CARCINOMA LUNG

Case Summary

A 42-year-old female diagnosed to have carcinoma lung with bone metastasis was referred with defective vision in her left eye of 3 months duration. Her best-corrected visual acuity in the left eye was 6/9. Fluorescein angiography in the early phase revealed areas of hypo- and hyperfluorescence surrounded by a ring of hypofluorescence and the late phase showed increasing hyperfluorescence with multiple hyperfluorescent dots on the surface of the lesion and evidence of serous fluid accumulation (Figures 7.3.1 and 7.3.2).

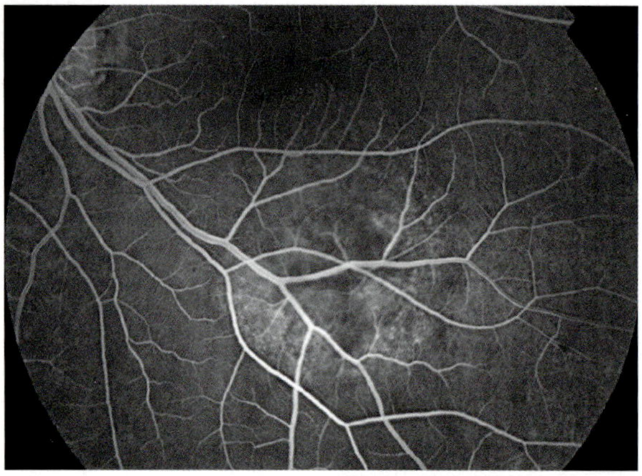

Figure 7.3.1: Early phase angiogram shows areas of hypo and hyperfluorescence within the lesion

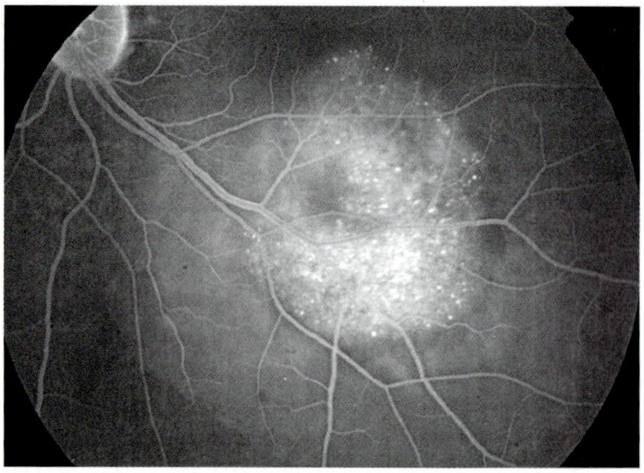

Figure 7.3.2: Late phase angiogram shows increasing hyperfluorescence with multiple hyperfluorescent dots and evidence of serous fluid accumulation

Optical Coherence Tomography–1

Horizontal line scan through the fovea showed loss of fovea contour, dome shaped elevation of the retina attached to the retinal pigment epithelium-choriocapillaris complex and a shallow neurosensory retinal detachment (Figures 7.3.3A and B).

Optical Coherence Tomography–2

Horizontal line scan through the lesion showed an elevated choroidal mass with adjoining serous retinal detachment (Figures 7.3.3C and D).

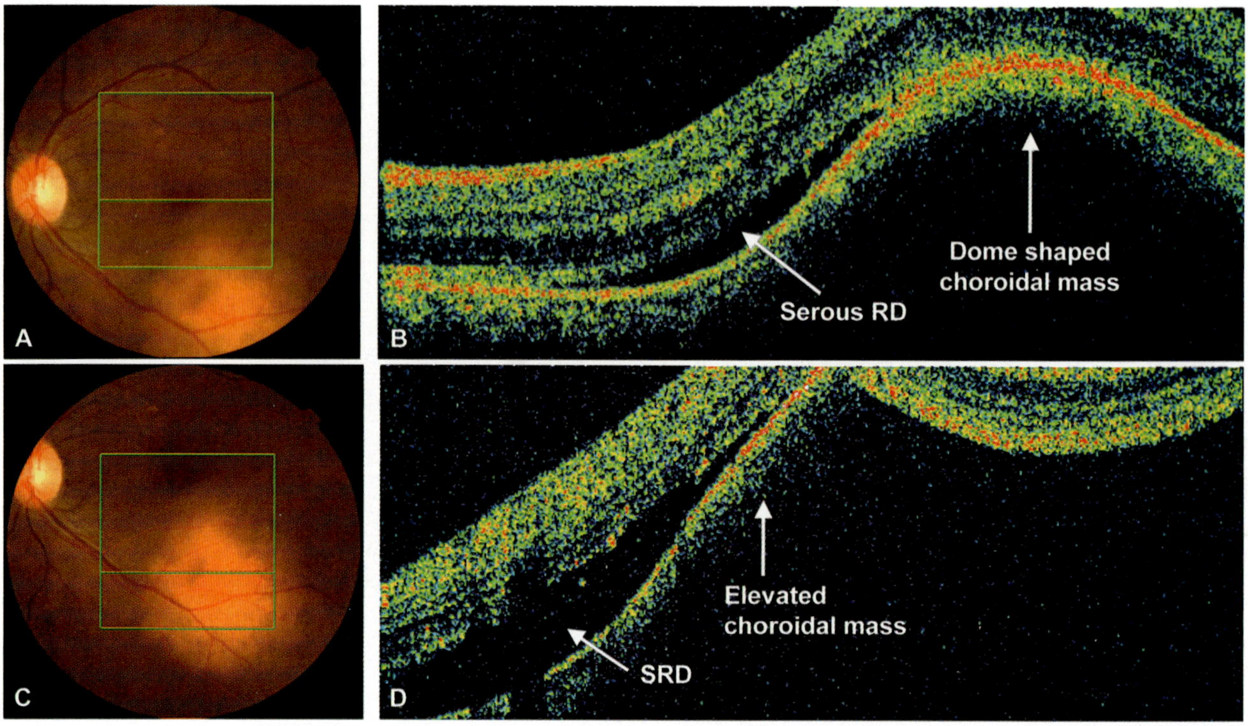

Figures 7.3.3A to D: (A) Color fundus photograph showing the horizontal line scan through the fovea. (B) Horizontal line scan through the fovea, 2D image showing loss of fovea contour, dome shaped elevation of the retina attached to the retinal pigment epithelium-choriocapillaris complex and a shallow neurosensory retinal detachment. (C) Color fundus photograph showing the horizontal line scan through the lesion. (D) Horizontal line scan through the lesion, 2D image showing an elevated choroidal mass with adjoining serous retinal detachment.

Ultrasonography

B-scan showed a choroidal mass with irregular echotexture and A-scan showed moderate anterior surface spike and high irregular internal reflectivity consistent with choroidal metastasis (Figure 7.3.4).

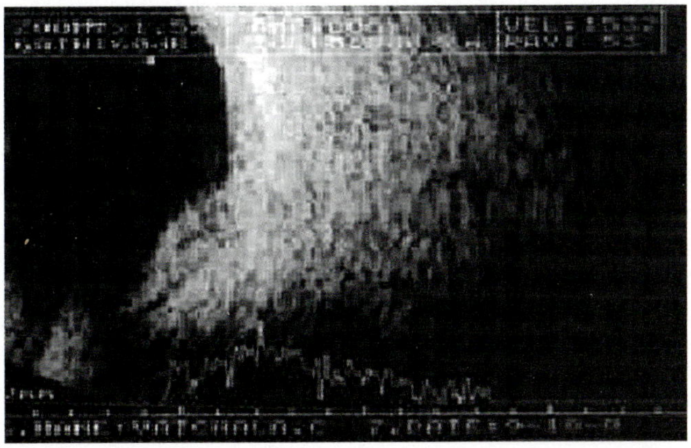

Figure 7.3.4: Ultrasound B scan shows a choroidal mass with irregular echotexture and A-scan shows moderate anterior surface spike and high irregular internal reflectivity consistent with choroidal metastasis

CONCLUSION

Optical coherence tomography is useful in demonstrating the secondary retinal and RPE changes and in evaluating the response of choroidal tumors to treatment.

CHOROIDAL HEMANGIOMA

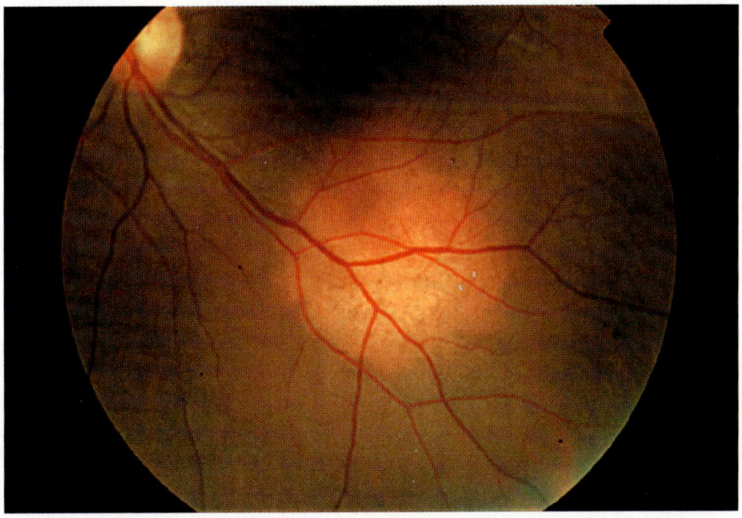

Choroidal hemangioma is a benign vascular tumor of the choroid which occurs in two distinct clinical forms: a circumscribed form that is almost always isolated and nonsyndromic and a diffuse form that is usually part of Sturge-Weber syndrome.

Fluorescein Angiography

Choroidal hemangioma shows early hyperfluorescence with late leakage of the dye and staining of the tumor.

Optical Coherence Tomography

Destruction of the overlying RPE by the choroidal hemangioma impairs the blood-retina barrier, which then allows the large incompetent choroidal vessels from within the substance of the tumor to leak into the surrounding tissues. OCT, therefore, is helpful in detecting the presence of serous retinal detachment, extent of the subretinal fluid and the presence of cystoid macular edema.

CASE 7.4: CIRCUMSCRIBED CHOROIDAL HEMANGIOMA ASSOCIATED WITH STURGE-WEBER SYNDROME

Case Summary

A 24-year-old male presented with defective vision in his right eye of two months duration. His best-corrected visual acuity in this eye was counting fingers at one metre. On examination, he was found to have facial nevus flammeus on the right side and normal intraocular pressure. Fluorescein angiography showed a circumscribed area of hyperfluorescence in the early phase with leakage of the dye and staining of the central portion of the tumor in the late phase. Retinal vascular tortuosity was also evident (Figures 7.4.1 and 7.4.2).

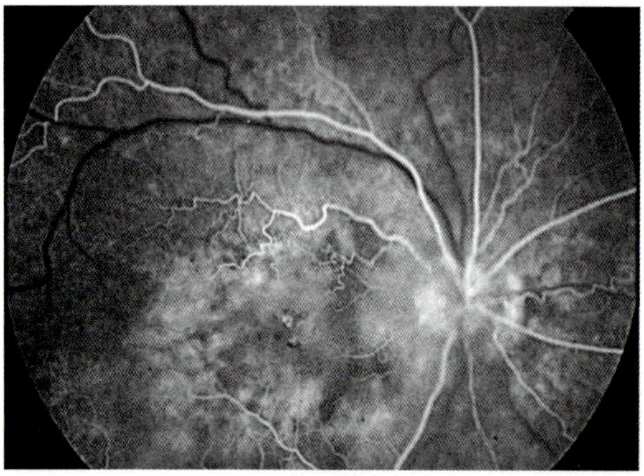

Figure 7.4.1: Early phase angiogram shows a circumscribed area of hyperfluorescence

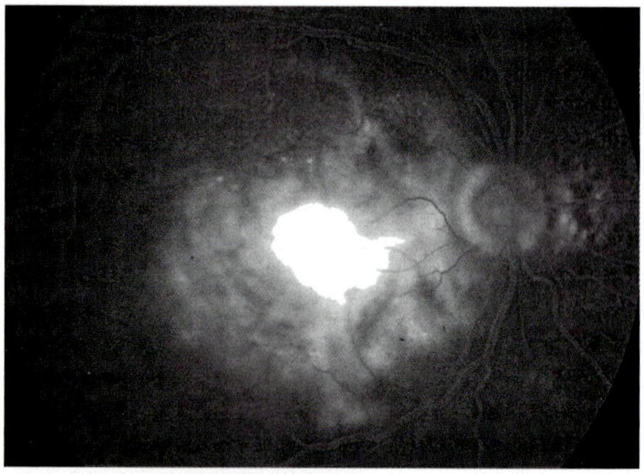

Figure 7.4.2: Late phase angiogram shows leakage of dye and staining of the central portion of the tumor

Optical Coherence Tomography

Horizontal line scan passing through the fovea showed loss of foveal contour, cystoid spaces and serous retinal detachment (Figures 7.4.3A to D).

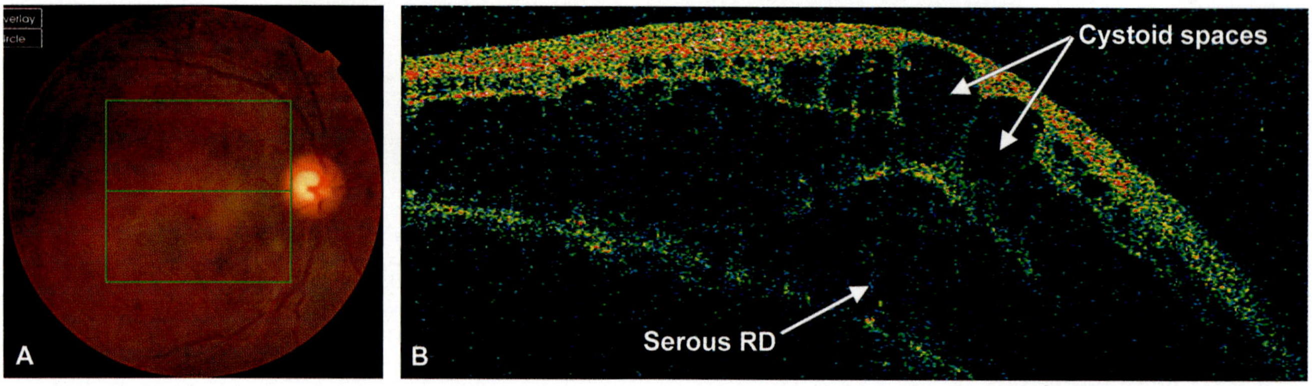

Figures 7.4.3A and B: (A) Color fundus photograph showing the horizontal line scan through the fovea. (B) Horizontal line scan through the fovea, 2D image showing loss of foveal contour, cystoid spaces and serous retinal detachment

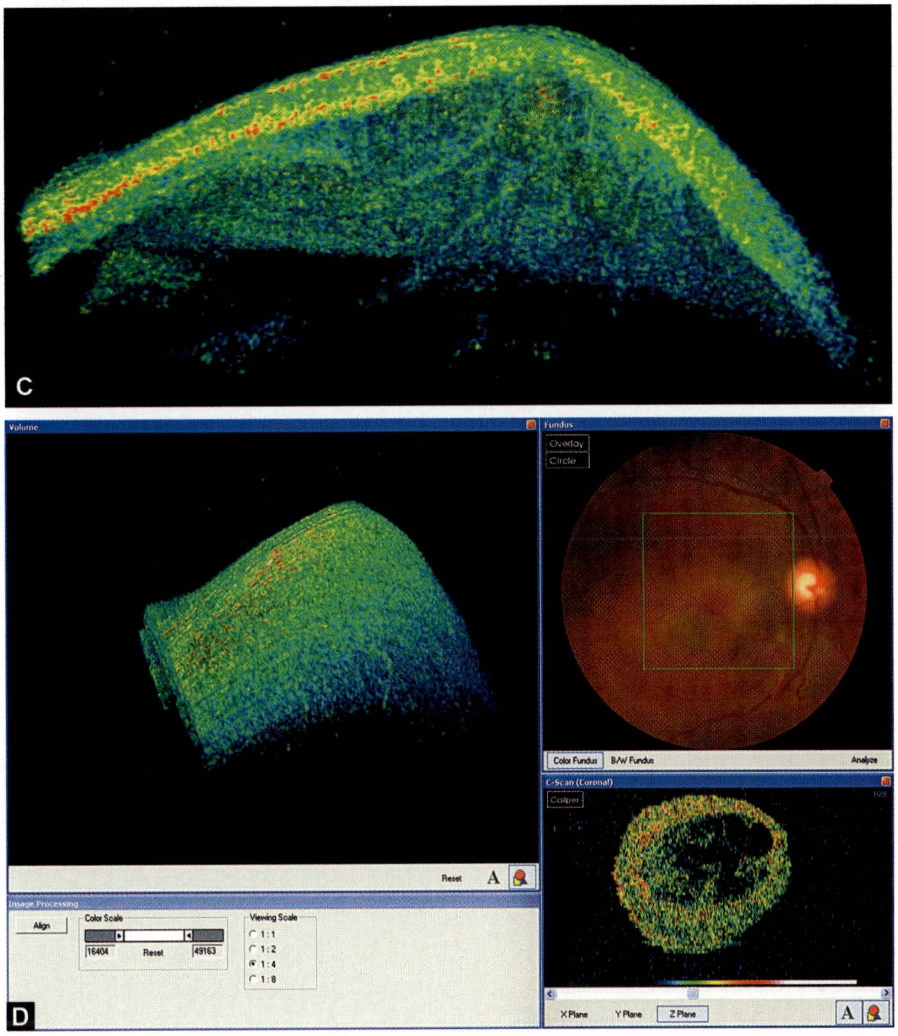

Figures 7.4.3C and D: (C) Cropped 3D image showing loss of foveal contour, cystoid spaces and serous retinal detachment. (D) 3D image of Case 7.4

Horizontal line scan passing through the optic disc showed evidence of serous retinal fluid surrounding the disc (Figures 7.4.4A and B).

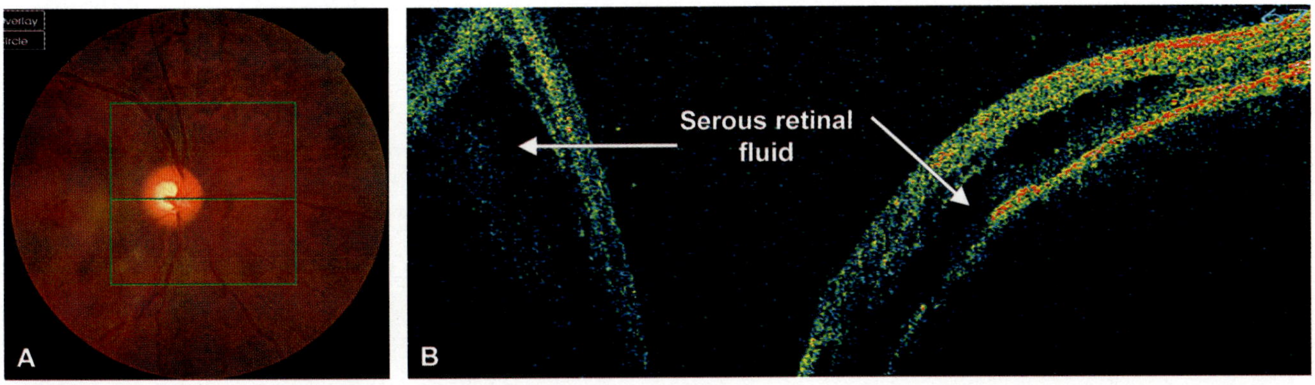

Figures 7.4.4A and B: (A) Color fundus photograph showing the horizontal line scan through the optic disc; (B) Horizontal line scan through the optic disc, 2D image showing evidence of serous retinal fluid surrounding the disc

Ultrasonography

B-scan showed a fusiform lesion with the internal brightness similar to orbital tissue. A-scan showed a high anterior surface spike and high irregular internal reflectivity consistent with choroidal hemangioma (Figure 7.4.5).

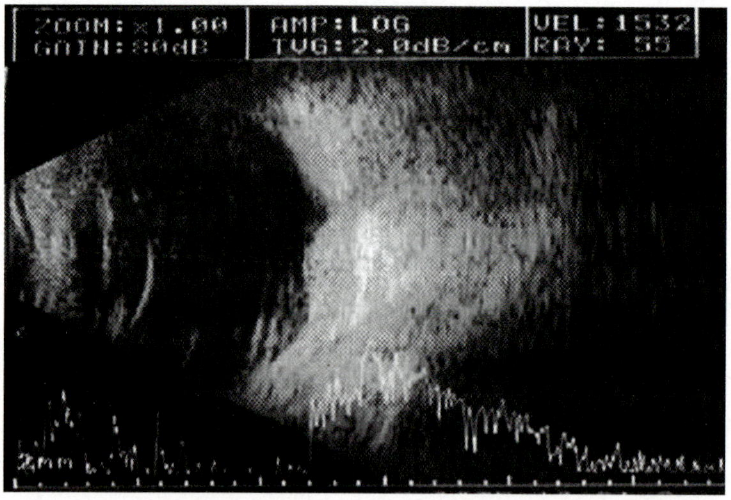

Figure 7.4.5: Ultrasound B scan shows a fusiform lesion with the internal brightness similar to orbital tissue. A-scan shows a high anterior surface spike and high irregular internal reflectivity consistent with choroidal hemangioma

CONCLUSION

Optical coherence tomography is useful in demonstrating the secondary retinal and RPE changes and in evaluating the response of the choroidal hemangioma to treatment.

SUGGESTED READING

1. Lingam Gopal, Balbir Khan, Sumeet Jain, Vilakkumadadhil S, Prakash. A clinical and optical coherence tomography study of the margins of choroidal colobomas. Ophthalmology 2007;114:571-80.
2. Giuseppe Giuffre, Mauro G. Distefano. Optical coherence tomography of chorioretinal and choriodal folds. Acta Ophthalmologica Scandinavica 2006.85(3) 333-6.
3. Schaudig U, Hassenstein A, Bernad A, et al. Limitations of imaging choroidal tumors in vivo by optical coherente tomography. Graefe's Arch Clin Exp Ophthalmol 1998;236:588-92.
4. J Fernando Arevalo, Carlos F Fernandez, Reinaldo A Garcia. Optical coherence tomography characteristics of choroidal metastasis. Ophthalmology 2005;112:1612-9.

8 Degenerative Myopia

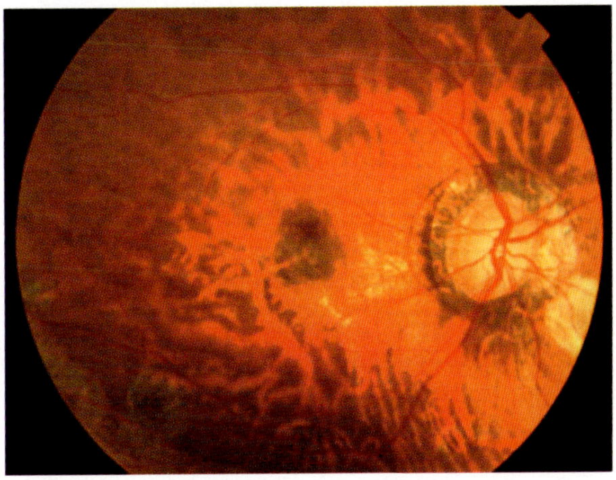

CASE 8.1: MYOPIA WITH CHOROIDAL NEOVASCULAR MEMBRANE (CNVM) TREATED WITH PHOTODYNAMIC THERAPY AND INTRAVITREAL RANIBIZUMAB

Case Summary

A 30-year-old male with high myopia presented with diminished vision and metamorphopsia in the right eye of one month duration. His best-corrected visual acuity in this eye was 6/24. Fluorescein angiography showed peripapillary atrophy with a classic subfoveal choroidal neovascular membrane and areas of RPE atrophy (Figures 8.1.1 and 8.1.2).

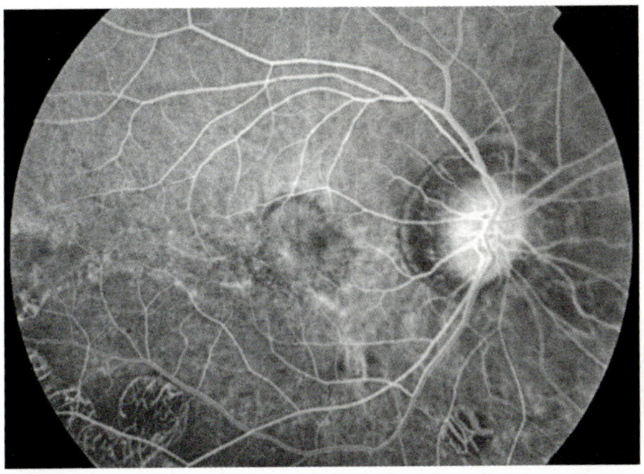

Figure 8.1.1: Early phase angiogram shows peripapillary atrophy with a classic subfoveal choroidal neovascular membrane and areas of RPE atrophy

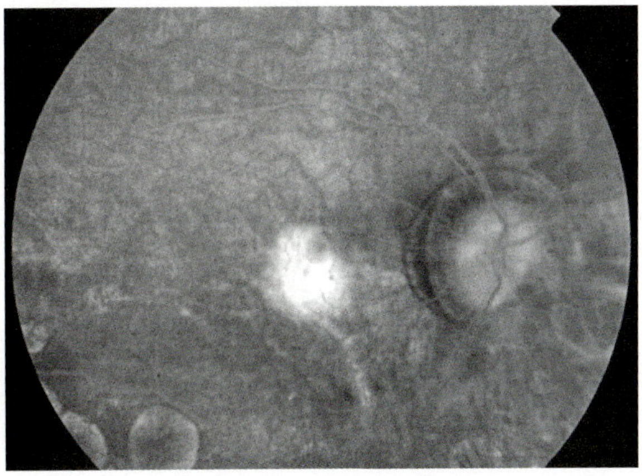

Figure 8.1.2: Late phase angiogram shows a classic subfoveal choroidal neovascular membrane

Indocyanine green angiography shows the extent of the CNVM (Figures 8.1.3 and 8.1.4).

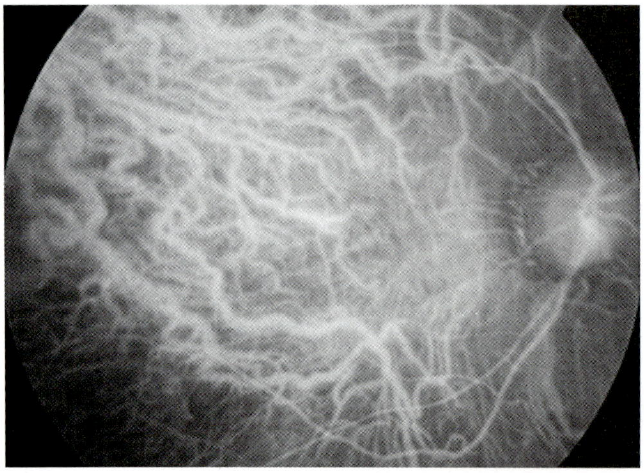

Figure 8.1.3: Early phase ICG shows CNVM

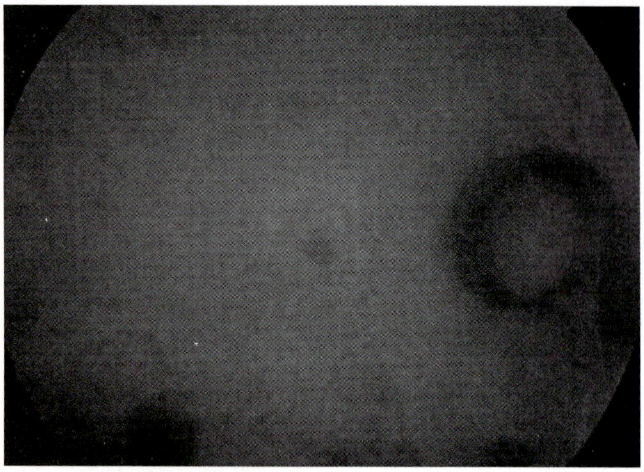

Figure 8.1.4: Late phase angiogram shows CNVM

Optical Coherence Tomography–1

Horizontal line scan showed increased retinal thickness (326 microns) with an area of moderate hyper-reflectivity in the outer retinal layers with small cystic spaces in the overlying retina suggestive of a predominantly classic CNVM (Figures 8.1.5A to D). The patient underwent photodynamic therapy followed by intravitreal Ranibizumab the next day. At one month follow-up, OCT showed reduction in retinal thickness (268 microns) with fibrous tissue formation (Figures 8.1.6A to D). The visual acuity had improved to 6/12.

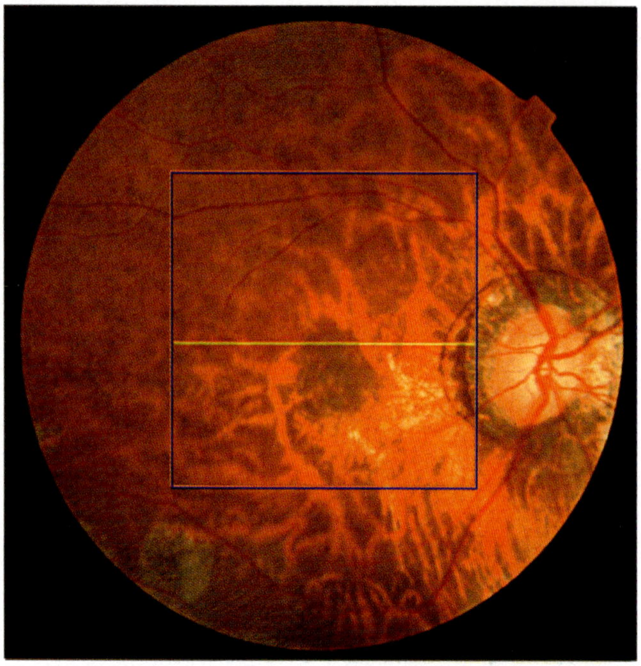

Figure 8.1.5A: Color fundus photograph showing the horizontal line scan through the CNVM

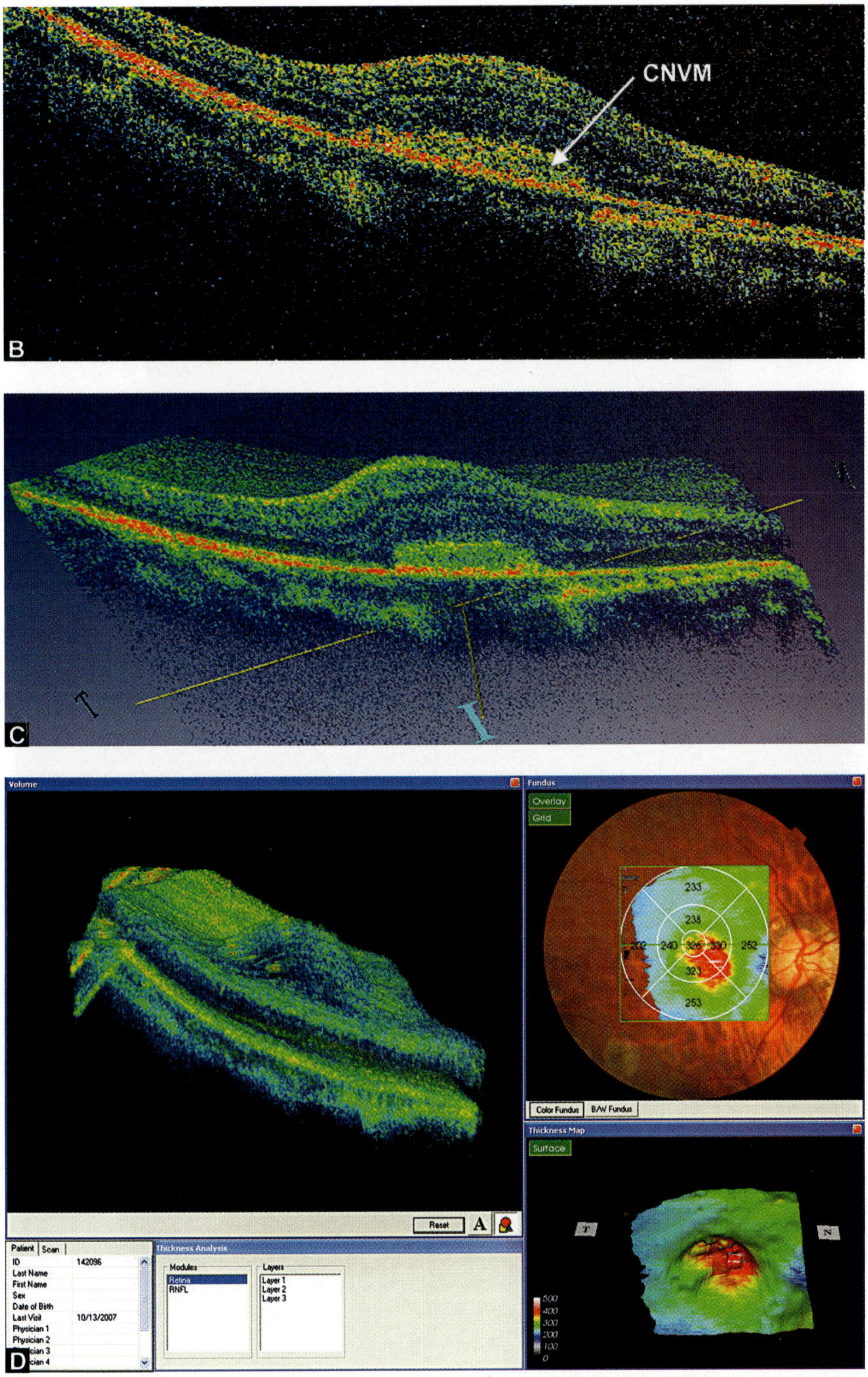

Figures 8.1.5B to D: (B) Horizontal line scan, 2D image showing increased retinal thickness (326 microns) with an area of moderate hyper-reflectivity in the outer retinal layers with small cystic spaces in the overlying retina suggestive of a predominantly classic CNVM. (C) Cropped 3D image showing an area of moderate hyper-reflectivity in the outer retinal layers with small cystic spaces in the overlying retina suggestive of a predominantly classic CNVM. (D) 3D image of Case 8.1

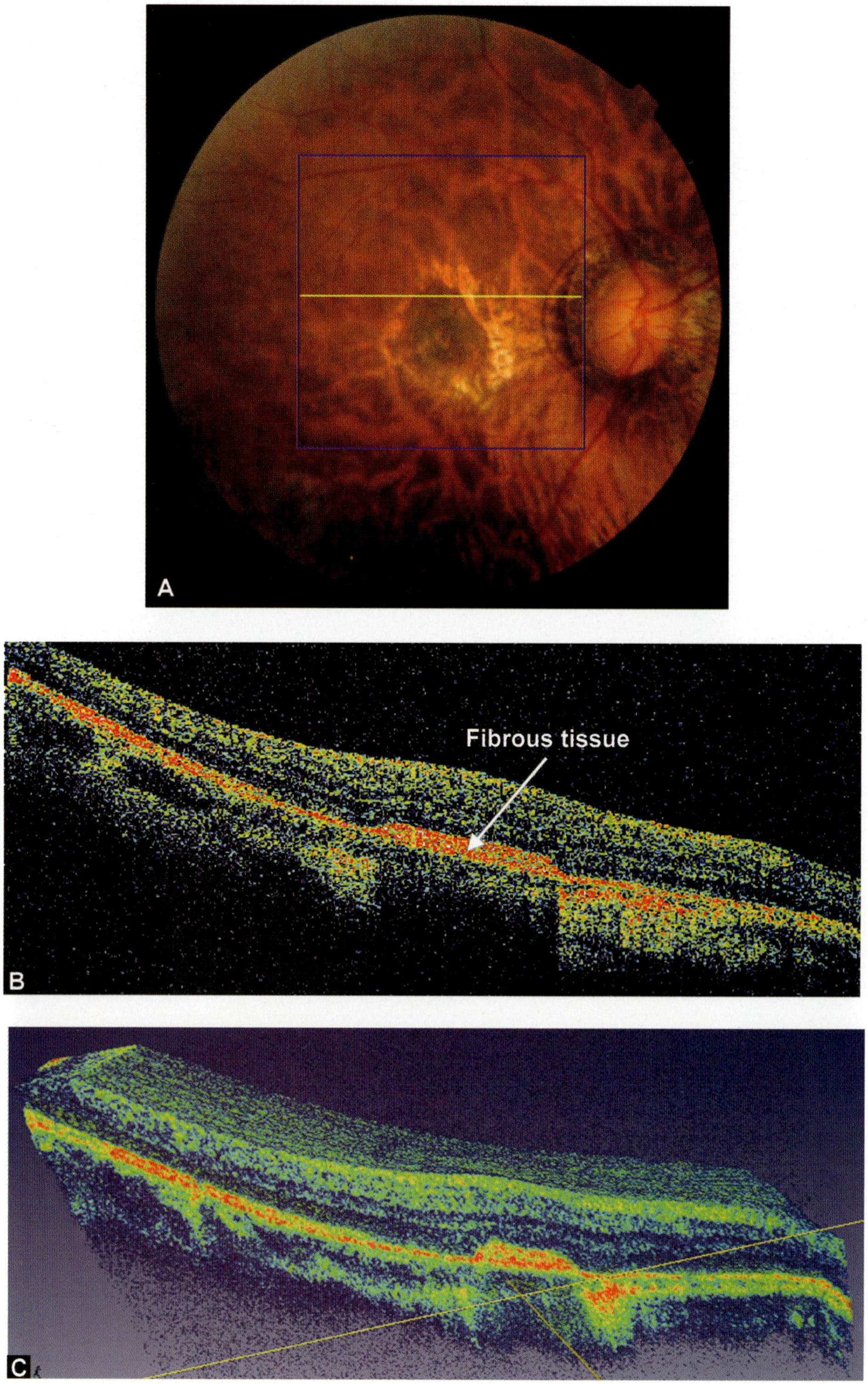

Figures 8.1.6A to C: (A) Color fundus photograph 1 month following PDT and intravitreal Ranibizumab showing the horizontal line scan. (B) Horizontal line scan, 2D image showing reduction in retinal thickness (268 microns) with fibrous tissue formation. (C) Cropped 3D image showing reduction in retinal thickness (268 microns) with fibrous tissue formation

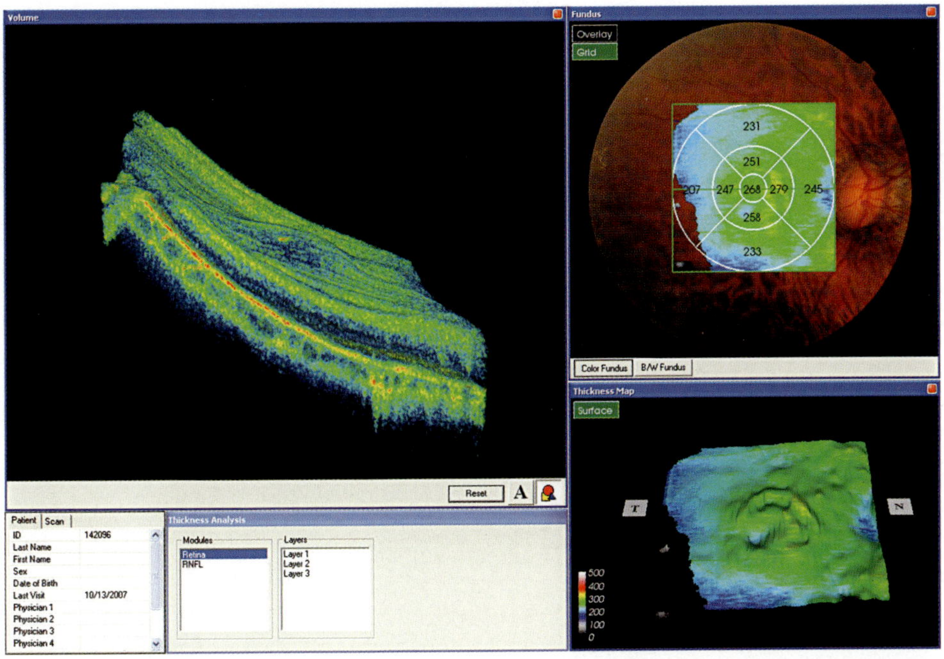

Figure 8.1.6D: 3D image of Case 8.1, one month following PDT and intravitreal Ranibizumab

Optical Coherence Tomography–2

At 2 months follow-up, OCT showed further reduction in retinal thickness (253 microns) (Figures 8.1.7A to D). The visual acuity had improved to 6/9.

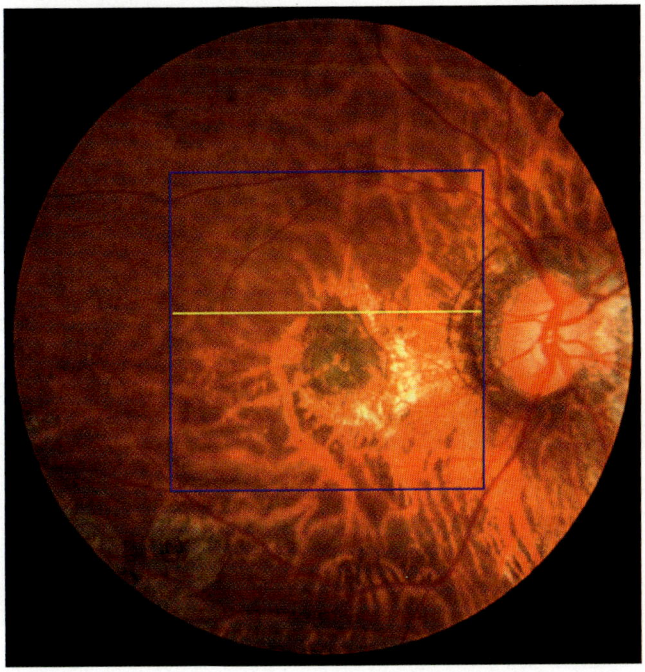

Figure 8.1.7A: Color fundus photograph 2 months following PDT and intravitreal Ranibizumab showing the horizontal line scan

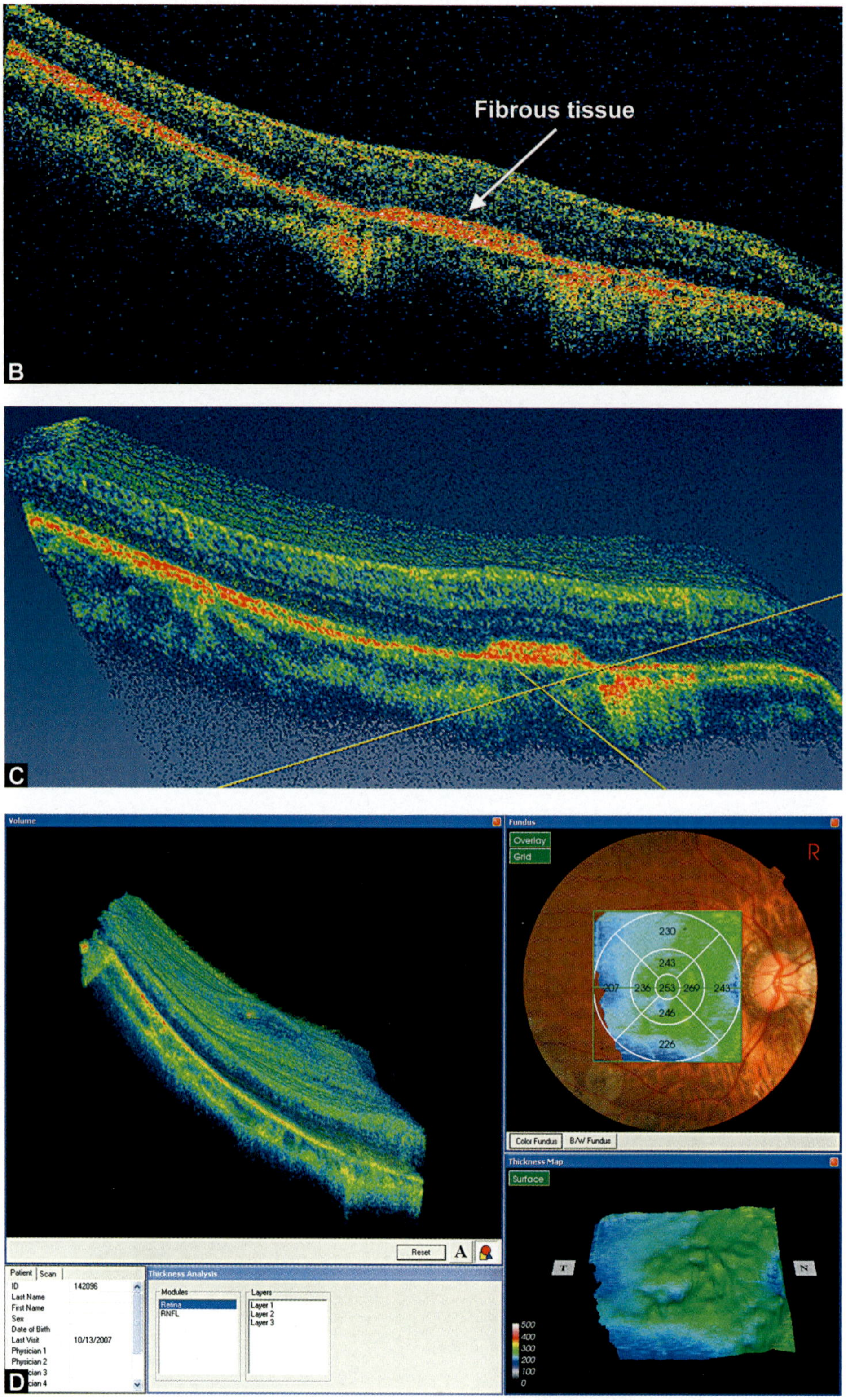

Figures 8.1.7B to D: (B) Horizontal line scan, 2D image showing further reduction in retinal thickness (253 microns). (C) Cropped 3D image showing further reduction in retinal thickness (253 microns). (D) 3D image of Case 8.1, two months following PDT and intravitreal Ranibizumab

CASE 8.2: POSTERIOR STAPHYLOMA

Case Summary

A 30-year-old male with high myopia presented with diminished vision in the left eye of 2 months duration. His best-corrected visual acuity in this eye was 6/12. Fluorescein angiography showed a ring of mottled hyperfluorescence corresponding to the posterior staphyloma (Figures 8.2.1 and 8.2.2).

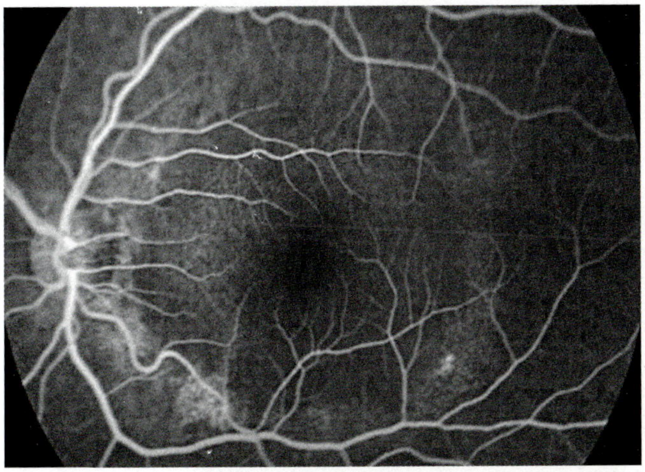

Figure 8.2.1: Early phase angiogram shows a ring of mottled hyperfluorescence corresponding to the posterior staphyloma

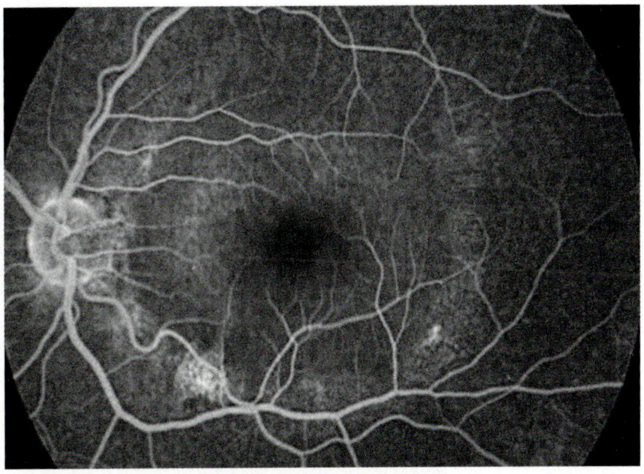

Figure 8.2.2: Late phase angiogram shows a ring of mottled hyperfluorescence corresponding to the posterior staphyloma

Optical Coherence Tomography

Horizontal line scan showed pronounced concavity of the retinal structure (Figures 8.2.3A to D)

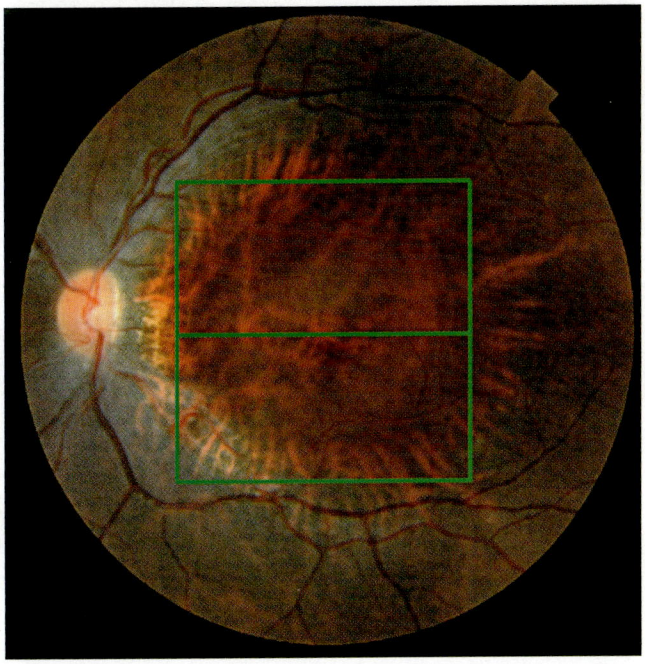

Figure 8.2.3A: Color fundus photograph showing the horizontal line scan through the fovea

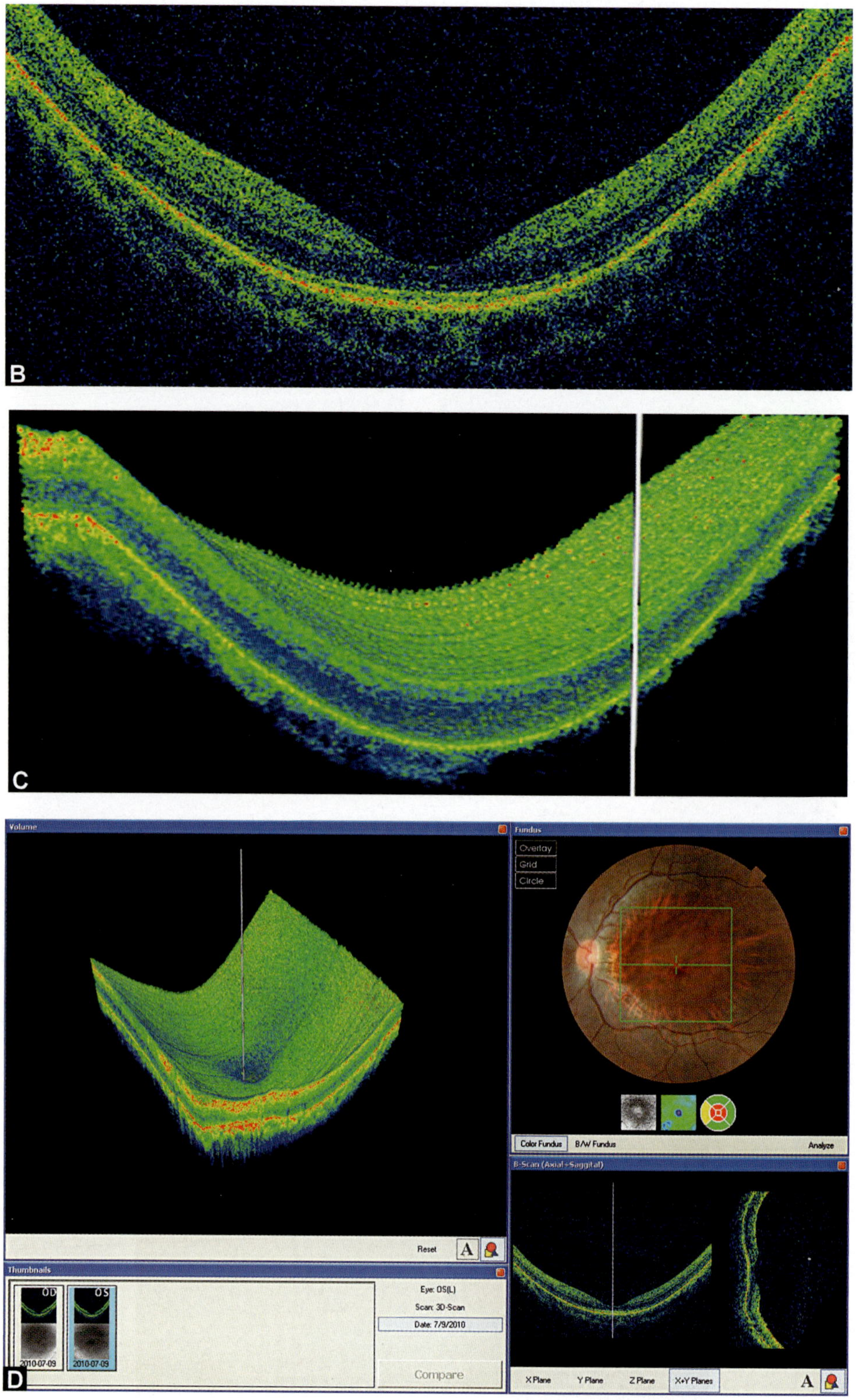

Figures 8.2.3B to D: (B) Horizontal line scan, 2D image showing pronounced concavity of the retinal structure. (C) Cropped 3D image showing pronounced concavity of the retinal structure. (D) 3D image of Case 8.2 **(Images with Topcon 3D OCT-2000)**

CONCLUSION

OCT makes it possible to monitor the evolution of the neovascular membrane following photodynamic treatment (PDT) and, above all, helps to decide if PDT should be repeated.

SUGGESTED READING

1. Blinder KJ, Blumenkranz MS, Bressler NM, Bressler SB, Donato G, Lewis H, et al. Verteporfin therapy of subfoveal choroidal neovascularization in pathological myopia: two-year results of a randomized clinical trial - VIP report no 3. Ophthalmology. 2003;110(4):667-73.
2. Zhanq MX, Yan M, Zhanq JJ, Tanq J, Wei CY, Menq D. The therapeutic effects of photodynamic therapy on choroidal neovascularization of pathological myopia. Zhonqhua Yan Ke Za Zhi. 2007;43(7):638-41. PubMed.

9 Diabetic Macular Edema

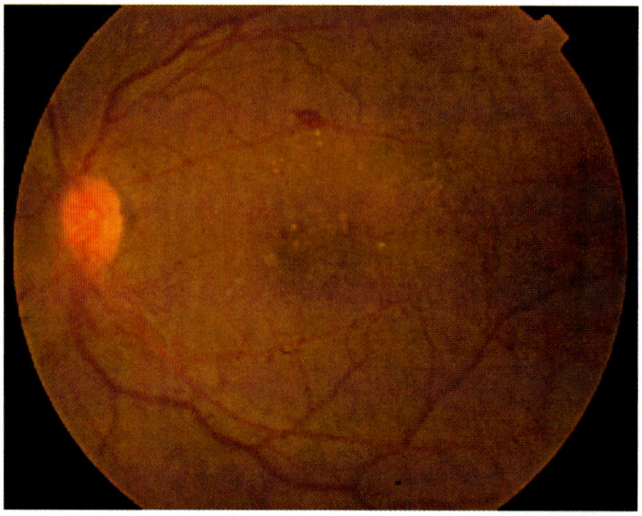

Diabetic macular edema (DME) is the most common cause of moderate visual loss in patients with diabetic retinopathy. Untreated, 25-30 percent of patients with clinically significant macular edema exhibit a doubling of the visual angle within 3 years and treated, the risk drops by 50 percent. It can occur at any stage of the disease, however, its incidence increases with the severity of the retinopathy.

Fluorescein angiography helps to distinguish and localize areas of focal versus diffuse leakage.

OPTICAL COHERENCE TOMOGRAPHY

The three main roles for OCT in DME are (i) defining the pattern of DME (ii) monitoring anatomical changes following treatment interventions (iii) defining indications for vitrectomy. OCT has been able to demonstrate a moderate correlation between retinal thickness and best-corrected visual acuity.

Five patterns of diabetic macular edema on OCT have been described. They are:

1. Sponge like retinal thickening.
2. Cystoid macular edema.
3. Serous retinal detachment.
4. Foveal tractional retinal detachment.
5. Taut posterior hyaloid membrane.

CASE 9.1: CSME WITH SPONGE LIKE THICKENING

Case Summary

A 67-year-old woman was seen with non-proliferative diabetic retinopathy and significant macular edema in the right eye. Her best-corrected visual acuity was 6/9 in this eye. Fluorescein angiography revealed late leakage consistent with macular edema (Figures 9.1.1 and 9.1.2).

Optical Coherence Tomography

Horizontal line scan revealed macular thickening temporal to the fovea with reduced optical backscatter due to accumulation of fluid in the outer retinal layers. The hyper-reflective areas are suggestive of hard exudates (Figures 9.1.3A to D).

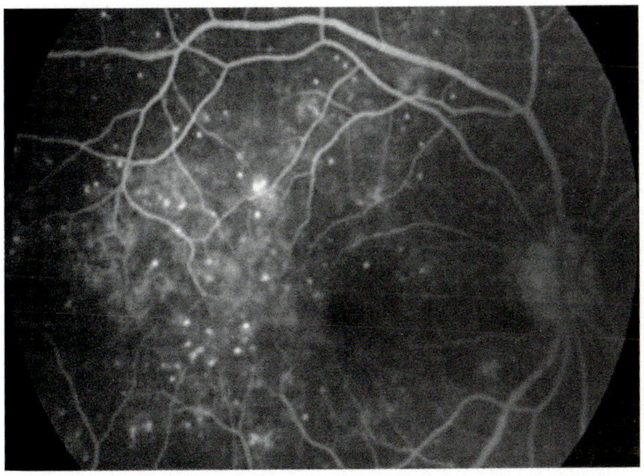

Figure 9.1.1: Early phase angiogram shows non-proliferative diabetic retinopathy

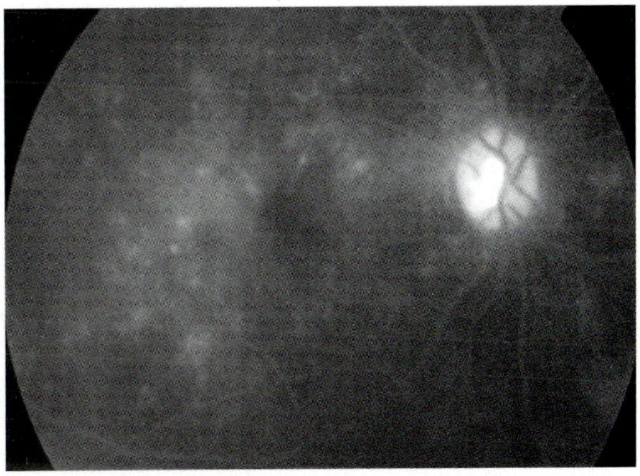

Figure 9.1.2: Late phase angiogram shows leakage consistent with macular edema

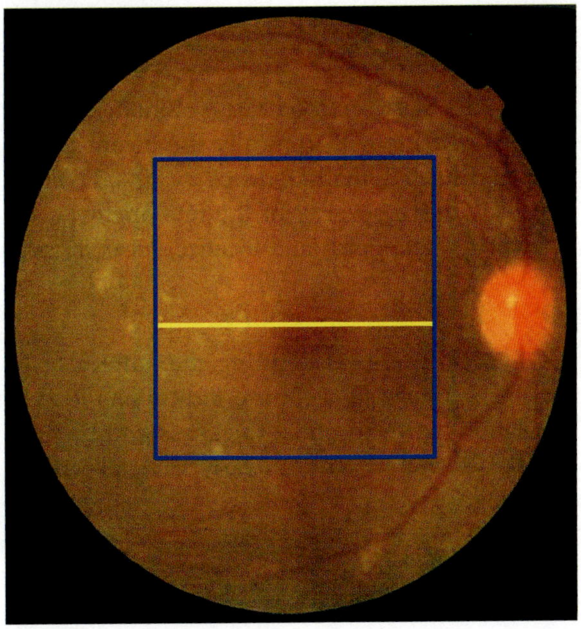

Figure 9.1.3A: Color fundus photograph showing the horizontal line scan through the fovea

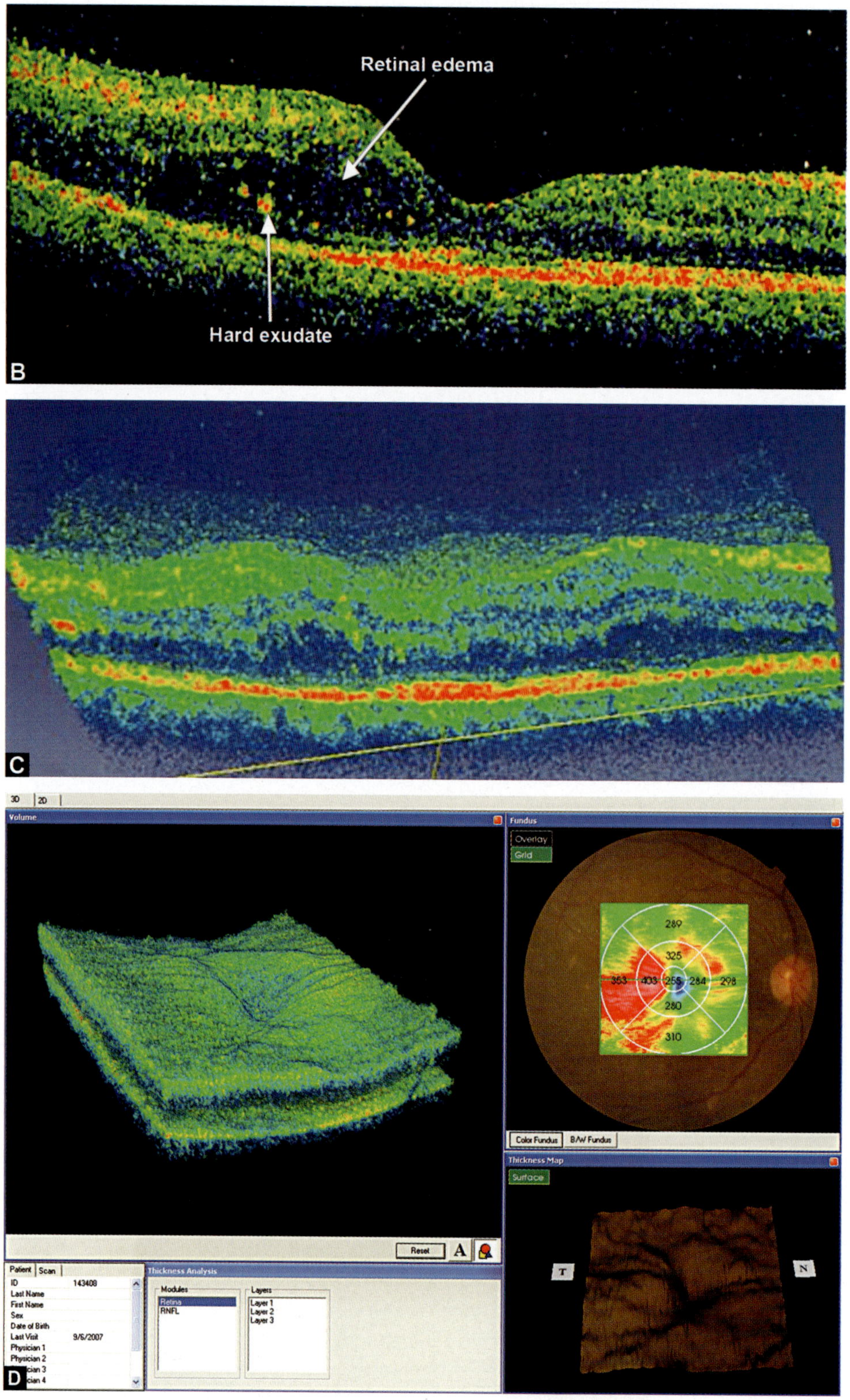

Figures 9.1.3B to D: (B) Horizontal line scan, 2D image showing macular thickening temporal to the fovea with reduced optical backscatter due to accumulation of fluid in the outer retinal layers. The hyper-reflective areas are suggestive of hard exudates. (C) Cropped 3D image showing macular thickening temporal to the fovea with reduced optical backscatter due to accumulation of fluid in the outer retinal layers. The hyper-reflective areas are suggestive of hard exudates. (D) 3D image of Case 9.1

CASE 9.2: CSME WITH CYSTOID MACULAR EDEMA

Case Summary

A 59-year-old woman with 25 years history of NIDDM who had undergone focal laser treatment previously was seen. Her best-corrected vision in the right eye was 6/18. Fluorescein angiography showed photocoagulation scars with late leakage (Figures 9.2.1 and 9.2.2).

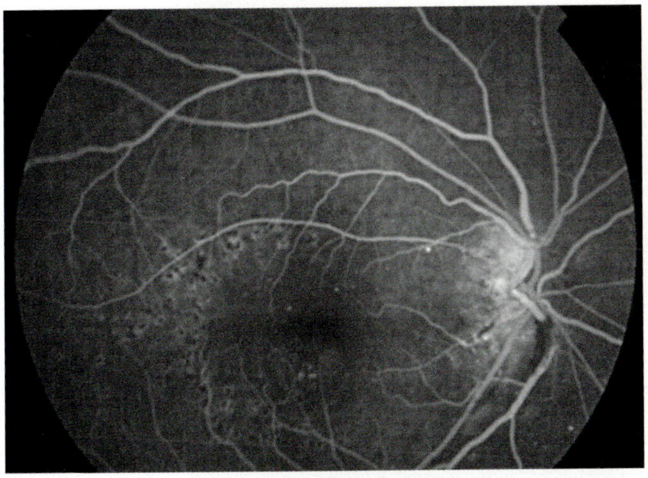

Figure 9.2.1: Early phase angiogram shows non-proliferative diabetic retinopathy with laser photocoagulation

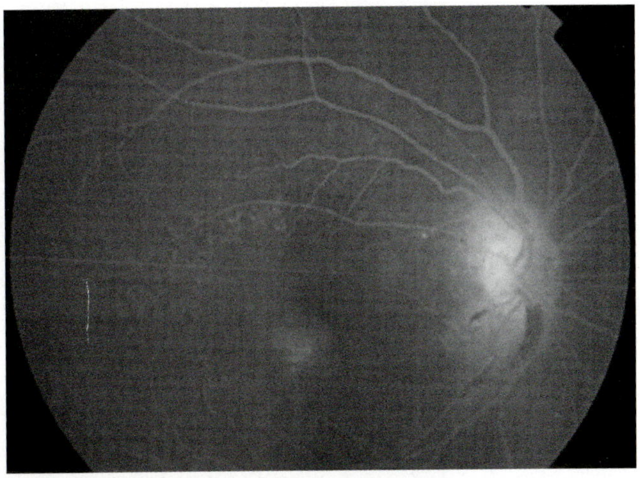

Figure 9.2.2: Late phase angiogram shows leakage consistent with macular edema

Optical Coherence Tomography

Horizontal line scan through the fovea showed macular thickening with two nearly full thickness cystoid spaces under the fovea with intervening septae. The cysts in the adjoining retina were smaller in size and were mainly in the outer retinal layers. Posterior hyaloid separation was seen nasal to the fovea (Figures 9.2.3A to D).

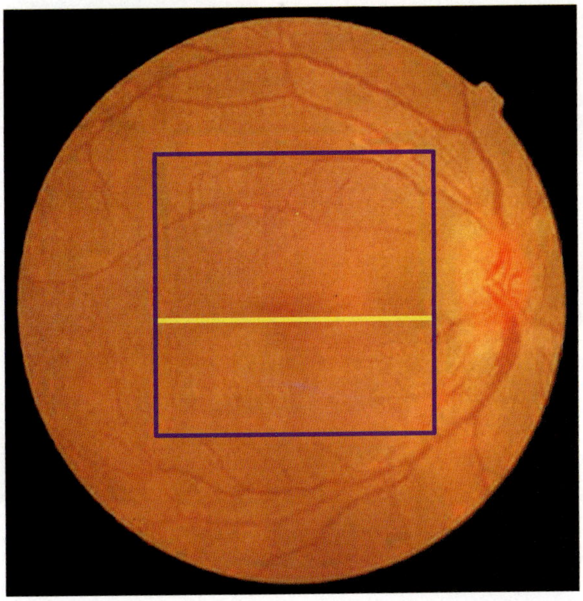

Figure 9.2.3A: Color fundus photograph showing the horizontal line scan through the fovea

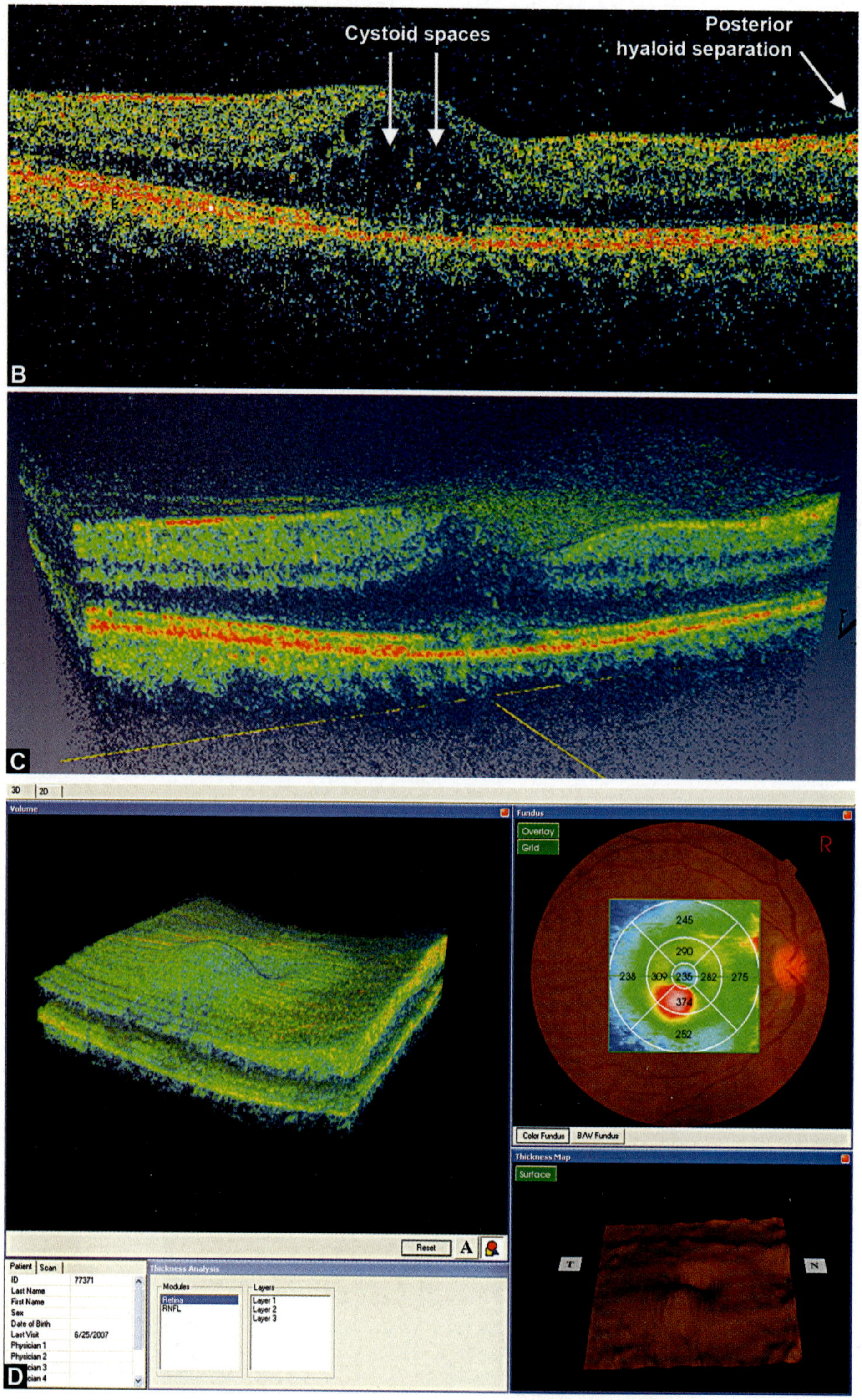

Figures 9.2.3B to D: (B) Horizontal line scan, 2D image showing macular thickening with two nearly full thickness cystoid spaces under the fovea with intervening septae. The cysts in the adjoining retina are smaller in size and are mainly in the outer retinal layers. Posterior hyaloid separation is seen nasal to the fovea. (C) Cropped 3D image showing macular thickening with two nearly full thickness cystoid spaces under the fovea with intervening septae. The cysts in the adjoining retina are smaller in size and are mainly in the outer retinal layers. Posterior hyaloid separation is seen nasal to the fovea. (D) 3D image of Case 9.2

CASE 9.3: CSME WITH CYSTOID MACULAR EDEMA AND SEROUS RETINAL DETACHMENT

Case Summary

A 59-year-old diabetic woman was seen with non-proliferative diabetic retinopathy and cystoid macular edema. She already had 3 sessions of focal laser photocoagulation. Her best-corrected vision in the left eye was 6/60. Fluorescein angiography revealed photocoagulation scars with cystoid spaces in the late phase (Figures 9.3.1 and 9.3.2).

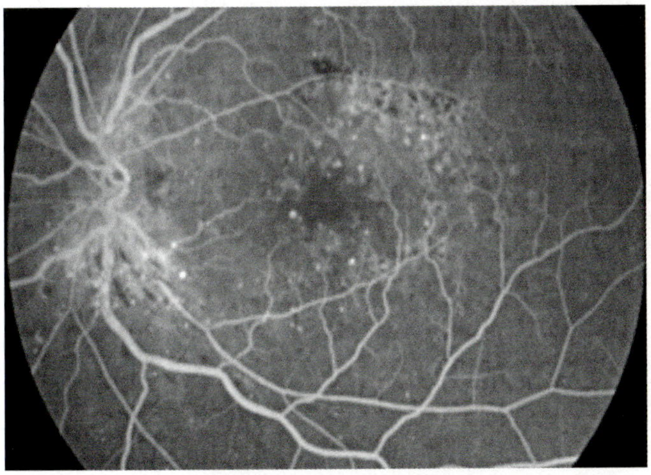

Figure 9.3.1: Early phase angiogram shows non-proliferative diabetic retinopathy with laser photocoagulation

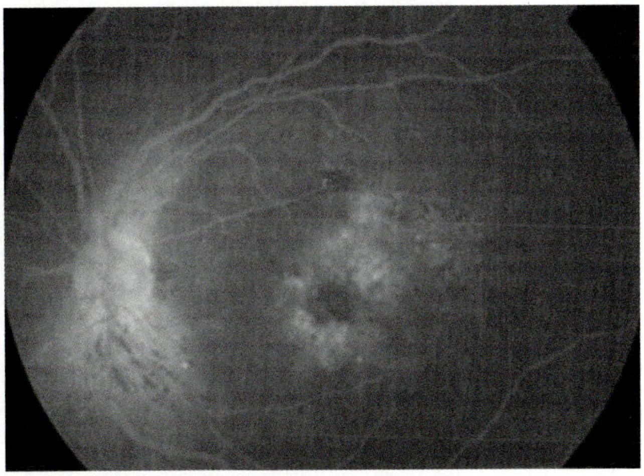

Figure 9.3.2: Late phase angiogram shows cystoid macular edema

Optical Coherence Tomography

Horizontal line scan confirmed the cystoid spaces under the fovea with intervening septae. In addition, there was an area of hyporeflectivity in the subfoveal region consistent with subfoveal serous retinal detachment. Posterior hyaloid separation was seen in the perifoveal region (Figures 9.3.3A to D).

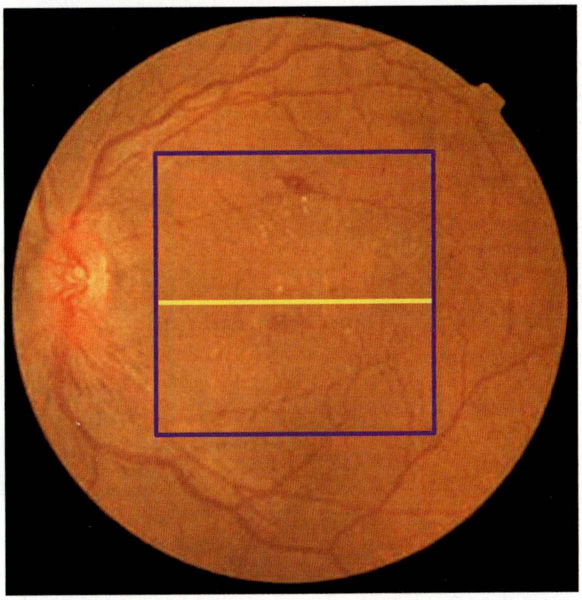

Figure 9.3.3A: Color fundus photograph showing the horizontal line scan through the fovea

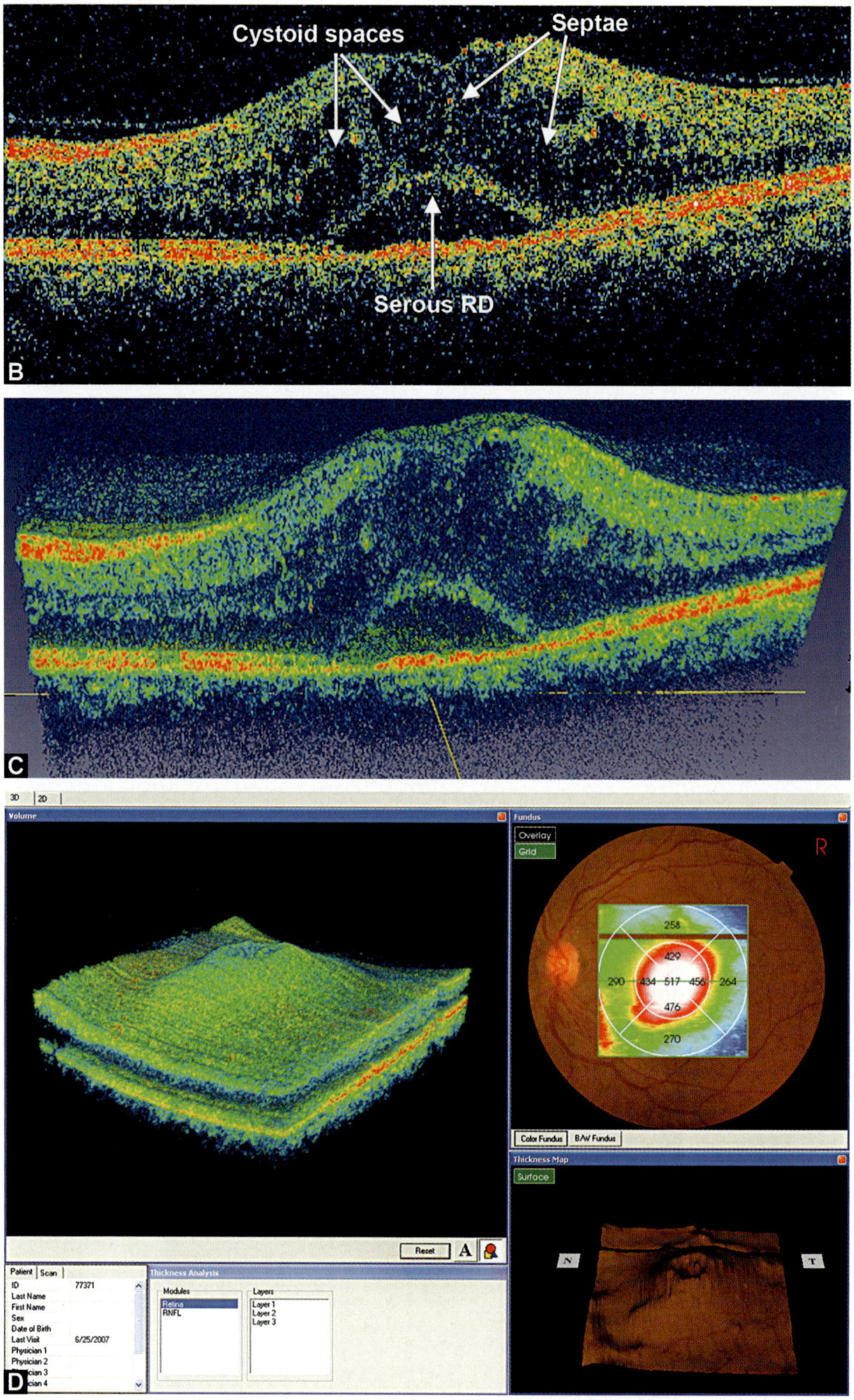

Figures 9.3.3B to D: (B) Horizontal line scan, 2D image showing cystoid spaces under the fovea with intervening septae. There is an area of hyporeflectivity in the subfoveal region consistent with subfoveal serous retinal detachment. Posterior hyaloid separation is seen in the perifoveal region. (C) Cropped 3D image showing cystoid spaces under the fovea with intervening septae. There is an area of hyporeflectivity in the subfoveal region consistent with subfoveal serous retinal detachment. Posterior hyaloid separation is seen in the perifoveal region. (D) 3D image of Case 9.3

CASE 9.4: CSME WITH CLINICALLY UNRECOGNIZABLE TAUT POSTERIOR HYALOID MEMBRANE

Case Summary

A 67-year-old woman with type 2 diabetes of 10 years duration was seen with proliferative diabetic retinopathy. Her best-corrected visual acuity was 6/60 in the left eye.

Optical Coherence Tomography

Horizontal line scan showed increased retinal thickening in the center of the macula with taut posterior hyaloid membrane (TPHM). The hyper-reflective areas seen in the retinal layers are due to hard exudates (Figures 9.4.1A to D).

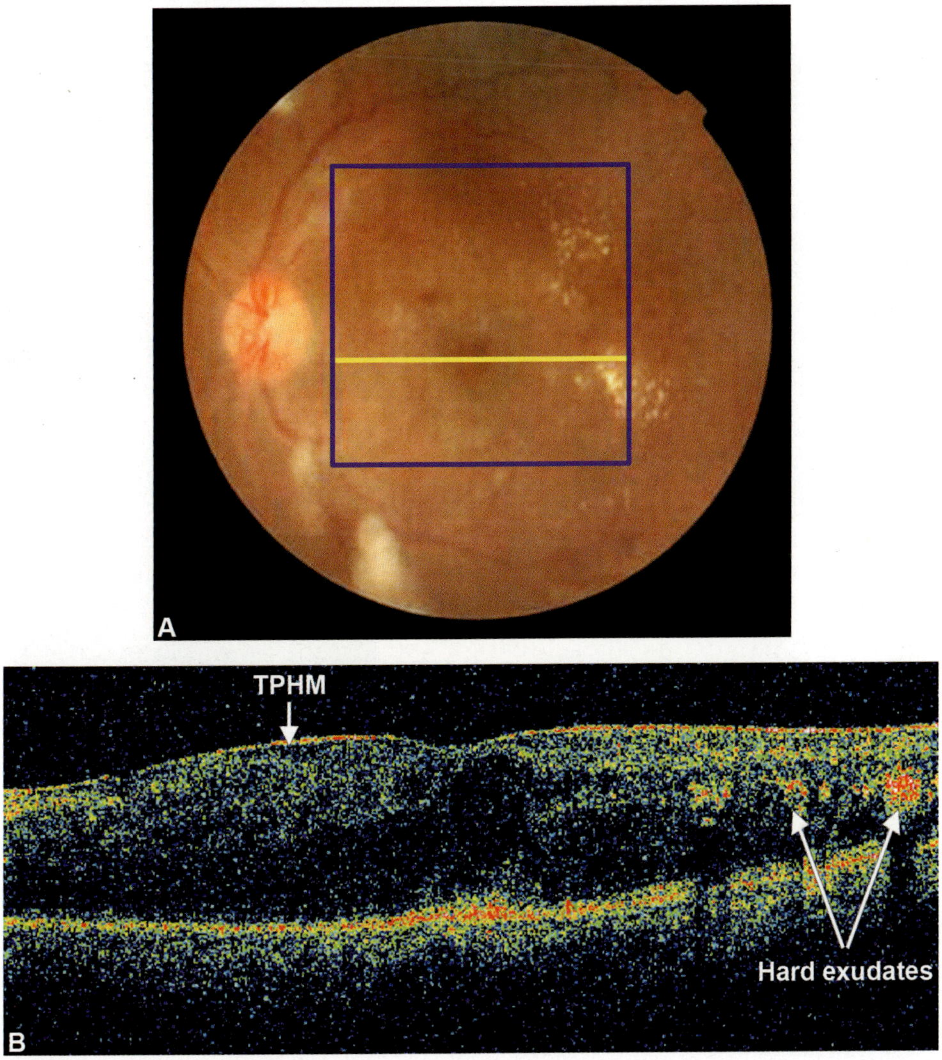

Figures 9.4.1A and B: (A) Color fundus photograph showing the horizontal line scan through the fovea. (B) Horizontal line scan, 2D image showing increased retinal thickening in the center of the macula with taut posterior hyaloid membrane (TPHM). The hyper-reflective areas seen in the retinal layers are due to hard exudates

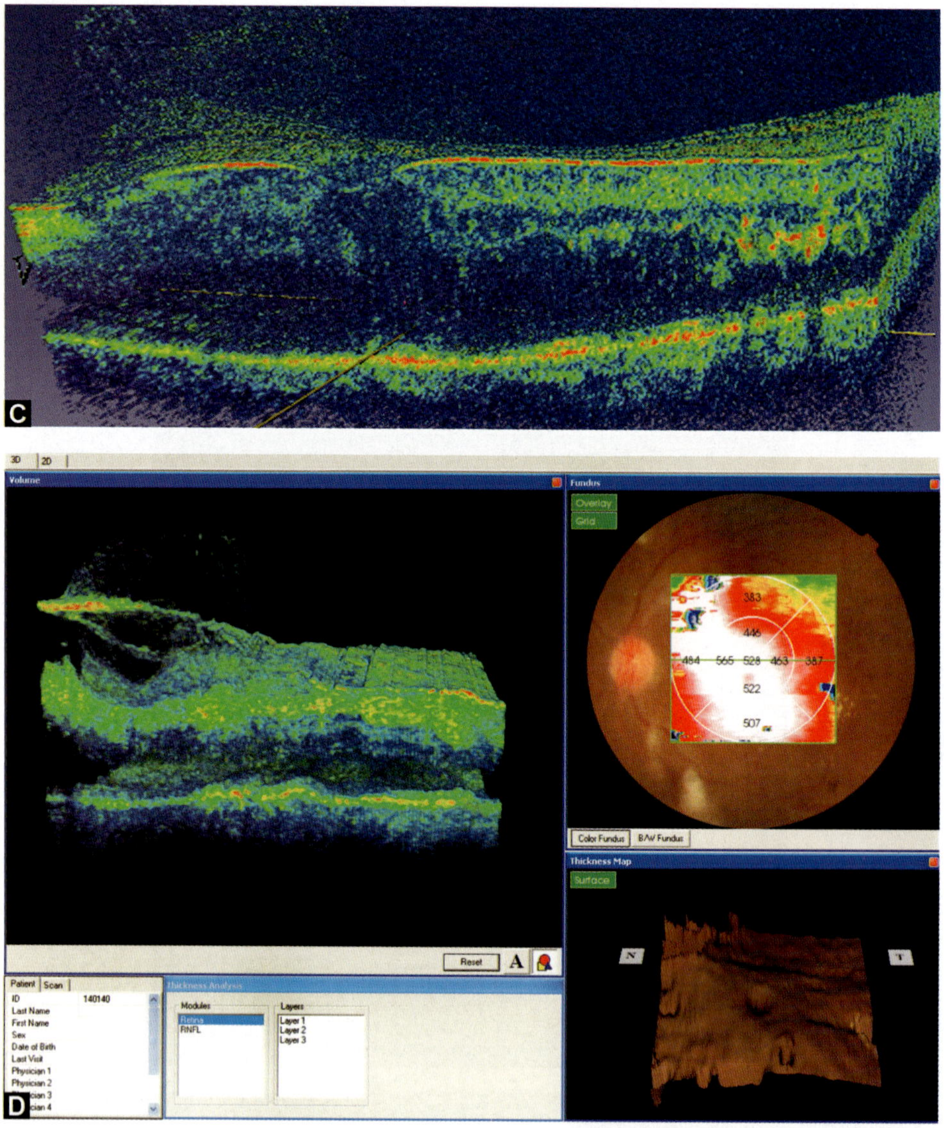

Figures 9.4.1C and D: (C) Cropped 3D image showing increased retinal thickening in the center of the macula with taut posterior hyaloid membrane (TPHM). The hyper-reflective areas seen in the retinal layers are due to hard exudates. (D) 3D image of Case 9.4

CASE 9.5: CSME WITH FOVEOVITREAL TRACTION

Case Summary

A 63-year-old woman with 27 years of diabetes was seen with proliferative diabetic retinopathy. Her best-corrected visual acuity was 3/60 in the right eye. She had received pan retinal photocoagulation. Fluorescein angiography revealed persistent neovascularization with macular edema. Clinically, a foveovitreal traction was not visible (Figures 9.5.1 and 9.5.2).

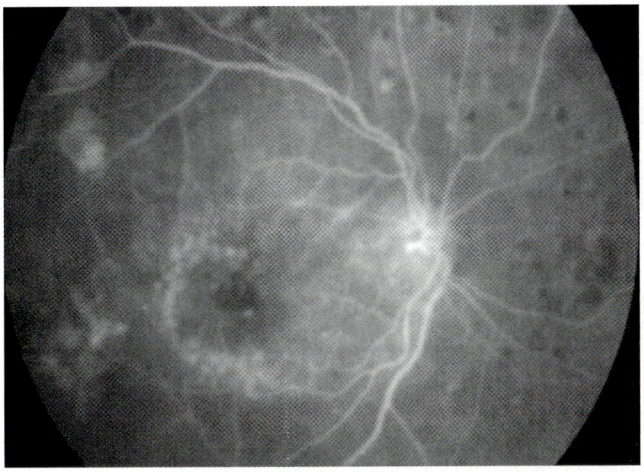

Figure 9.5.1: Early phase angiogram shows proliferative diabetic retinopathy with laser photocoagulation

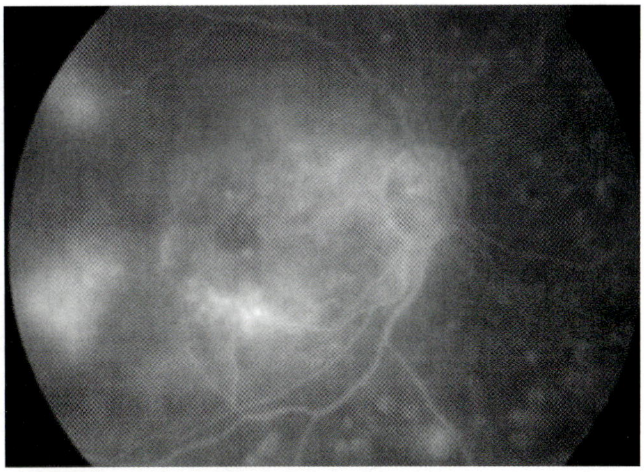

Figure 9.5.2: Late phase angiogram shows macular edema

Optical Coherence Tomography

Horizontal line scans showed increased retinal thickening with vitreoschisis, i.e. splitting of posterior vitreous phase into two lamellae. This caused focal traction on the fovea with resultant cystoid macular edema (Figures 9.5.3A to D). Laser photocoagulation in this setting would certainly worsen the edema. On the other hand, this would be an ideal case for pars plana vitrectomy. This case highlights the importance of OCT in recalcitrant diabetic macular edema, without which proper management would not have been possible.

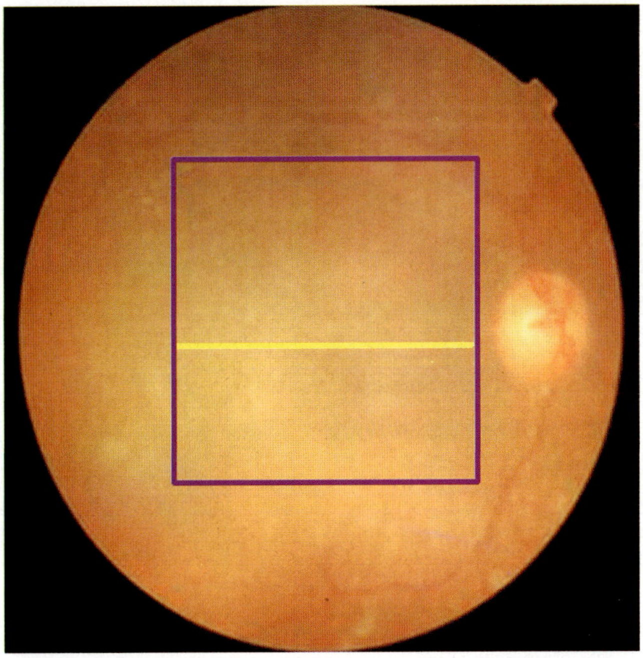

Figure 9.5.3A: Color fundus photograph showing the horizontal line scan through the fovea

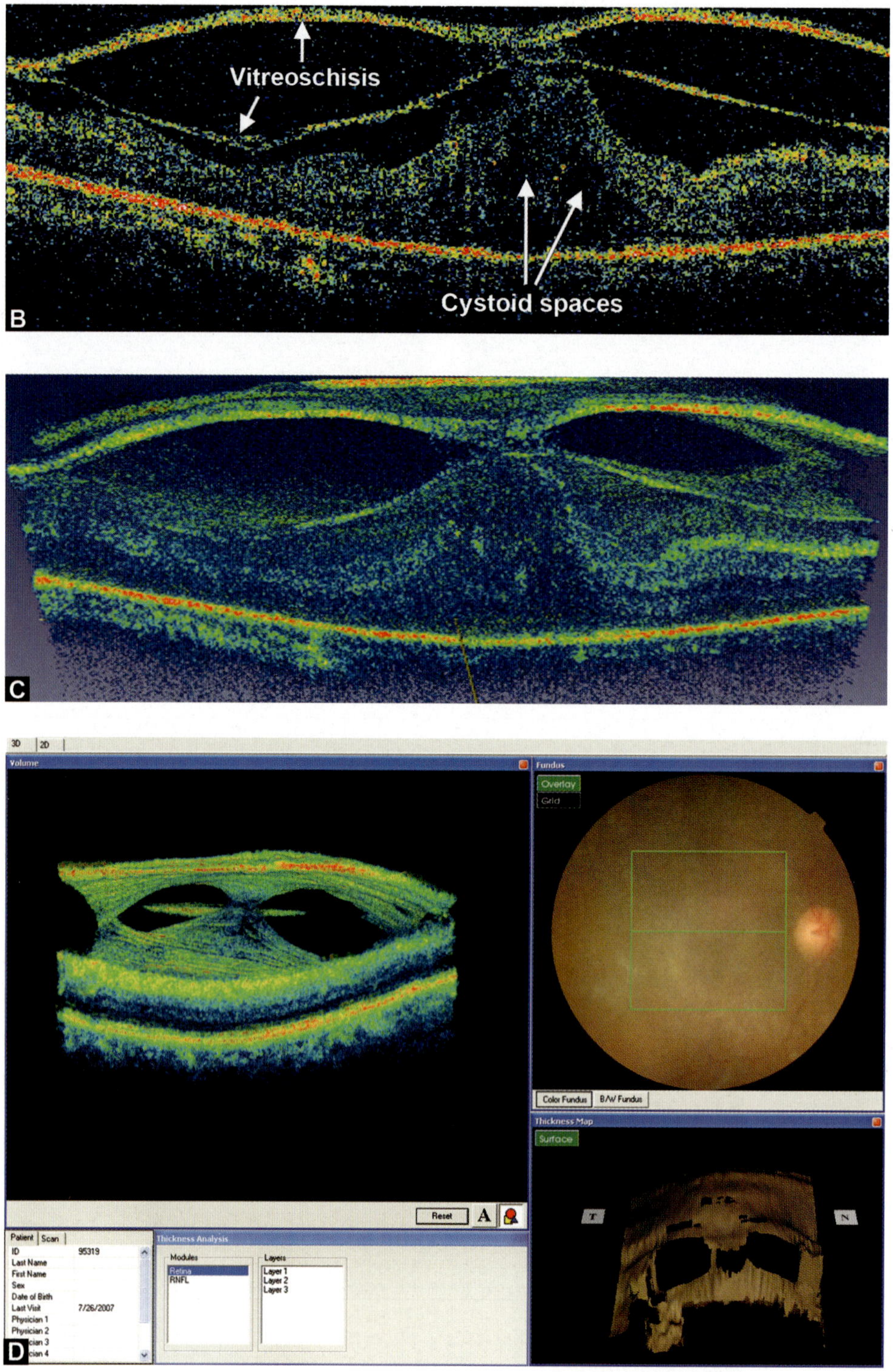

Figures 9.5.3B to D: (B) Horizontal line scan, 2D image showing increased retinal thickening with vitreoschisis, i.e splitting of posterior vitreous phase into two lamellae and cystoid macular edema. (C) Cropped 3D image showing increased retinal thickening with vitreoschisis, i.e splitting of posterior vitreous phase into two lamellae and cystoid macular edema. (D) 3D image of Case 9.5

CASE 9.6: INTRAVITREAL TRIAMCINOLONE ACETONIDE IN DIABETIC MACULAR EDEMA

Case Summary

A 56-year-old man with non-insulin-dependent diabetes mellitus of 12 years duration was seen with recalcitrant CSME in the left eye that had not responded to laser photocoagulation. His best-corrected visual acuity was 6/36 in this eye. Fluorescein angiography revealed cystoid macular edema (Figures 9.6.1 and 9.6.2).

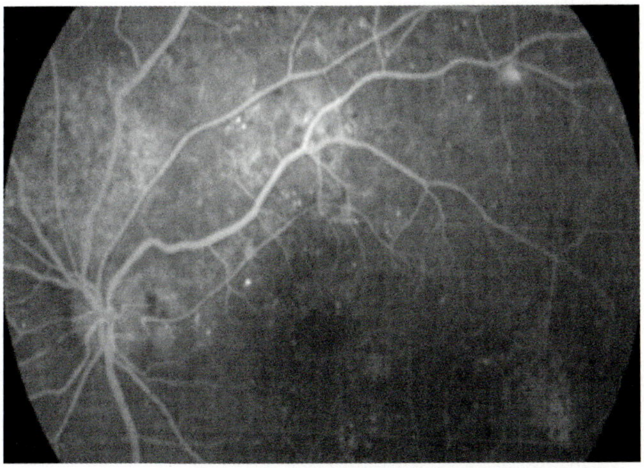

Figure 9.6.1: Early phase angiogram shows non-proliferative diabetic retinopathy with laser photocoagulation

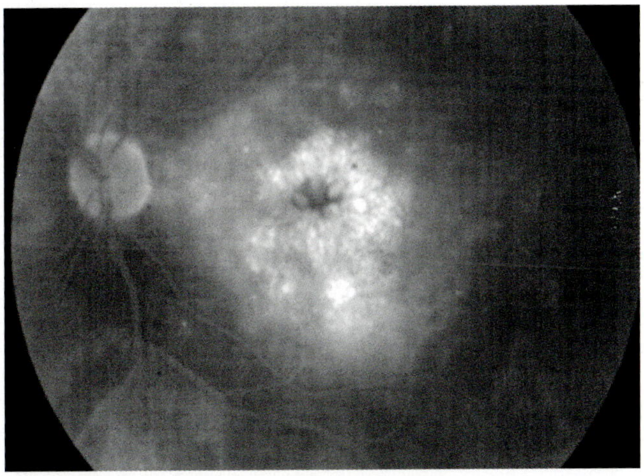

Figure 9.6.2: Late phase angiogram shows cystoid macular edema

Optical Coherence Tomography

Horizontal line scan showed loss of foveal contour with retinal thickness measuring 572 microns in the foveal center and multiple hyporeflective areas with intervening hyper-reflective septae consistent with cystoid macular edema. Another hyporeflective area under the fovea was suggestive of serous retinal detachment (Figures 9.6.3A to D). The patient received intravitreal triamcinolone acetonide (4 mg). Follow-up scan at one month showed reduction in the foveal thickness to 175 microns and the visual acuity improved to 6/18. OCT demonstrated return of foveal contour with disappearance of retinal cysts and serous retinal detachment (Figures 9.6.4A to D).

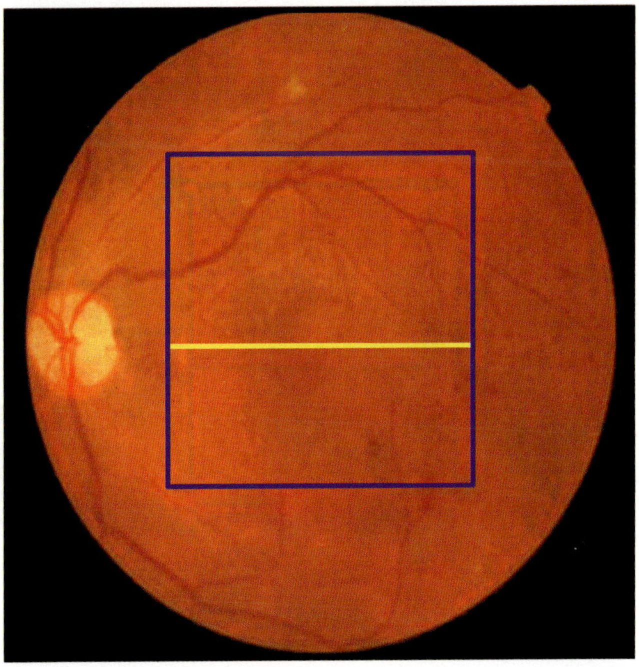

Figure 9.6.3A: Color fundus photograph showing the horizontal line scan through the fovea

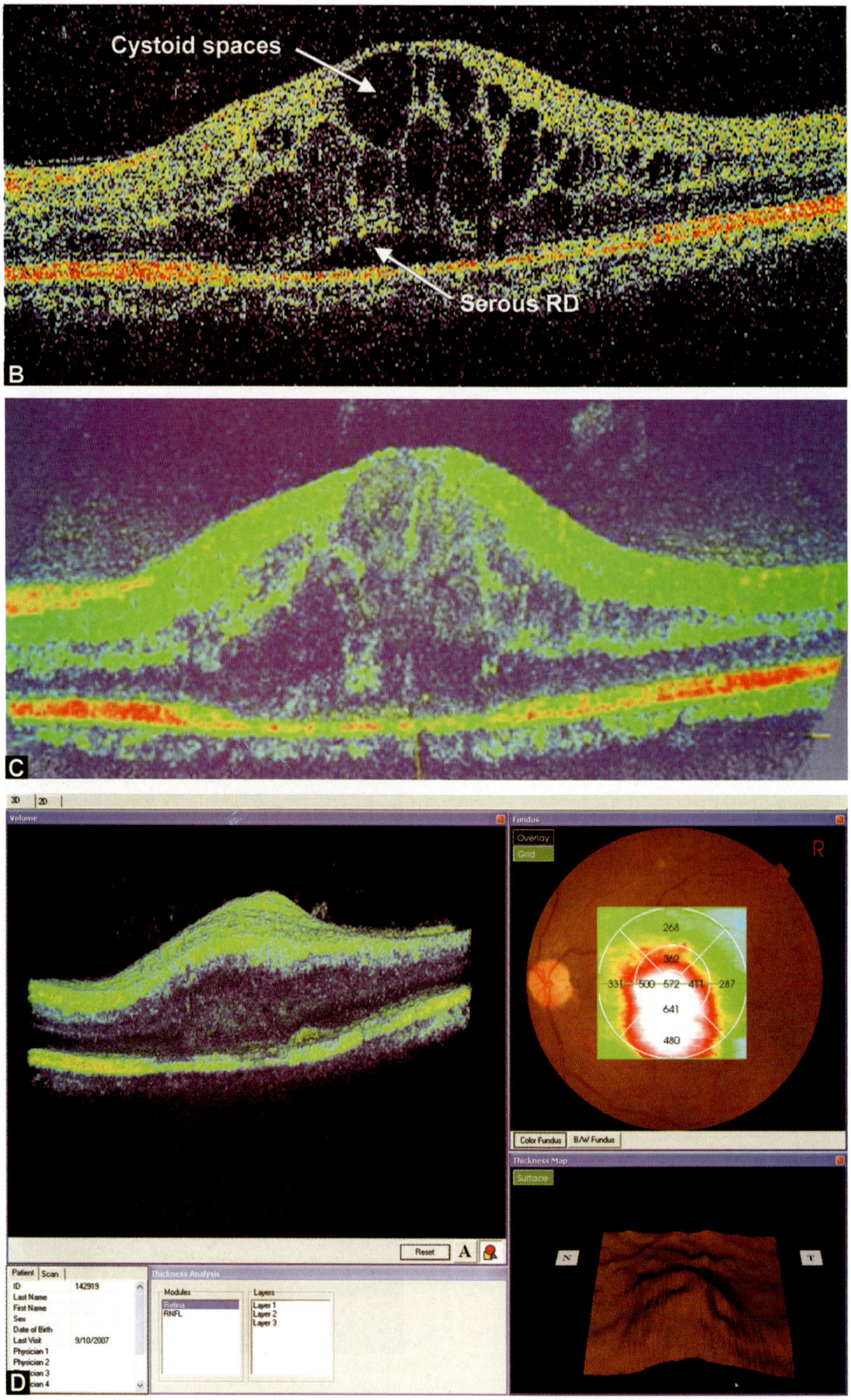

Figures 9.6.3B to D: (B) Horizontal line scan, 2D image showing loss of foveal contour and multiple hypo-reflective areas with intervening hyper-reflective septae consistent with cystoid macular edema. A hyporeflective area under the fovea is suggestive of serous retinal detachment. (C) Cropped 3D image showing loss of foveal contour and multiple hypo-reflective areas with intervening hyper-reflective septae consistent with cystoid macular edema. A hyporeflective area under the fovea is suggestive of serous retinal detachment. (D) 3D image of Case 9.6

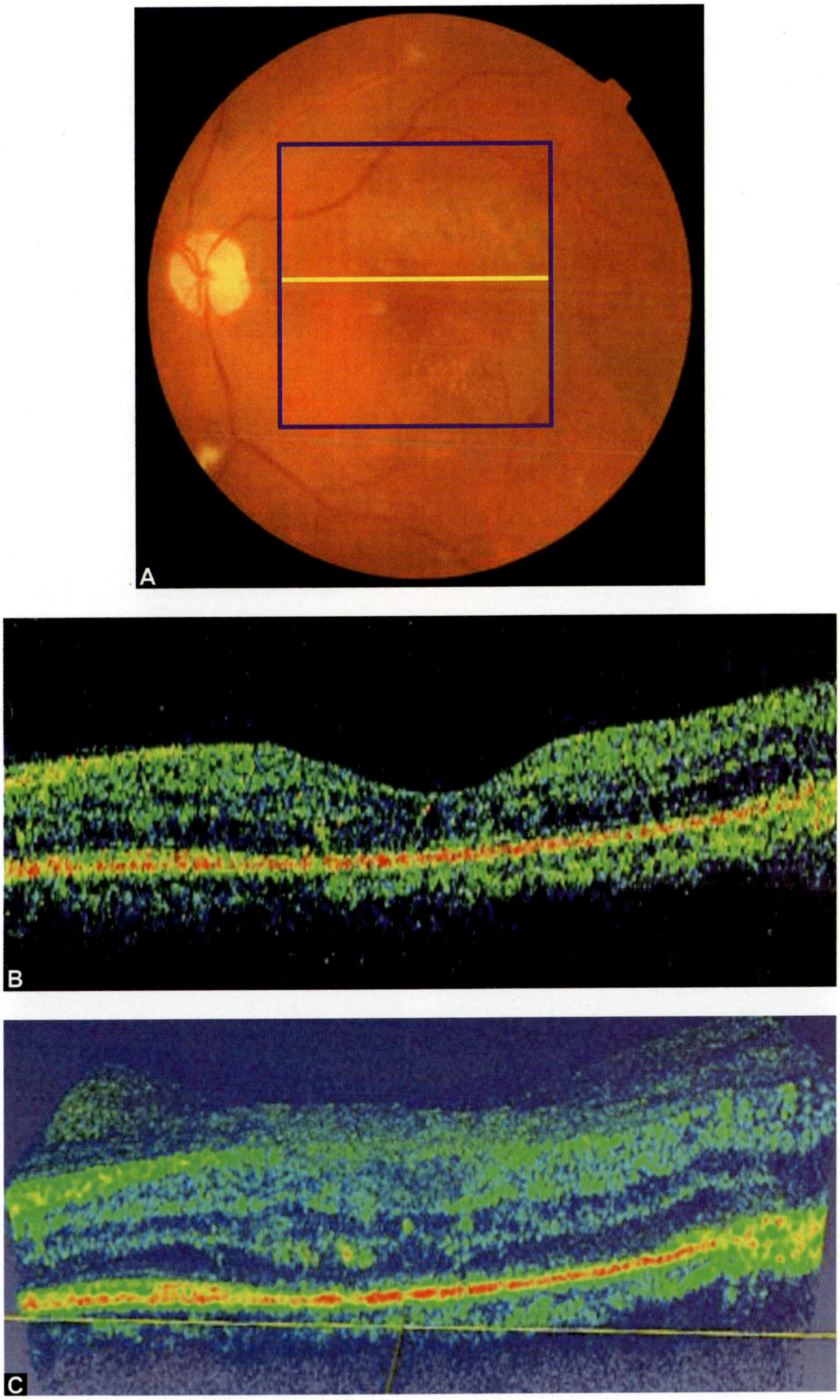

Figures 9.6.4A to C: (A) Color fundus photograph following intravitreal triamcinolone showing the horizontal line scan through the fovea. (B) Horizontal line scan, 2D image showing return of foveal contour with disappearance of retinal cysts and serous retinal detachment. (C) Cropped 3D image showing. return of foveal contour with disappearance of retinal cysts and serous retinal detachment

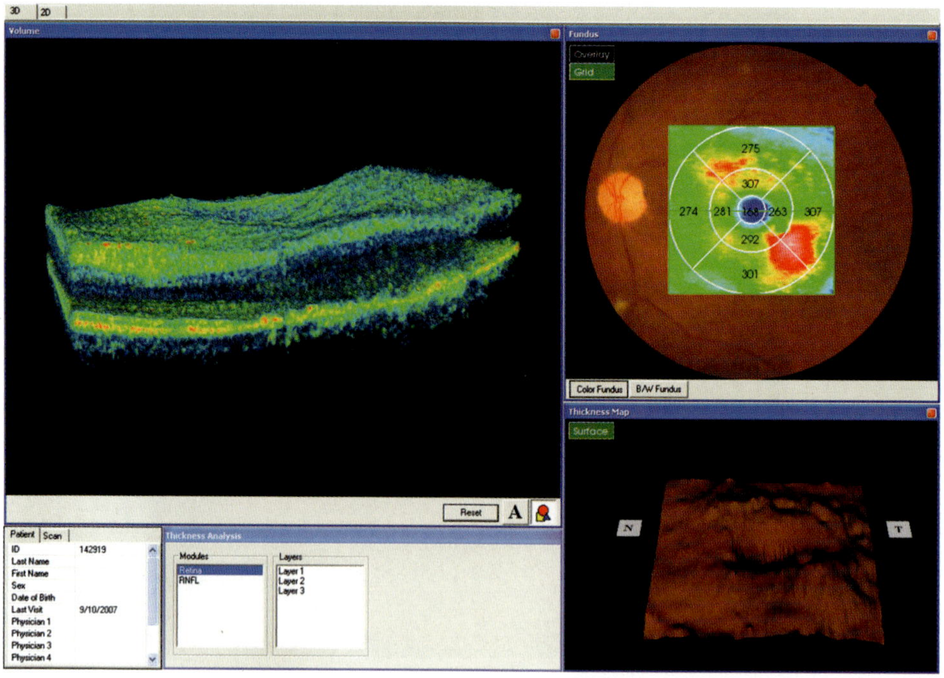

Figure 9.6.4D: 3D image of Case 9.6 following intravitreal triamcinolone

CASE 9.7: CSME WITH SEROUS RETINAL DETACHMENT

Case Summary

A 50-year-old woman, a known diabetic for the past 20 years presented with distortion in the right eye for 2 months. Her best-corrected visual acuity was 6/24; N8 in the right eye. Fluorescein angiography showed diffuse leaks in the late phase (Figures 9.7.1 and 9.7.2).

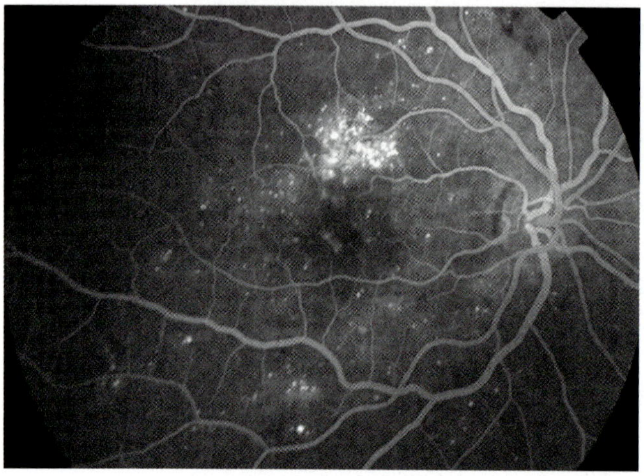

Figure 9.7.1: Early phase angiogram shows non-proliferative diabetic retinopathy

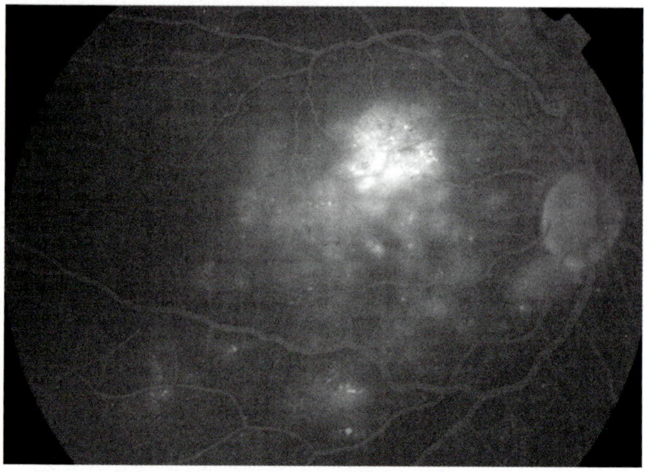

Figure 9.7.2: Late phase angiogram shows macular edema

Optical Coherence Tomography

Horizontal line scan showed ERM with retinal thickening, hard exudates and the presence of serous retinal detachment (Figures 9.7.3A to D).

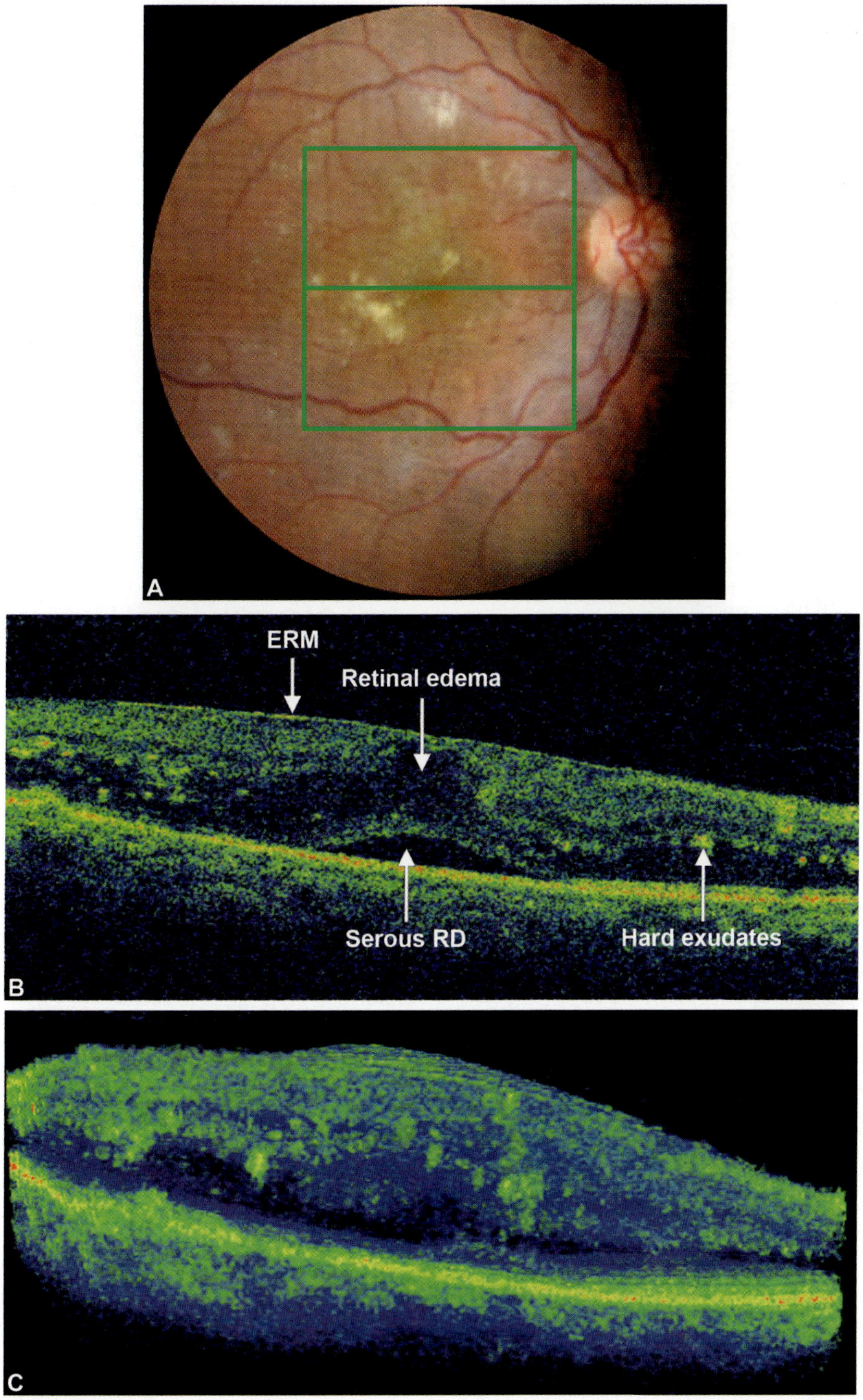

Figures 9.7.3A to C: (A) Color fundus photograph showing the horizontal line scan through the fovea. (B) Horizontal line scan, 2D image showing ERM with retinal thickening, hard exudates and the presence of serous retinal detachment. (C) Cropped 3D image showing ERM with retinal thickening, hard exudates and the presence of serous retinal detachment

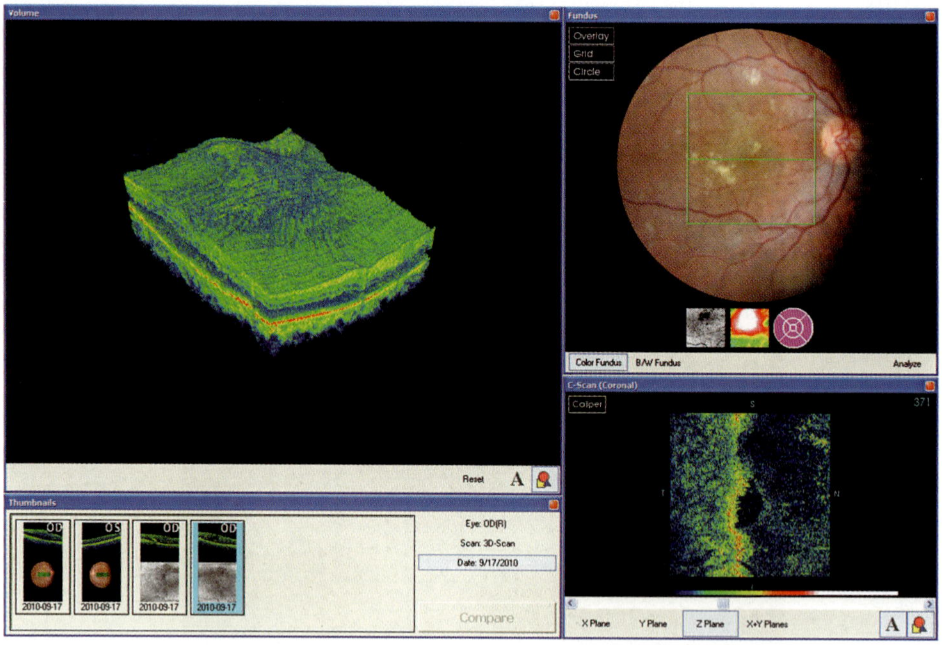

Figure 9.7.3D: 3D image of Case 9.7 **(Images with Topcon 3D OCT-2000)**

SUGGESTED READING

1. Thomas D, Bunce C, Moorman C, Laaidlan AH. Frequency and association of a taut thickened posterior hyaloid, partial vitreomacular separation and subretinal fluid in patients with diabetic macular edema. Retina.2005 Oct-Nov; 25(7):883-8.
2. Kim BY, Smith SD, Kaiser PK. Optical coherence tomography patterns of diabetic macular edema. Am J Ophthalmol 2006 Sept; 142(3):405-12.
3. Gibran SK, Khan K, Jungkim S, Cleary PE. Optical coherence tomography pattern may predict visual outcome after intravtreal triamcinolone acetonide for diabetic macular edema. Ophthalmolog.2007 May;114(5):890-4.
4. Solimon W, Sauder B, Hasler PW, Larsen M. Correlation between intraretinal changes in diabetic macular edema seen in fluorescein angiography and optical coherence tomography. Acta Ophthalmol Scand.2007 Jul 25;[Epub ahead of print]

10 Epiretinal Membranes

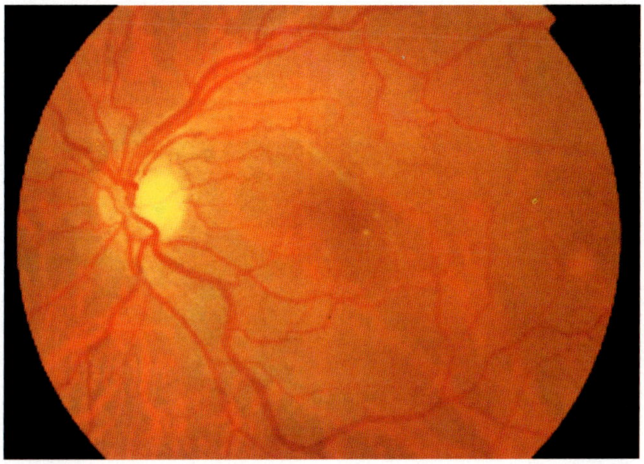

Epiretinal membranes (ERMs) are avascular, fibrocellular membranes that proliferate on the surface of the retina. These membranes have contractile properties and patients can present with metamorphopsia and visual changes because of their effect on the underlying retina.

ERMs can be associated with a variety of ocular conditions, such as posterior vitreous detachments (PVD), retinal tears, retinal detachments, retinal vascular occlusive diseases, ocular inflammatory diseases, and vitreous hemorrhage. However, a large proportion does not occur in the context of any associated disease or known history and therefore are classified as idiopathic epiretinal membranes.

Gass has formulated a classification system based on the appearance of the membrane and the underlying retinal tissue and vessels.

Grade 0 membranes are translucent membranes not associated with any retinal distortion. These ERMs are also known as cellophane maculopathy owing to the cellophane like sheen coming from the inner retinal surface as it is seen ophthalmoscopically.

Grade 1 membranes cause an irregular wrinkling of the inner retinal surface. Fine, superficial, radiating folds extend outward from the margins of the contracted membrane. Wrinkling may be sufficient to produce tortuosity of the paramacular vessels pulling them toward the fovea. Cystoid macular edema, retinal hemorrhage, exudates, and RPE disturbances are typically absent.

Grade 2 membranes have an opaque, thick appearance. Gross, full-thickness puckering of the macula may be present along with retinal edema, small hemorrhages, cotton-wool spots, and infrequently, a localized detachment of the retina. These membranes are also called macular puckers.

Optical Coherence Tomography can elucidate the presence or absence of an ERM. It can objectively measure other effects of the ERM on the retina, such as macular thickening, cystoid macular edema and any associated vitreous traction on the retina. It also allows the monitoring of the postoperative return of the normal retinal architecture as well as the presence of persistent traction or folds of the retina.

Based on OCT, epiretinal membranes are of two types:

1. Focally adherent membranes.
2. Globally adherent membranes.

CASE 10.1: GRADE 1 ERM: CRINKLED CELLOPHANE MACULOPATHY

Case Summary

A 72-year-old man was seen with complaints of defective near vision of one year duration. His best-corrected visual acuity in the right eye was 6/18. Fluorescein angiography showed distorted paramacular vessels which appeared pulled towards the fovea (Figures 10.1.1 and 10.1.2).

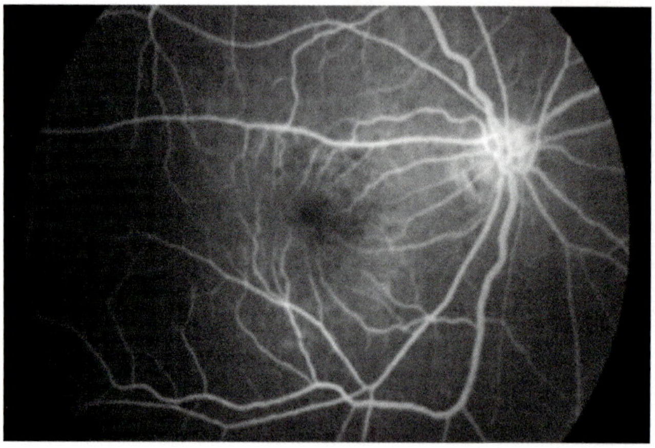

Figure 10.1.1: Early phase angiogram shows distorted paramacular vessels which appeared pulled towards the fovea

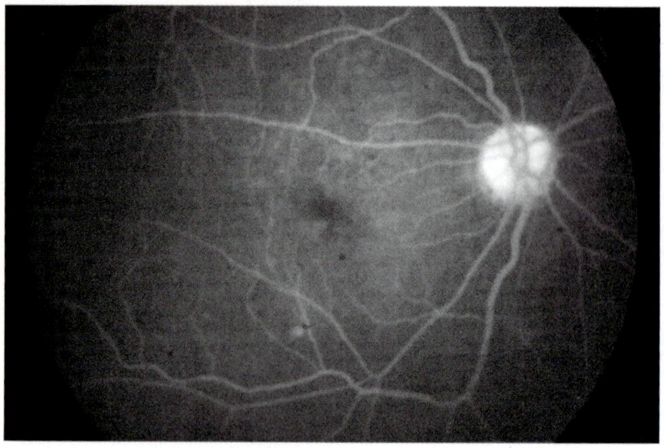

Figure 10.1.2: Late phase angiogram shows distorted paramacular vessels which appeared pulled towards the fovea

Optical Coherence Tomography

Horizontal line scan showed the presence of a hyper-reflective band at the vitreoretinal interface with traction on the underlying retina that was seen as in-foldings suggestive of ERM with focal adherence (Figures 10.1.3A to D). OCT helped in giving information regarding the status of underlying retinal traction in this patient that would justify surgery at this stage.

CASE 10.2: GRADE 2 ERM: MACULAR PUCKER

Case Summary

A 60-year-old man presented with diminished vision in both eyes of one year duration. His best-corrected visual acuity in the left eye was 6/60. Fluorescein angiography showed distorted and tortuous paramacular vessels which appeared dragged towards the fovea with leakage of dye from the retinal vessels (Figures 10.2.1 and 10.2.2).

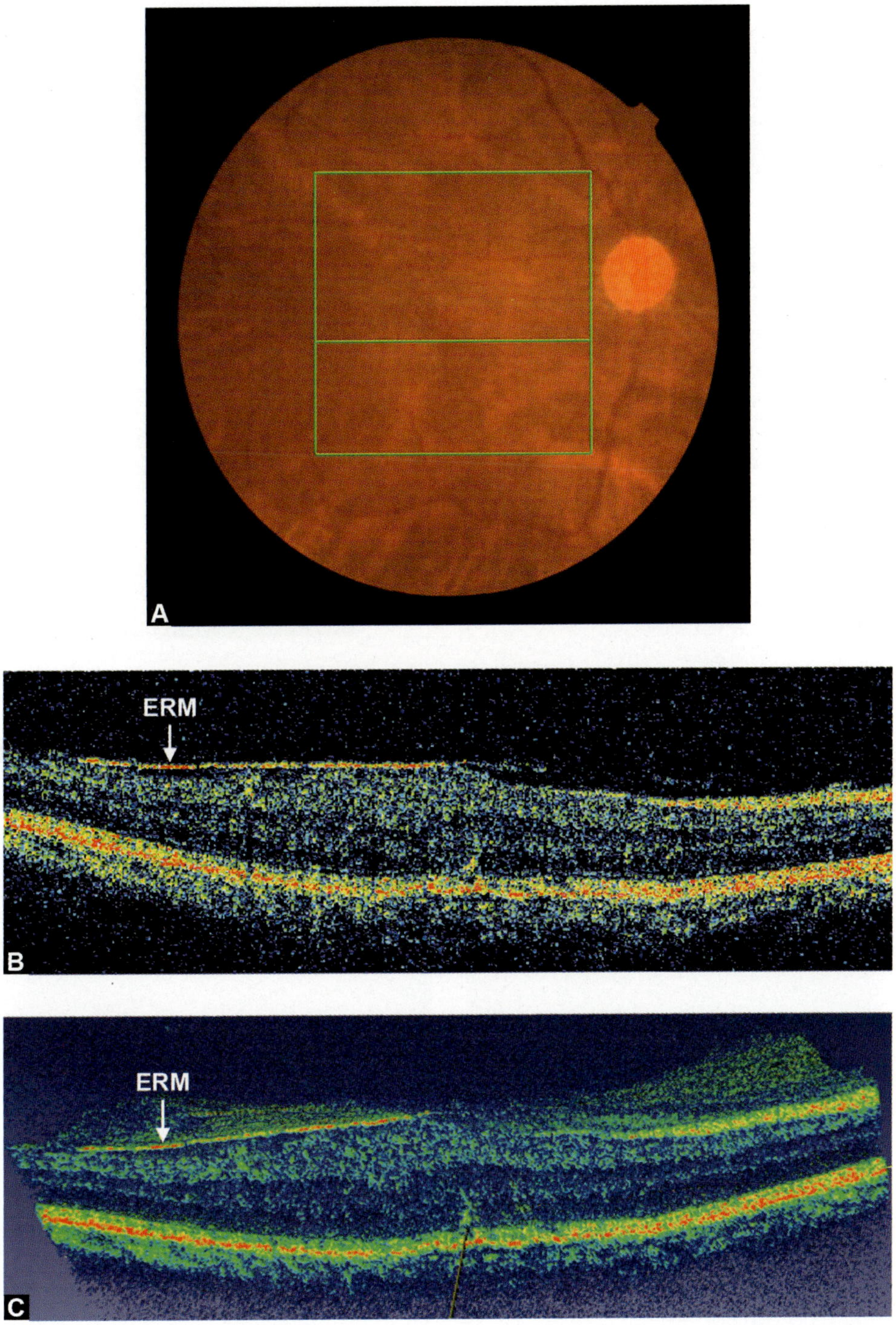

Figures 10.1.3A to C: (A) Color fundus photograph showing the horizontal line scan below the fovea. (B) Horizontal line scan below the fovea, 2D image showing the presence of a hyper-reflective band at the vitreo-retinal interface with traction on the underlying retina that is seen as in-foldings suggestive of ERM with focal adherence. (C) Cropped 3D image showing the presence of a hyper-reflective band at the vitreo-retinal interface with traction on the underlying retina that is seen as in-foldings suggestive of ERM with focal adherence

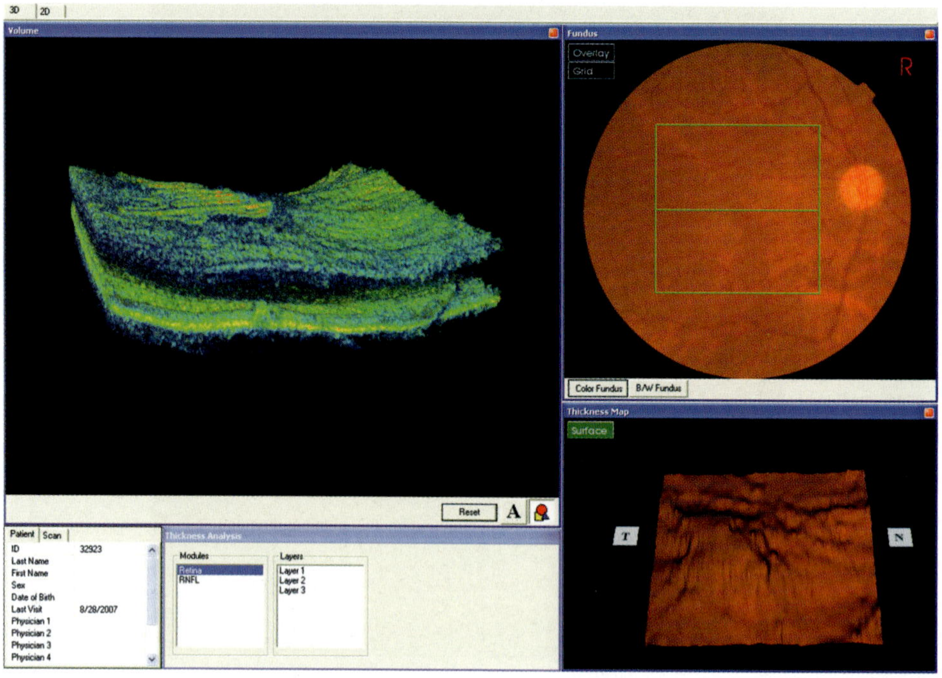

Figure 10.1.3D: 3D image of Case 10.1

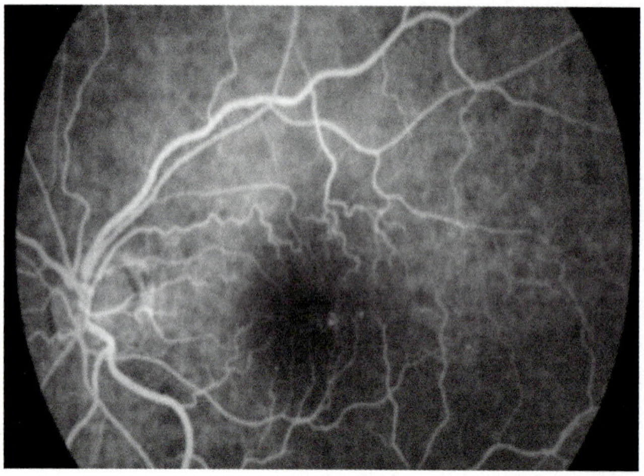

Figure 10.2.1: Early phase angiogram shows distorted and tortuous paramacular vessels which appeared dragged towards the fovea

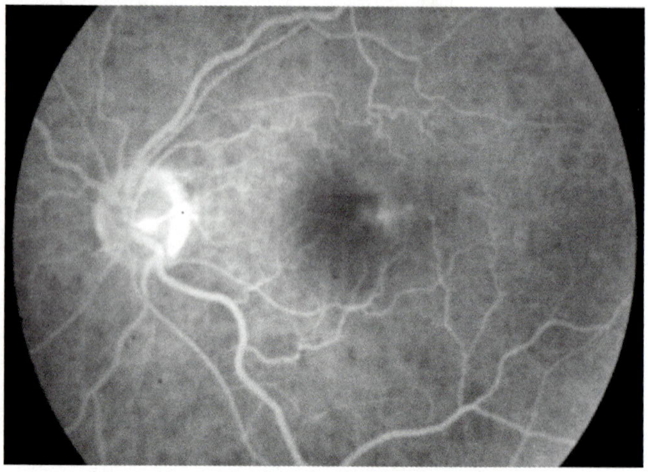

Figure 10.2.2: Late phase angiogram shows leakage of dye from the retinal vessels

Optical Coherence Tomography–1

Horizontal line scan showed the presence of a hyper-reflective band at the vitreo-retinal interface with traction on the underlying retina that was seen as in-foldings. In some areas, the membrane was clearly detached from the retina (Figures 10.2.3A to D). In addition, there was reduced backscatter from the outer retinal layers suggesting underlying retinal edema that corresponded to the leakage seen on fluorescein angiography. OCT was helpful in diagnosing underlying retinal edema that could give the prognosis following surgery.

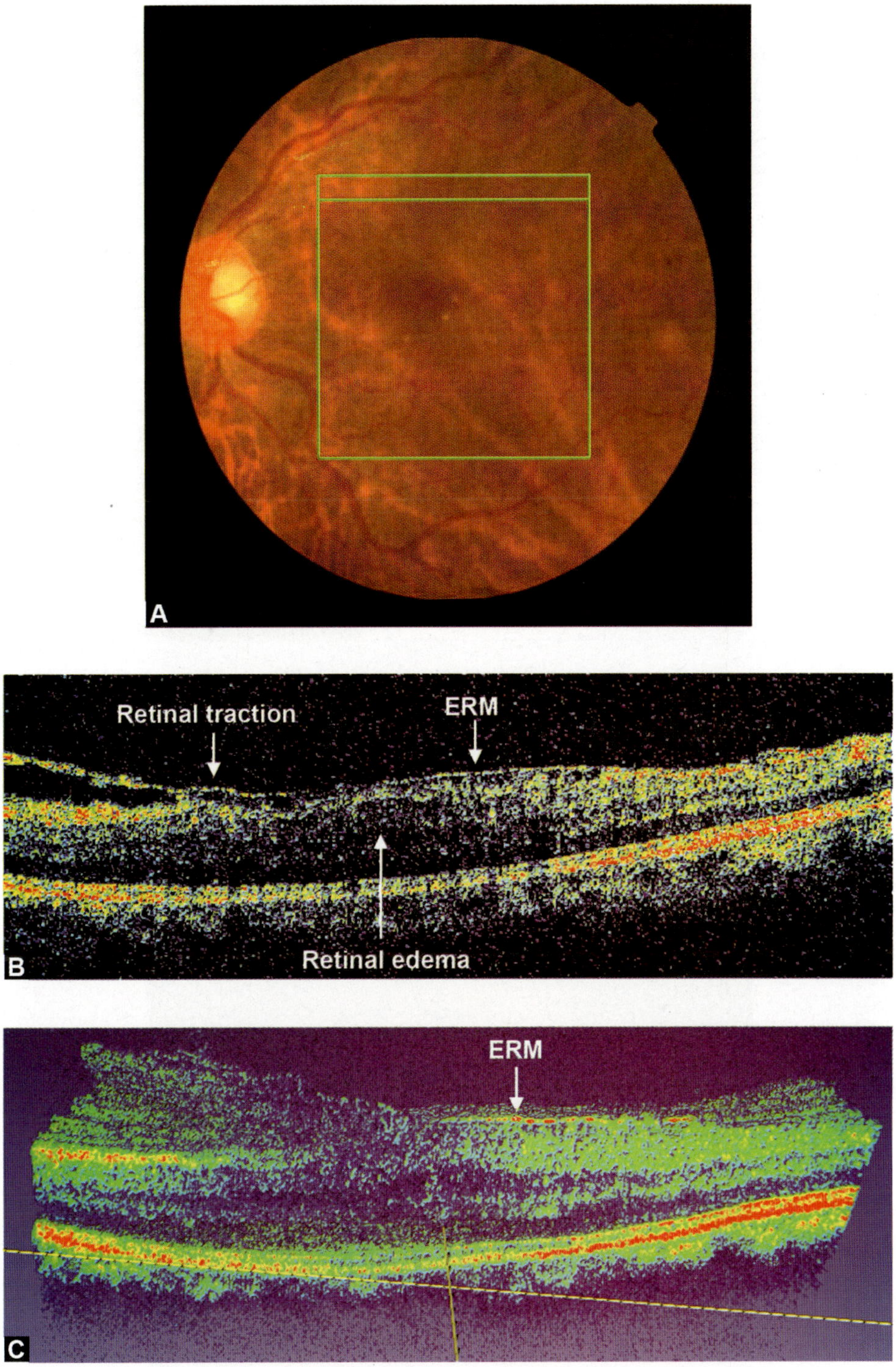

Figures 10.2.3A to C: (A) Color fundus photograph showing the horizontal line scan above the fovea. (B) Horizontal line scan above the fovea, 2D image showing the presence of a hyper-reflective band at the vitreo-retinal interface with traction on the underlying retina that is seen as in-foldings. In some areas, the membrane is clearly detached from the retina. The reduced backscatter from the outer retinal layers is suggestive of underlying retinal edema. (C) Cropped 3D image showing the presence of a hyper-reflective band at the vitreo-retinal interface with traction on the underlying retina that is seen as in-foldings. In some areas, the membrane is clearly detached from the retina. The reduced backscatter from the outer retinal layers is suggestive of underlying retinal edema

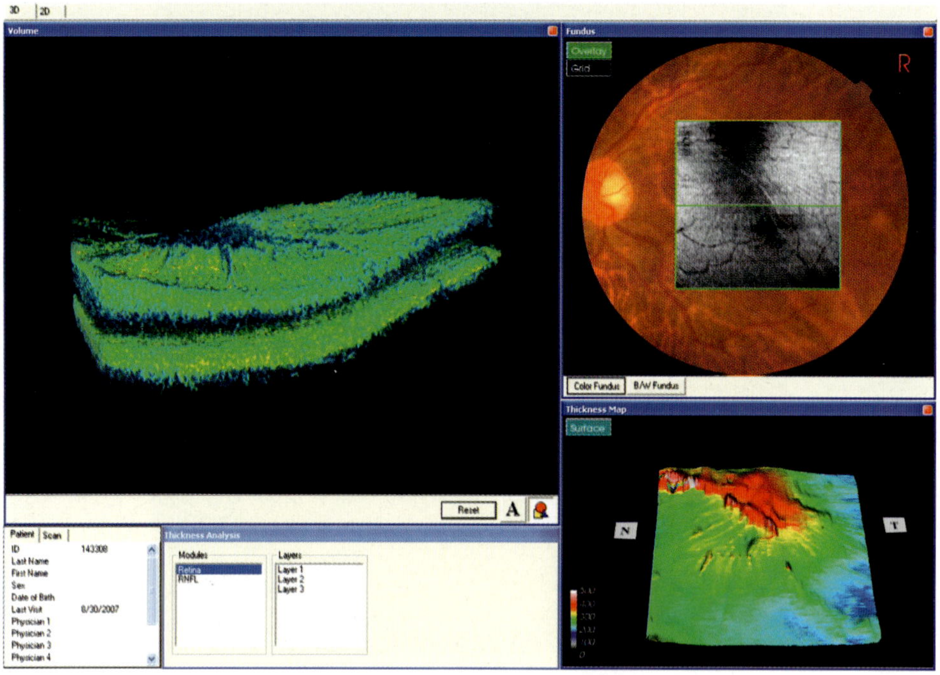

Figure 10.2.3D: 3D image of Case 10.2

Optical Coherence Tomography–2

Horizontal line scan passing just above the fovea showed small cystic spaces in the inner retinal layers and ERM causing retinal traction (Figures 10.2.3E to G). Thus, the 3D OCT with its ability to perform a continuous raster scan is capable of demonstrating the full extent of the ERM.

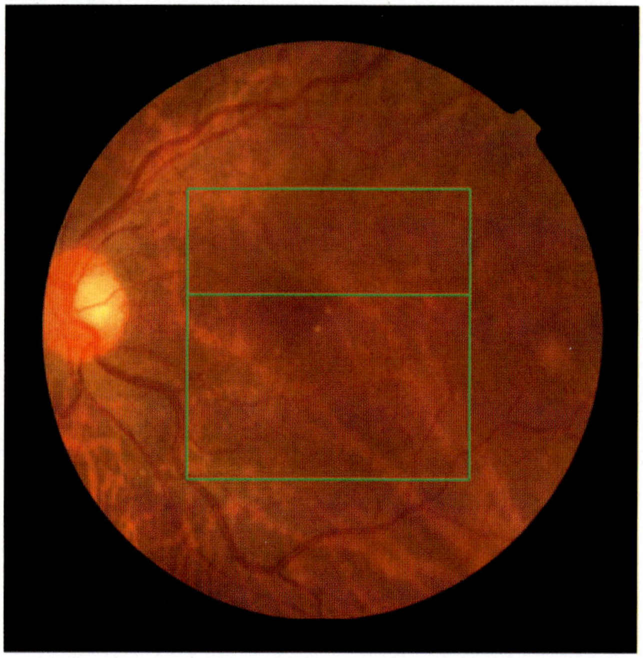

Figure 10.2.3E: Color fundus photograph showing the horizontal line scan just above the fovea

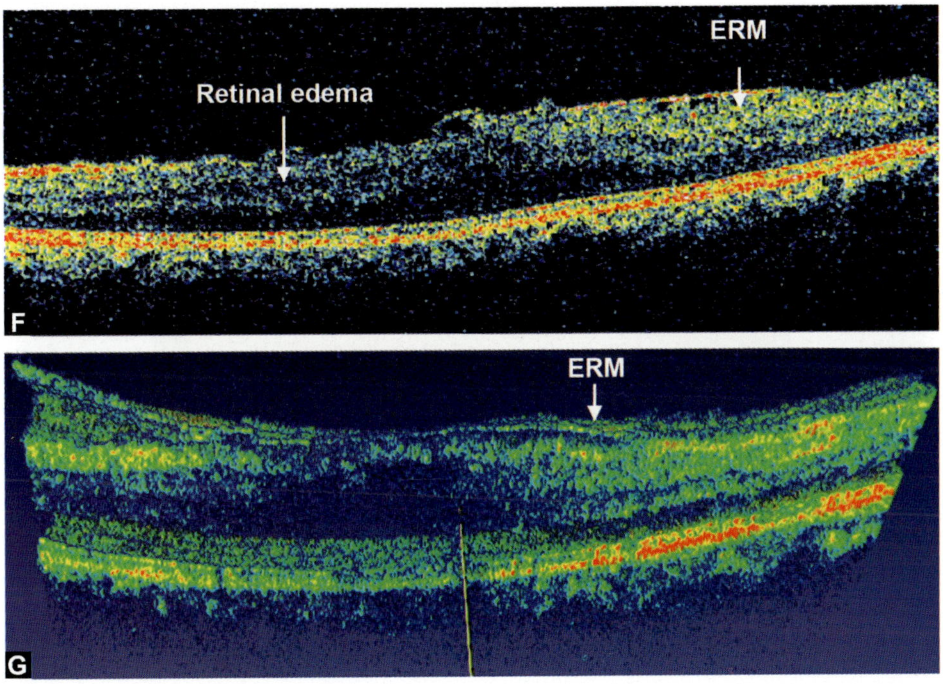

Figures 10.2.3F and G: (F) Horizontal line scan just above the fovea, 2D image showing small cystic spaces in the inner retinal layers and ERM causing retinal traction. (G) Cropped 3D image showing small cystic spaces in the inner retinal layers and ERM causing retinal traction

CASE 10.3: ERM IN EALES DISEASE

Case Summary

A 31-year-old man who had received laser photocoagulation for Eales disease in the right eye was seen with a best-corrected visual acuity of 6/12 in this eye. Fluorescein angiography showed distorted paramacular vessels which appeared pulled towards the fovea with leakage of dye (Figures 10.3.1 and 10.3.2).

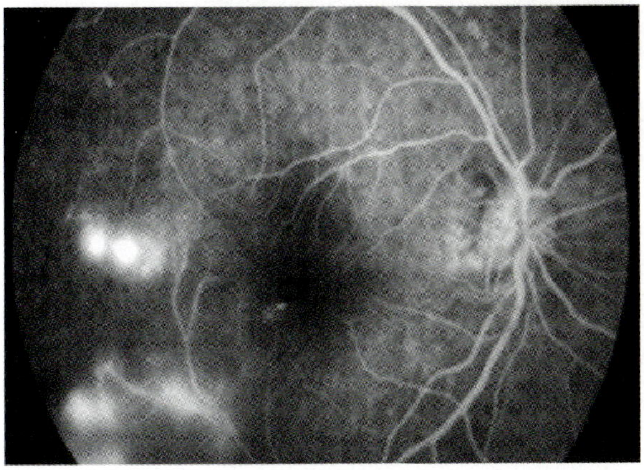

Figure 10.3.1: Early phase angiogram shows distorted paramacular vessels which appears pulled towards the fovea, NVE and photocoagulation scars

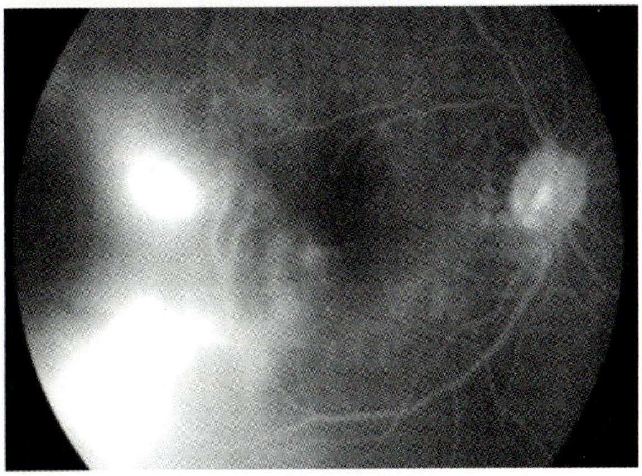

Figure 10.3.2: Late phase angiogram shows leakage of dye from the retinal vessels

Optical Coherence Tomography

Horizontal line scan passing above the fovea showed corrugations on the inner surface of the retina suggestive of globally adherent ERM (Figures 10.3.3A to C).

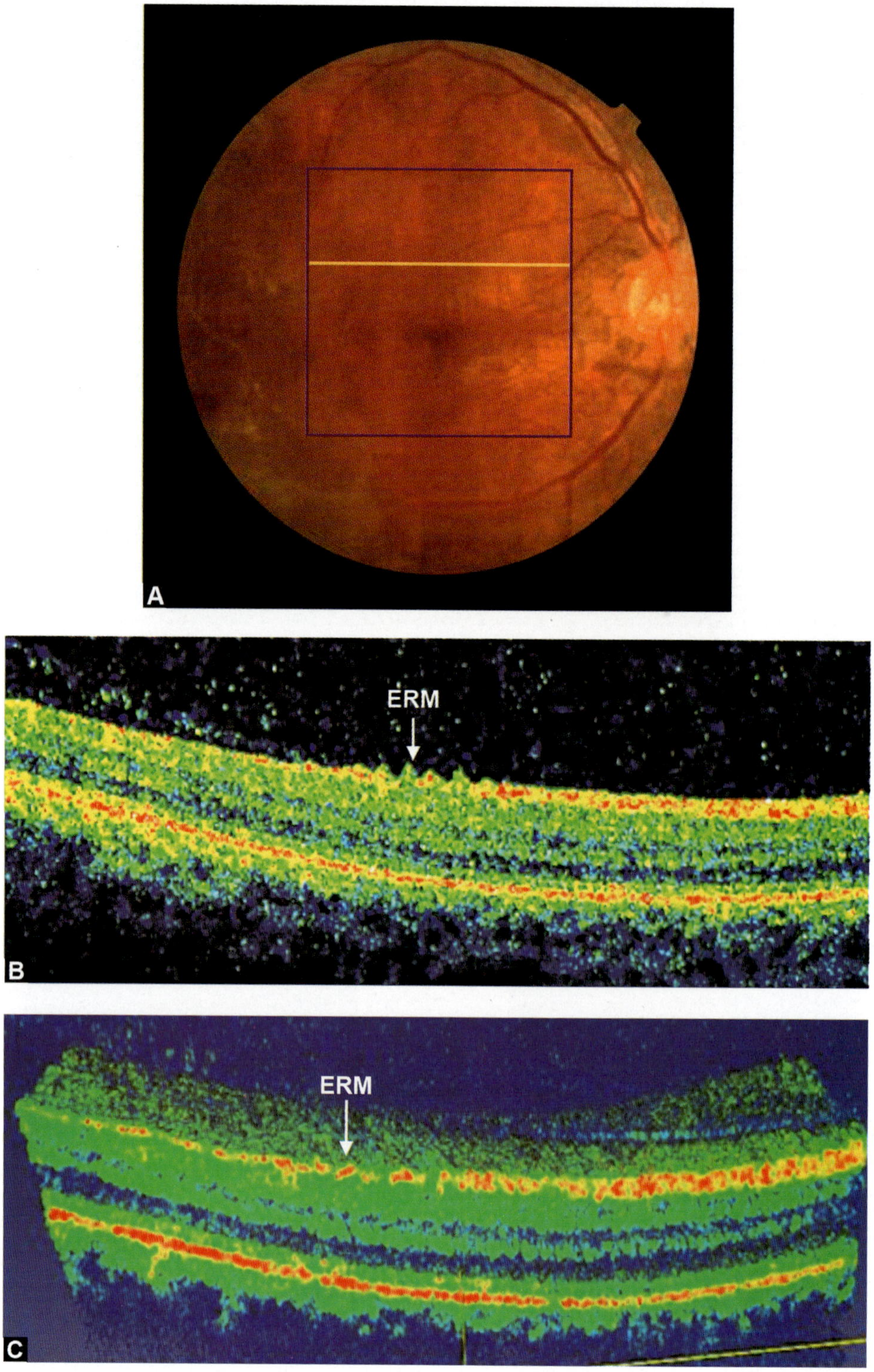

Figures 10.3.3A to C: (A) Color fundus photograph showing the horizontal line scan above the fovea. (B) Horizontal line scan above the fovea, 2D image showing corrugations on the inner surface of the retina suggestive of globally adherent ERM. (C) Cropped 3D image showing corrugations on the inner surface of the retina suggestive of globally adherent ERM

CASE 10.4: GRADE 1 ERM

Case Summary

A 60-year old lady was seen with complaints of defective vision in the right eye of 5 months duration. Her best-corrected visual acuity in this eye was 6/12 .

Optical Coherence Tomography

Horizontal line scan passing through the fovea showed the presence of a hyper-reflective band at the vitreoretinal interface with traction on the underlying retina that was seen as in-foldings. In addition, there was reduced backscatter from the outer retinal layers suggesting underlying retinal edema (Figures 10.4.1A to D).

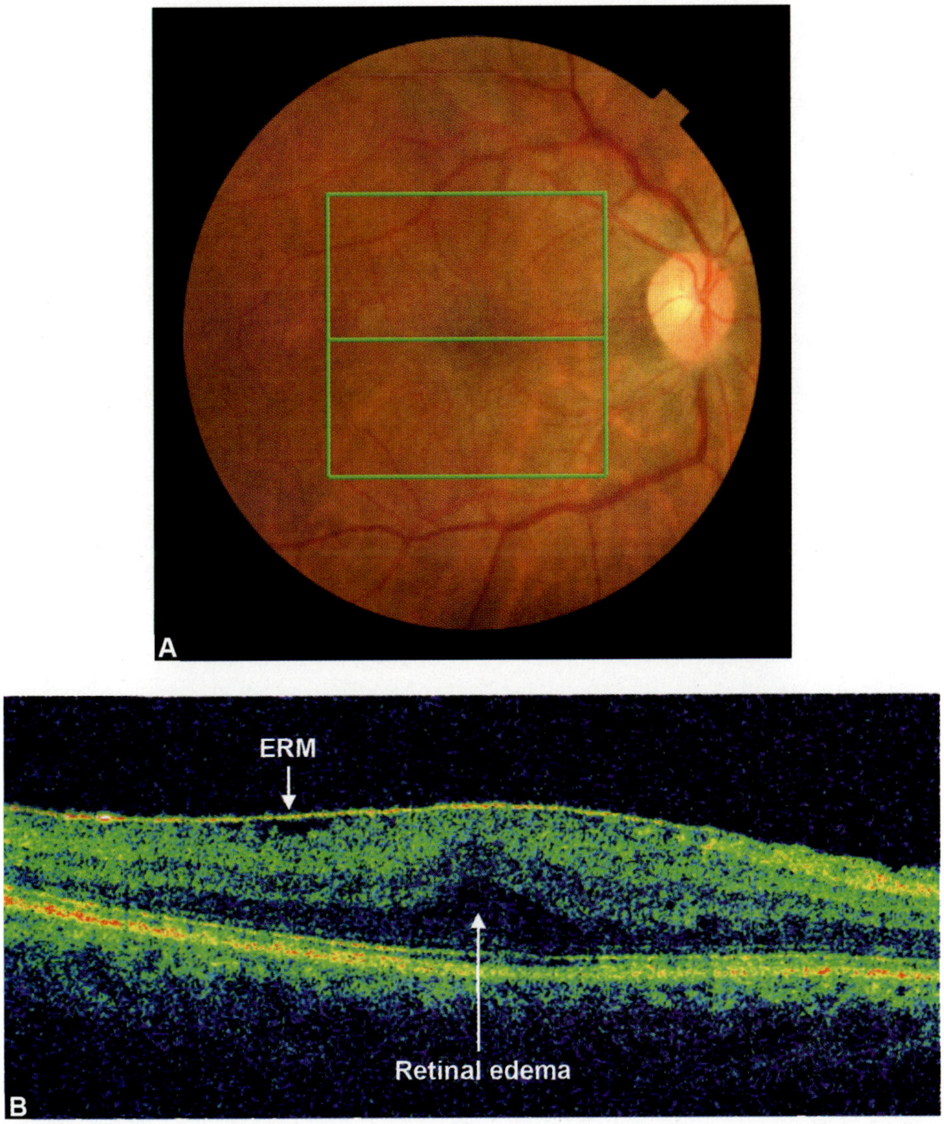

Figures 10.4.1A and B: (A) Color fundus photograph showing the horizontal line scan through the fovea. (B) Horizontal line scan through the fovea, 2D image showing the presence of a hyper-reflective band at the vitreoretinal interface with traction on the underlying retina that is seen as in-foldings. The reduced backscatter from the outer retinal layers is suggestive of underlying retinal edema

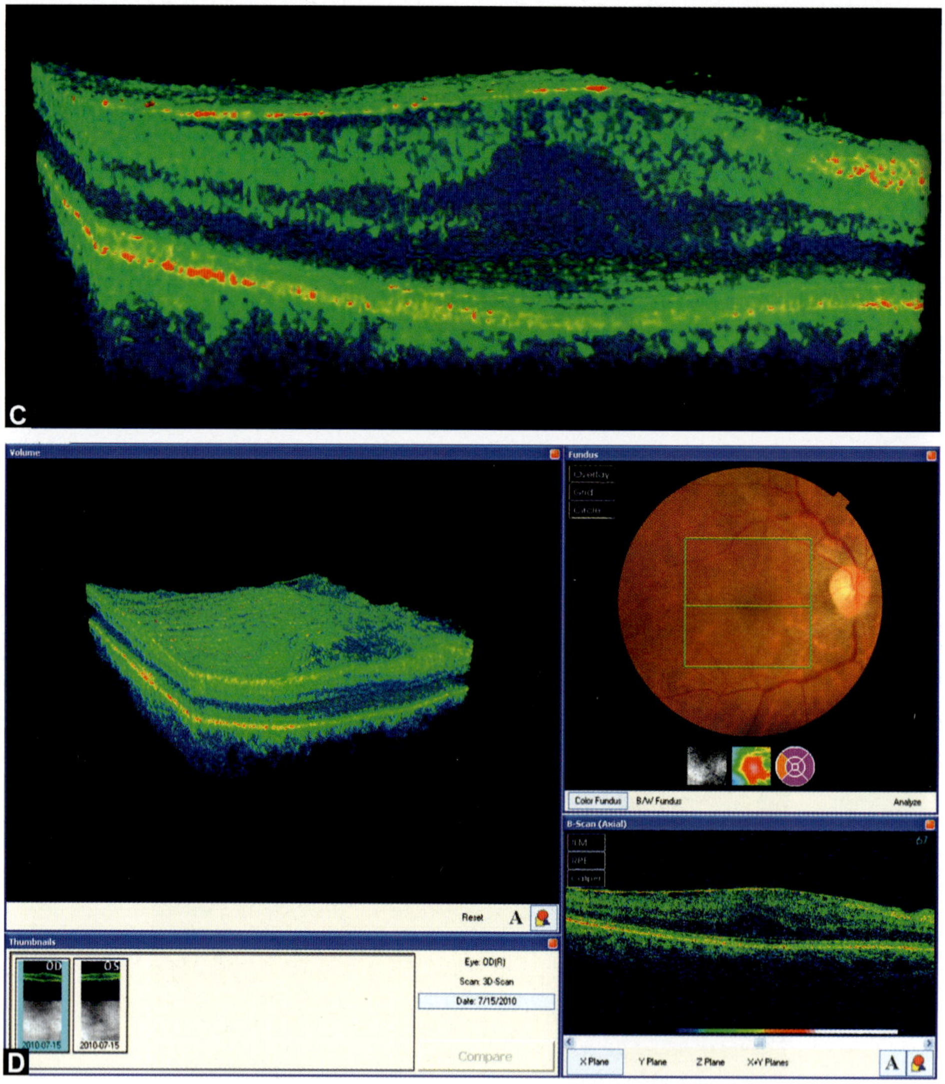

Figures 10.4.1C and D: (C) Cropped 3D image showing the presence of a hyper-reflective band at the vitreoretinal interface with traction on the underlying retina that is seen as in-foldings. The reduced backscatter from the outer retinal layers is suggestive of underlying retinal edema. (D) 3D image of Case 10.4 **(Images with TOPCON 3D OCT-2000)**

SUGGESTED READING

1. Do Dv, Cho M.Nguyen O.D, Shah SM, Handa JT, Campochiars PA, et al. The impact of optical coherence tomography on surgical decision making in epiretinal membrane and vitreomacular traction. Retina.2007 Jun;27(5):552-6.
2. Massin P, Allouch C, Haouchine B, Metge F, Paques M, Tangui L, et al. Optical coherence tomography of idiopathic macular epiretinal membranes before and after surgery. Am J Ophthalmol.2000 Dec;130(6):732-9.
3. Mori K, Gehlbach PL, Sano A, Deguchi T, Yoneya S. Comparison of epiretinal membranes of differing pathogenesis using optical coherence tomography. Retina.2004 Feb;24(1):57-62.

11 Foveal Hemorrhage

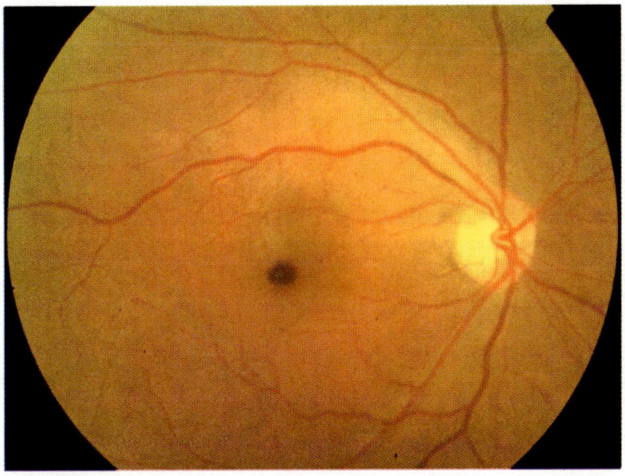

CASE 11.1: FOVEAL HEMORRHAGE

Case Summary

A 68-year-old woman with mild non-proliferative diabetic retinopathy presented with sudden loss of vision in the right eye of two days duration. Her best-corrected vision in this eye was counting fingers. Fundus showed the presence of a dark red spot at the fovea. Fluorescein angiography revealed blocked fluorescence at the fovea, confirming the presence of a hemorrhage (Figures 11.1.1 and 11.1.2).

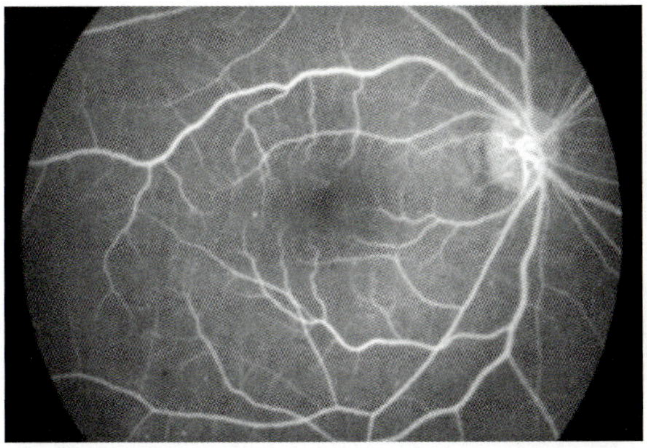

Figure 11.1.1: Early phase angiogram shows blocked fluorescence due to hemorrhage

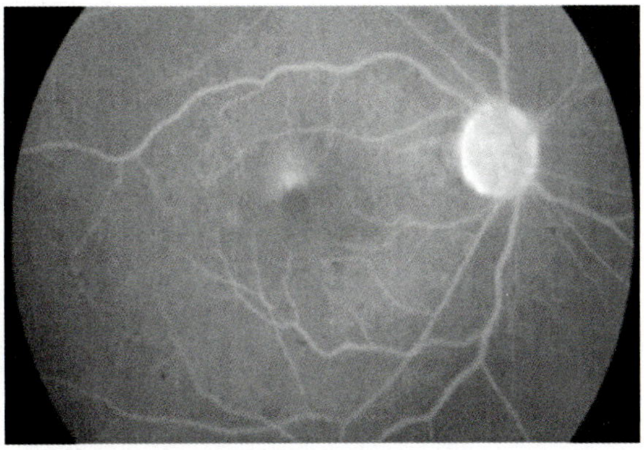

Figure 11.1.2: Late phase angiogram shows blocked fluorescence due to hemorrhage

Optical Coherence Tomography–1

Horizontal lines scan above the fovea showed the presence of a hyper-reflective band at the vitreoretinal interface with traction on the underlying retina that was seen as in-foldings (Figures 11.1.3A to C).

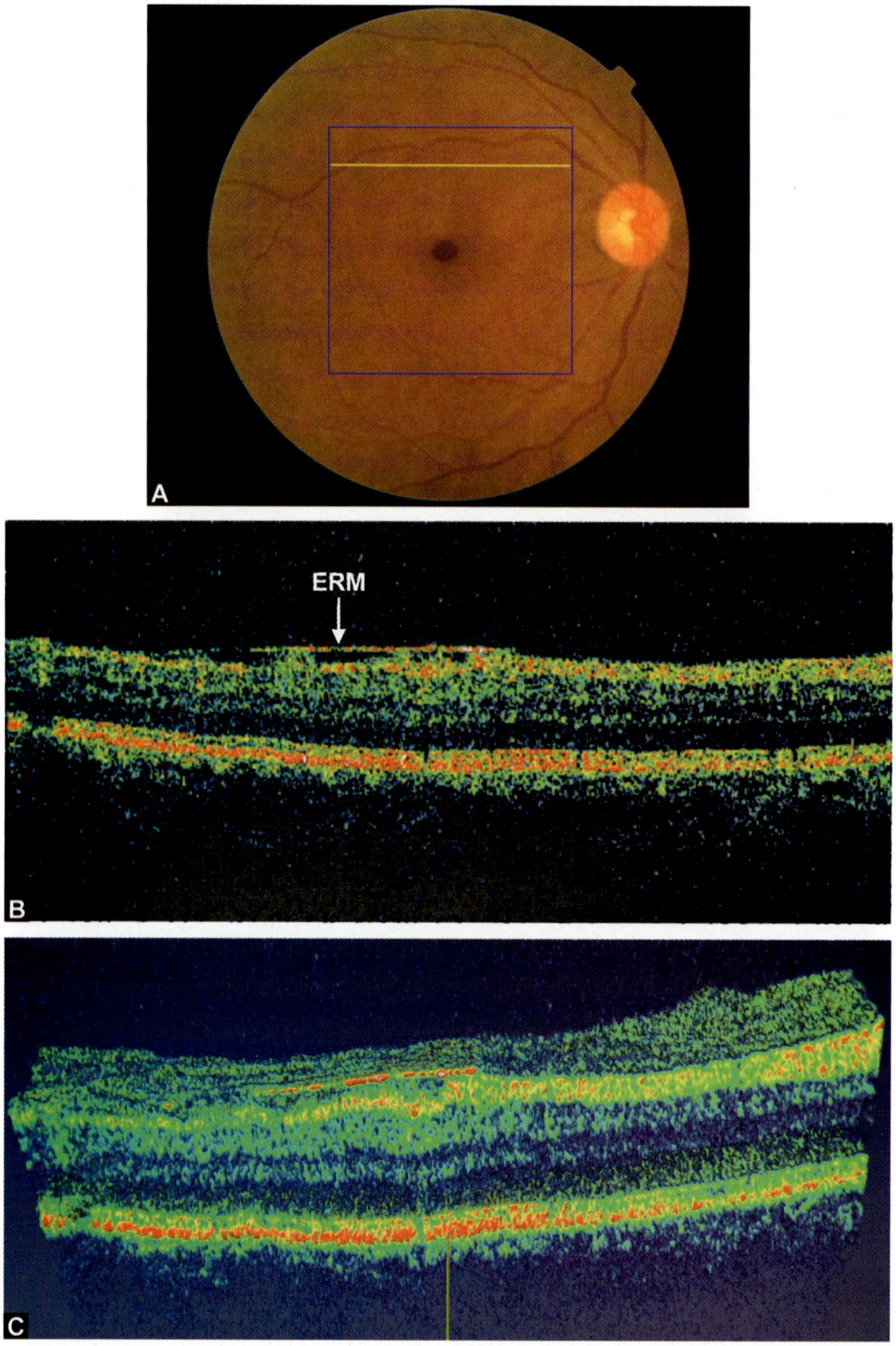

Figures 11.1.3A to C: (A) Color fundus photograph showing the horizontal line scan above the fovea. (B) Horizontal line scan above the fovea, 2D image showing the presence of a hyper-reflective band at the vitreo-retinal interface with traction on the underlying retina that is seen as in-foldings. (C) Cropped 3D image showing the presence of a hyper-reflective band at the vitreo-retinal interface with traction on the underlying retina that is seen as in-foldings

Optical Coherence Tomography–2

Horizontal lines scan through the foveal center showed the presence of a focal area of enhanced backscatter, corresponding to the area of blood seen clinically. The shadow that is created masks all retinal layers beneath it (Figures 11.1.4A to D). OCT helped in showing the presence of the epiretinal membrane which probably caused traction on the retina resulting in the superficial foveal hemorrhage.

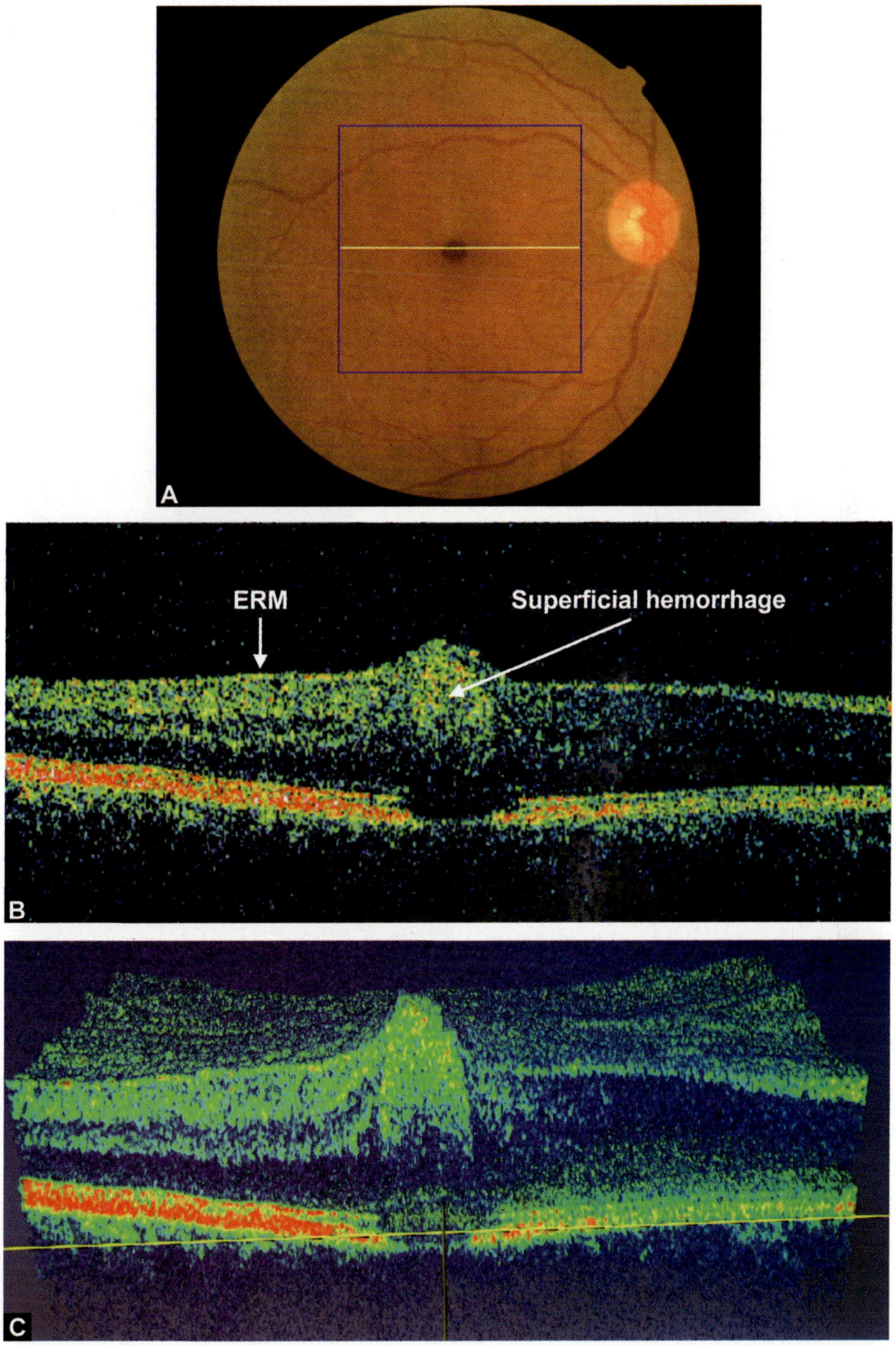

Figures 11.1.4A to C: (A) Color fundus photograph showing the horizontal line scan through the fovea. (B) Horizontal line scan through the fovea, 2D image showing the presence of a focal area of enhanced backscatter corresponding to the area of blood seen clinically. The shadow that is created masks all retinal layers beneath it. ERM is also evident. (C) Cropped 3D image showing the presence of a focal area of enhanced backscatter corresponding to the area of blood seen clinically. The shadow that is created masks all retinal layers beneath it. ERM is also evident

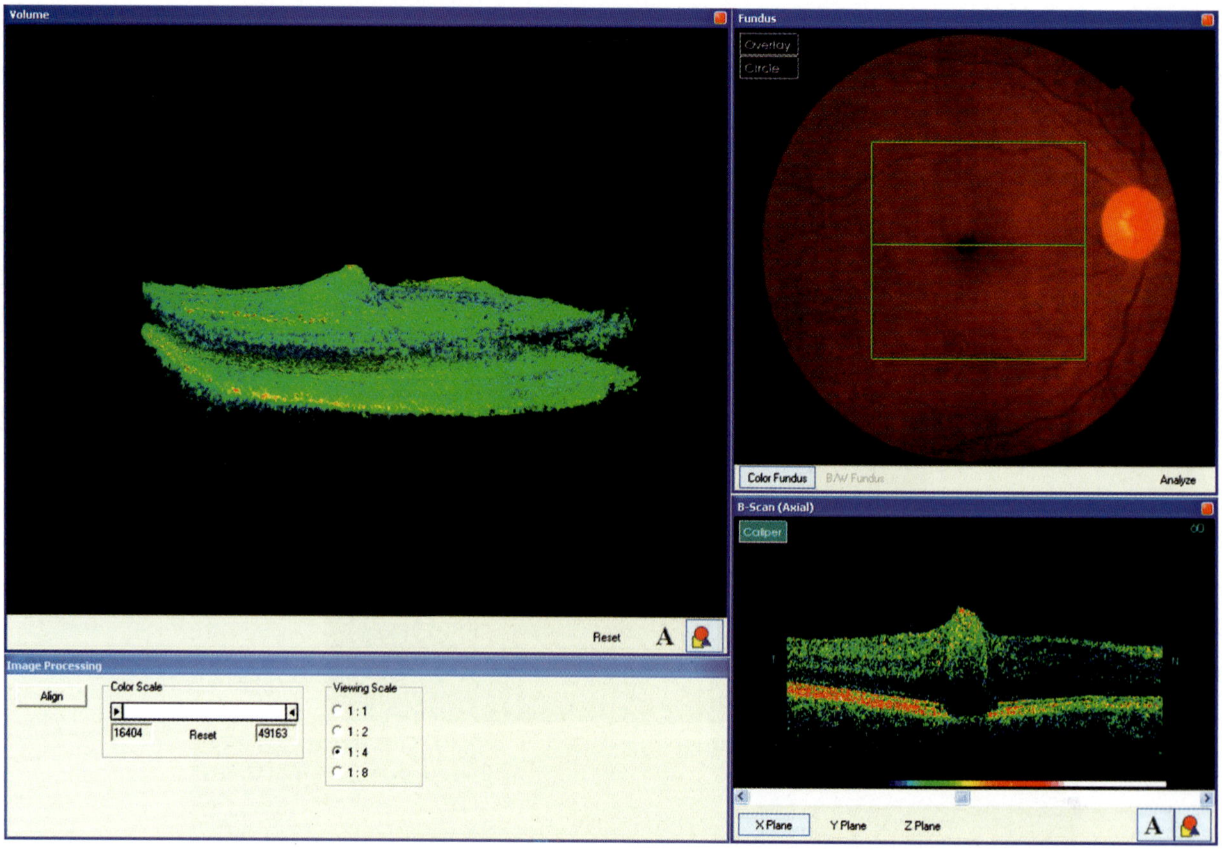

Figure 11.1.4D: 3D image of Case 11.1

CASE 11.2: ORGANIZED FOVEAL HEMORRHAGE

Case Summary

A 46-year old male patient presented with diminished vision in the left eye of one month duration. His best-corrected visual acuity in this eye was counting fingers 5 meters.

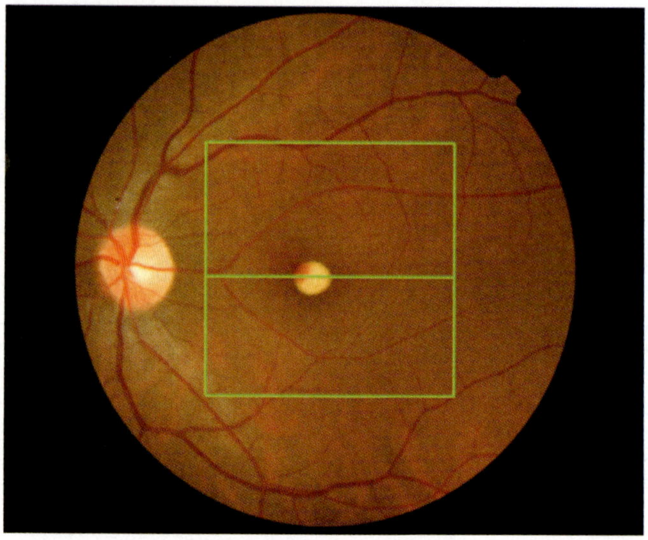

Figure 11.2.1A: Color fundus photograph showing the horizontal line scan through the fovea

Optical Coherence Tomography

Horizontal line scan through the fovea showed an area of increased reflectivity just beneath the ILM corresponding to the area of organized blood seen clinically. The shadow that is created masks all the retinal layers beneath it (Figures 11.2.1A to D).

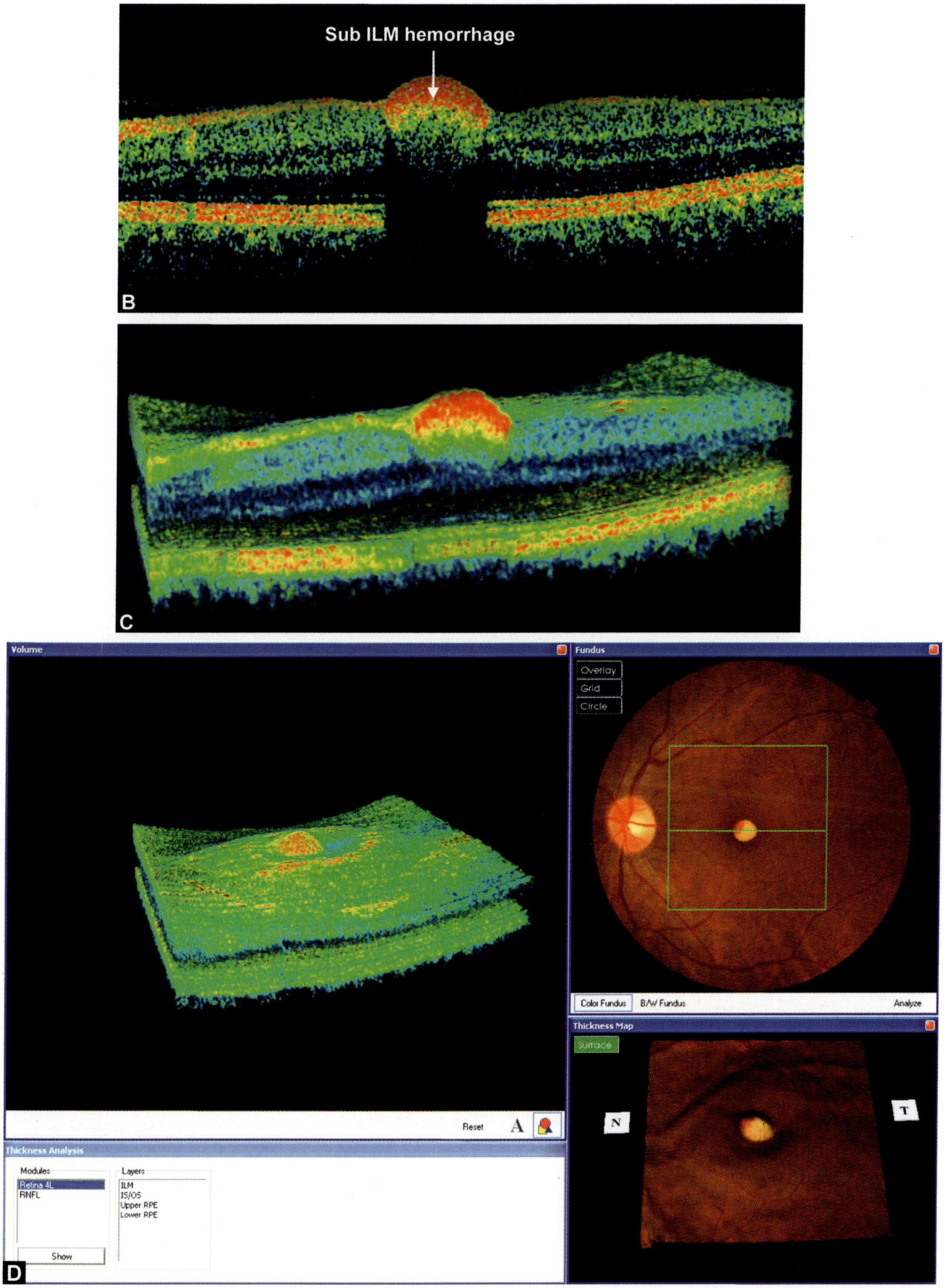

Figures 11.2.1B to D: (B) Horizontal line scan through the fovea, 2D image showing an area of increased reflectivity just beneath the ILM corresponding to the area of organized blood seen clinically. The shadow that is created masks all the retinal layers beneath it. (C) Cropped 3D image showing an area of increased reflectivity just beneath the ILM corresponding to the area of organized blood seen clinically. The shadow that is created masks all the retinal layers beneath it. (D) 3D image of Case 11.2

CONCLUSION

In patients with foveal hemorrhage, OCT helps in delineating the precise location and depth of the hemorrhage and may help in finding the cause of the hemorrrhage.

12 Heredomacular Disorders

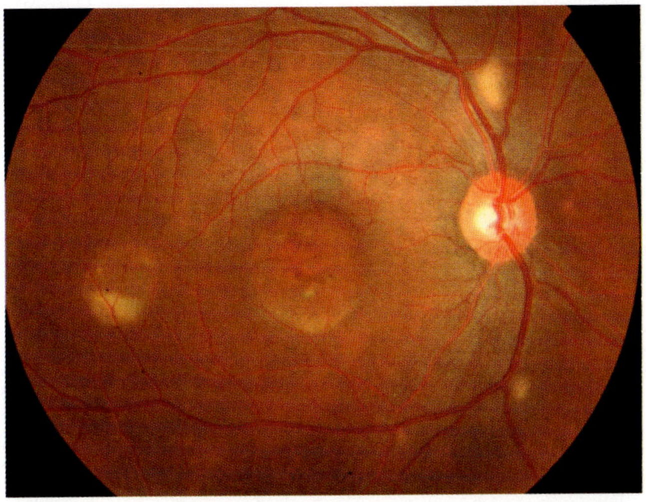

BEST'S DISEASE

Best's disease is an extremely rare autosomal dominant disorder with the gene responsible for the disease mapped to chromosome11q13. It is characterized by a large, yellow, yolk like (vitelliform) lesion that is bilateral and symmetric in the central macula and that appears during childhood. Later in life, the lesion breaks down with resultant scarring and atrophy and visual acuity drops. Late lesions often are difficult to diagnose correctly on the basis of their clinical appearance alone, the definitive diagnosis is made on the basis of an abnormal electro-oculogram (EOG). Less commonly, the lesions may be multifocal. Choroidal neovascularization can arise adjacent to old vitelliform scars. Histopathologic studies show an accumulation of lipofuschin-like material throughout the retinal pigment epithelium.

Optical coherence tomography shows separation of the inner RPE layer from the outer RPE layer with moderate reflectivity within corresponding to the accumulation of lipofuschin. An optically clear space was seen within the separated RPE layers where the lipofuschin was absent.

CASE 12.1: BEST'S DISEASE

Case Summary

A 31-year-old male presented with defective vision in both eyes of 3 years duration. His best-corrected visual acuity was 6/18; N6 in the right eye and 6/9; N6 in the left eye. Fluorescein angiography showed multifocal yellowish vitelliform lesions (Figures 12.1.1 and 12.1.2).

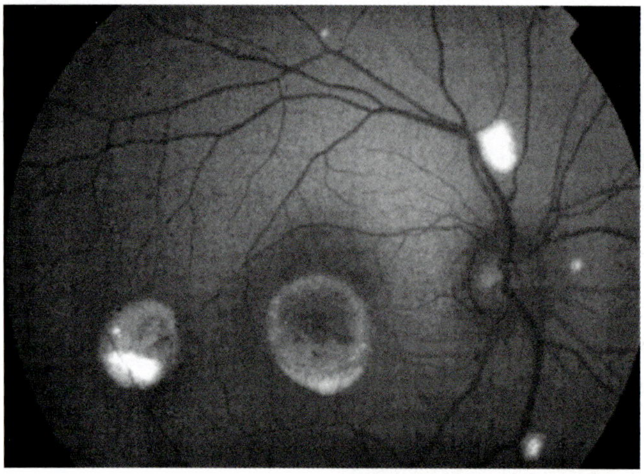

Figure 12.1.1: Early phase angiogram of the right eye shows multifocal vitelliform lesions

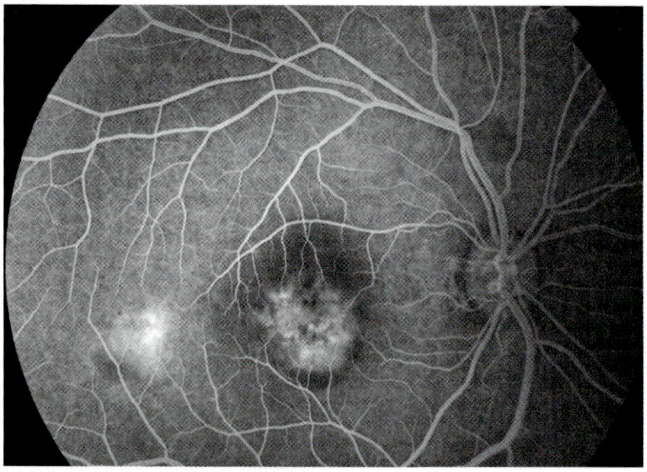

Figure 12.1.2: Late phase angiogram shows fading of some lesions

Optical Coherence Tomography–1

Horizontal line scan through the fovea showed separation of the inner RPE layer from the outer RPE layer with a hyporeflective space between the two layers (Figures 12.1.3A to D).

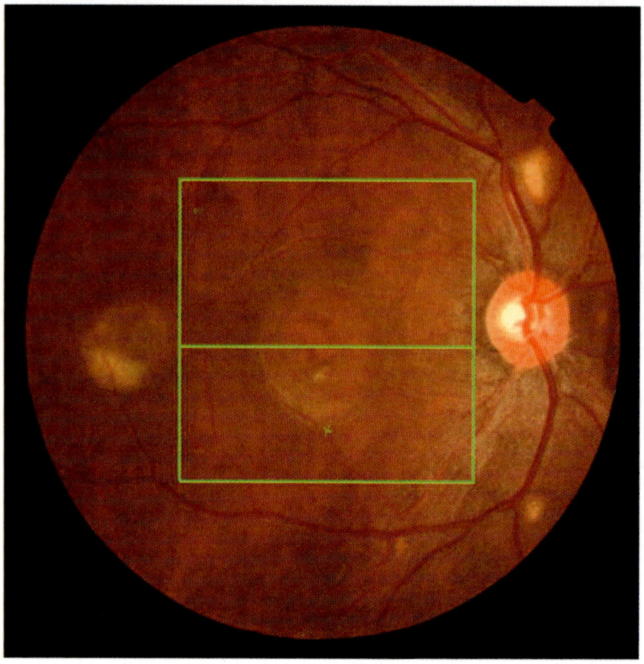

Figure 12.1.3A: Color fundus photograph showing the horizontal line scan through the fovea

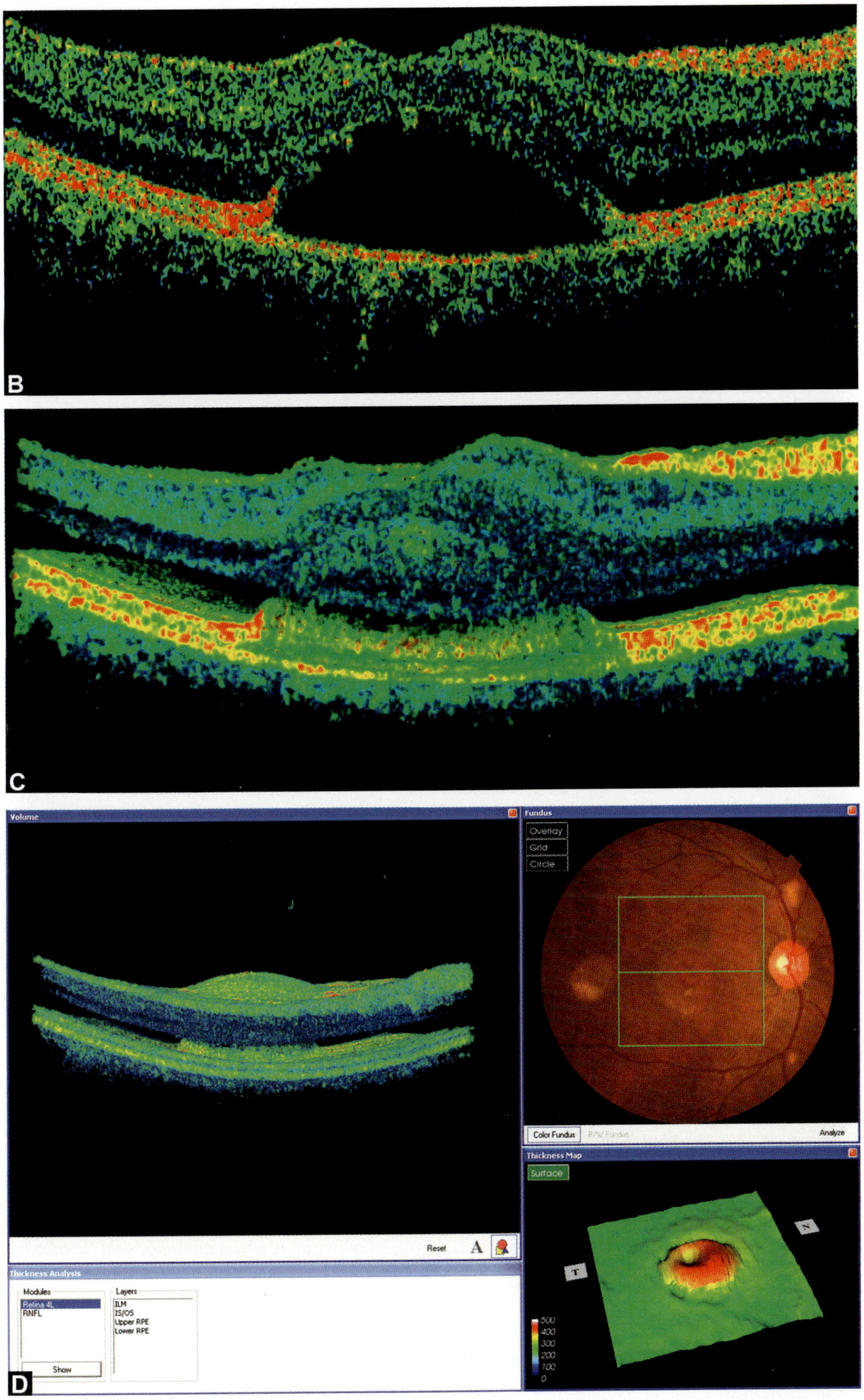

Figures 12.1.3B to D: (B) Horizontal line scan, 2D image showing separation of the inner RPE layer from the outer RPE layer with a hyporeflective space between the two layers. (C) Cropped 3D image showing separation of the inner RPE layer from the outer RPE layer with a hyporeflective space between the two layers. (D) 3D image of the right eye of Case 12.1

Optical Coherence Tomography–2

Horizontal line scan through the inferior portion of the lesion showed moderate reflectivity between the separated inner and outer RPE layers corresponding to the presence of lipofuschin (Figures 12.1.4A and B).

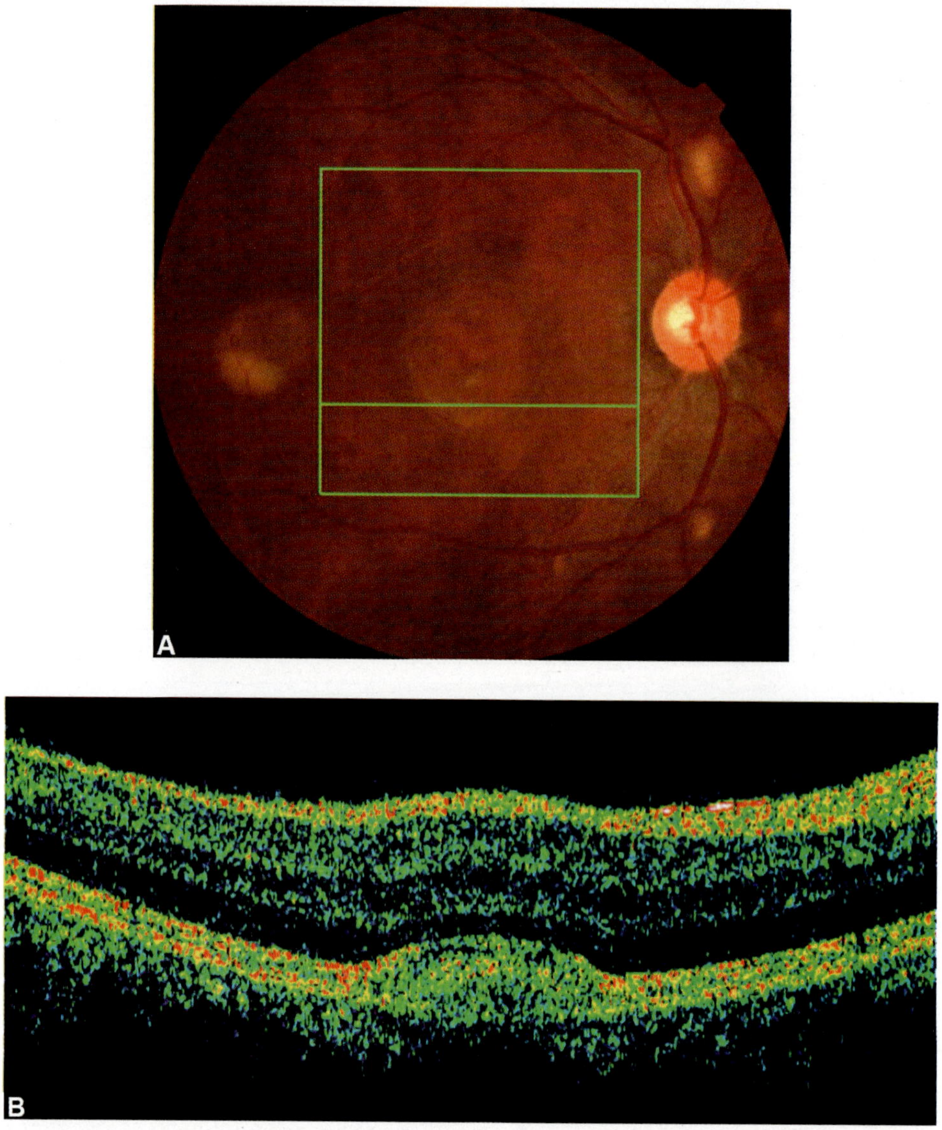

Figures 12.1.4A and B: (A) Color fundus photograph showing the horizontal line scan through the inferior portion of the lesion. (B) Horizontal line scan scan through the inferior portion of the lesion, 2D image showing moderate reflectivity between the separated inner and outer RPE layers corresponding to the presence of lipofuschin

Optical Coherence Tomography–3

Horizontal line scan through the upper portion of the lesion located temporal to the macula showed separation of the inner RPE layer from the outer RPE layer with a hyporeflective space between the two layers (Figures 12.1.5A and B).

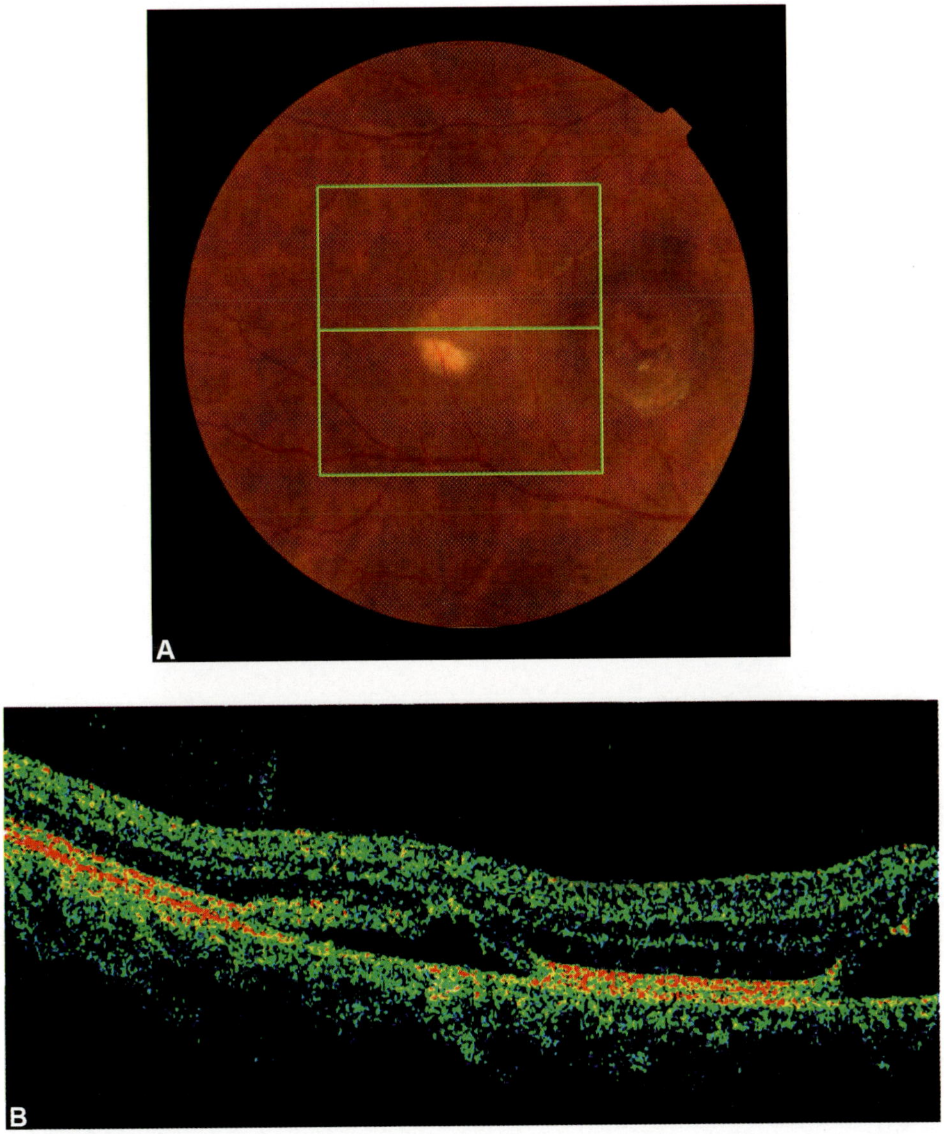

Figures 12.1.5A and B: (A) Color fundus photograph showing the horizontal line scan through the upper portion of the lesion located temporal to the macula. (B) Horizontal line scan through the upper portion of the lesion located temporal to the macula showing separation of the inner RPE layer from the outer RPE layer with a hyporeflective space between the two layers

Optical Coherence Tomography–4

Horizontal line scan through the inferior portion of the lesion located temporal to the macula lesion showed moderate reflectivity between the separated inner and outer RPE layers corresponding to the presence of lipofuschin (Figures 12.1.5C and D).

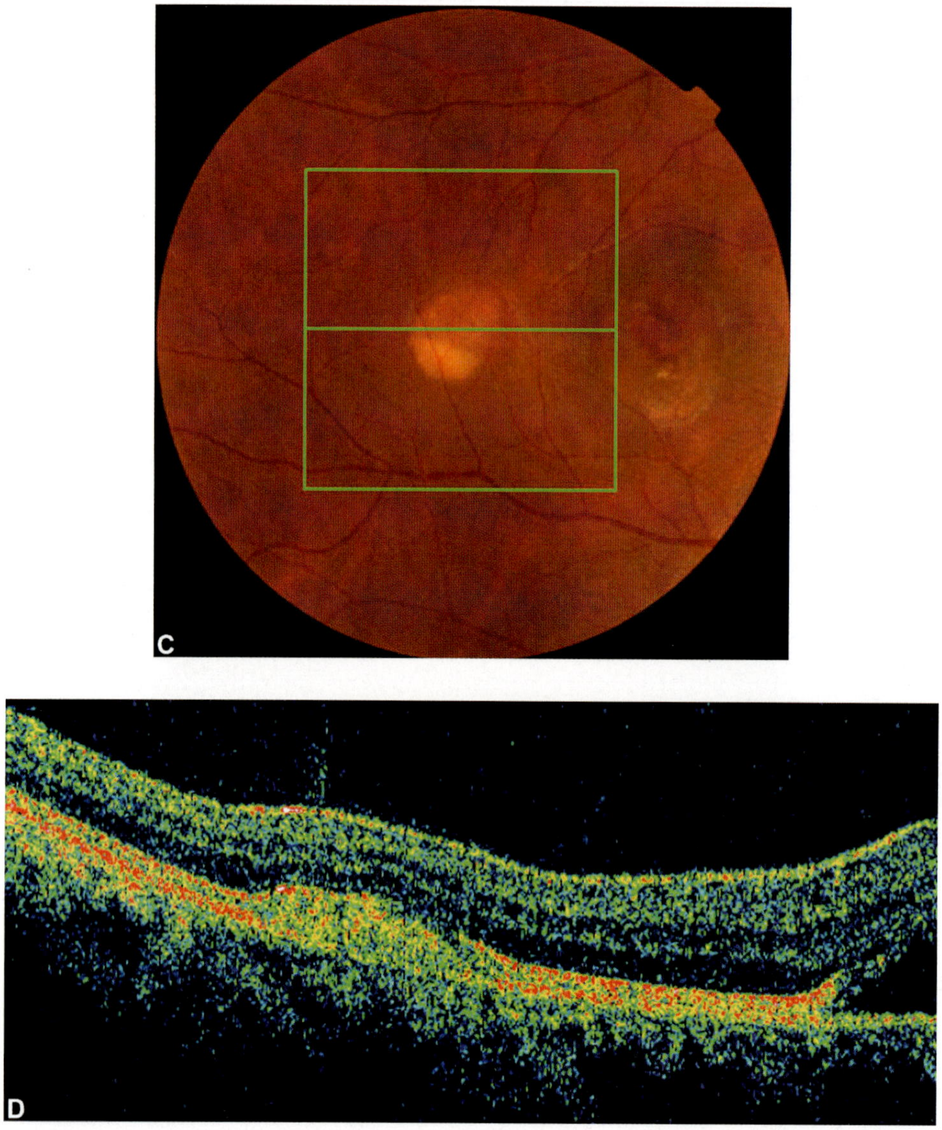

Figures 12.1.5C and D: (C) Color fundus photograph showing the horizontal line scan through the inferior portion of the lesion located temporal to the macula lesion. (D) Horizontal line scan through the inferior portion of the lesion located temporal to the macula showed moderate reflectivity between the separated inner and outer RPE layers corresponding to the presence of lipofuschin

Fluorescein angiography of the left eye showed a vitelliform lesion (Figures 12.1.6 and 12.1.7).

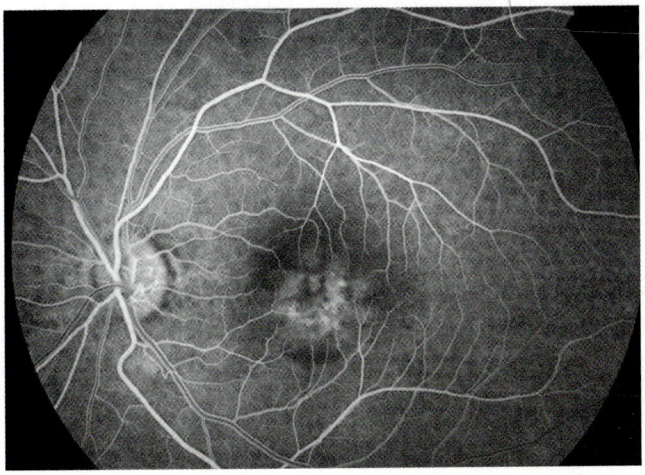

Figure 12.1.6: Early phase angiogram of the left eye shows a vitelliform lesion

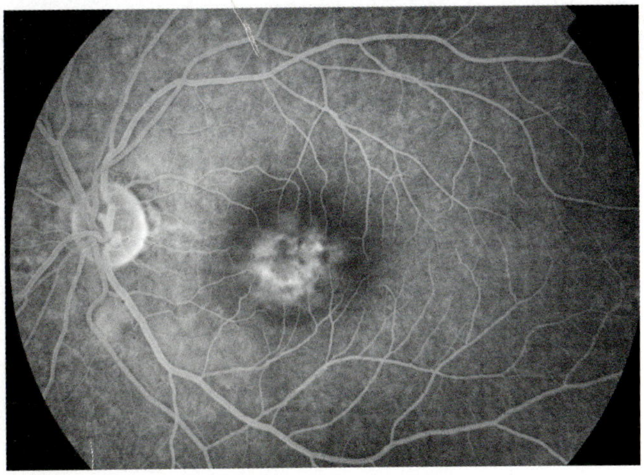

Figure 12.1.7: Late phase angiogram shows a vitelliform lesion

Optical Coherence Tomography–5

Horizontal line scan of the left eye through the fovea showed separation of the inner RPE layer from the outer RPE layer with a hyporeflective space between the two layers (Figures 12.1.8A to D).

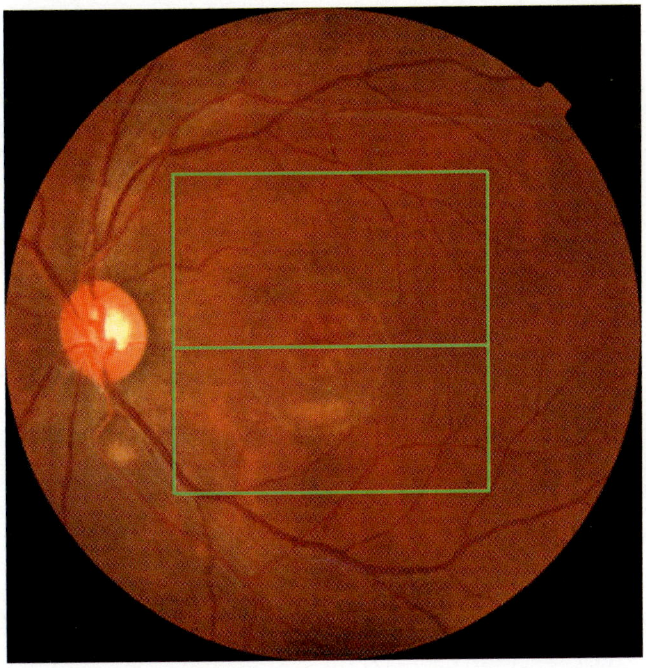

Figure 12.1.8A: Color fundus photograph showing the horizontal line scan through the fovea

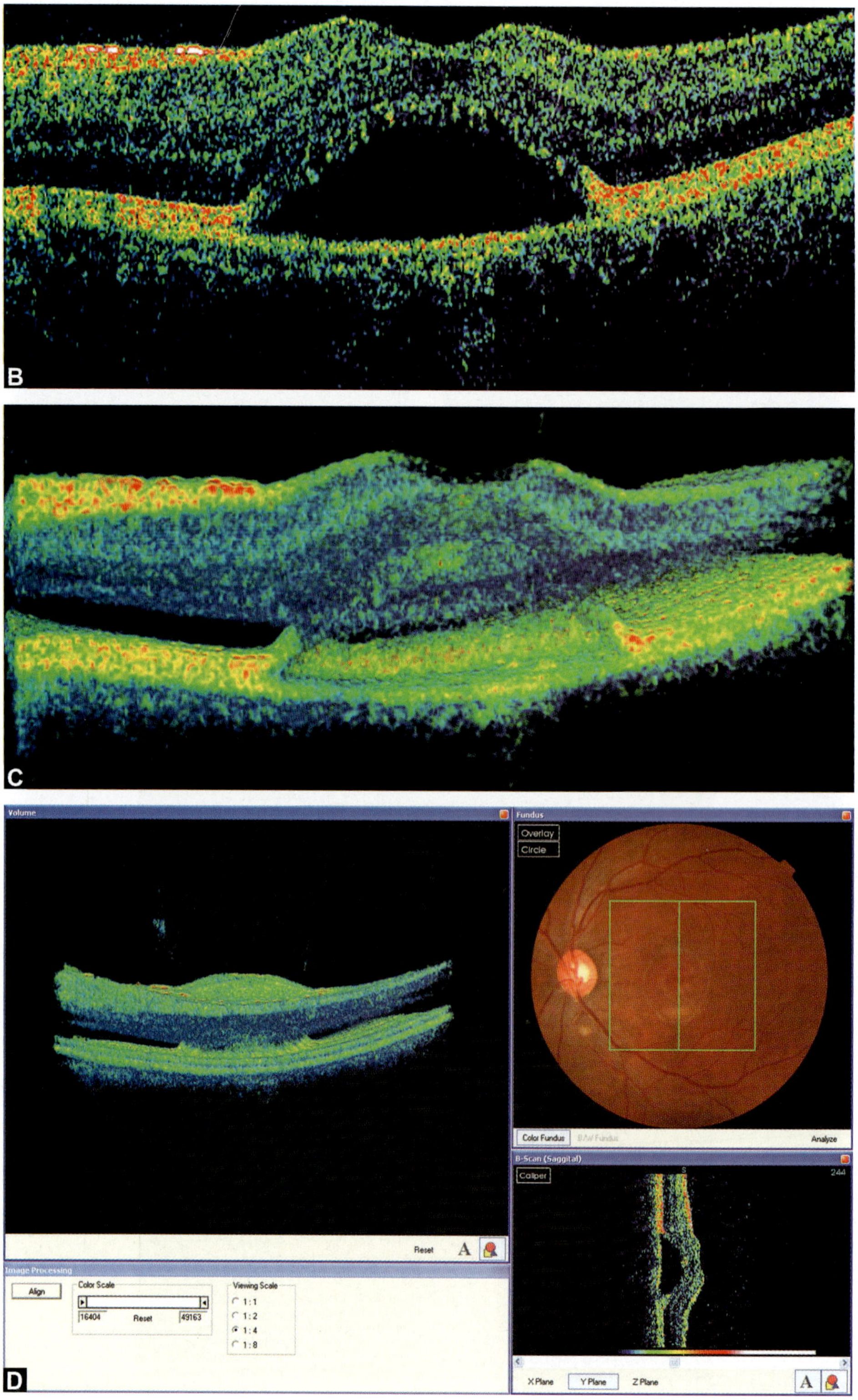

Figures 12.1.8B to D: (B) Horizontal line scan, 2D image showing separation of the inner RPE layer from the outer RPE layer with a hyporeflective space between the two layers. (C) Cropped 3D image showing separation of the inner RPE layer from the outer RPE layer with a hyporeflective space between the two layers. (D) 3D image of the left eye of Case 12.1

Optical Coherence Tomography–6

Horizontal line scan of the left eye through the inferior portion of the lesion showed moderate reflectivity between the separated inner and outer RPE layers corresponding to the presence of lipofuschin (Figures 12.1.9A and B).

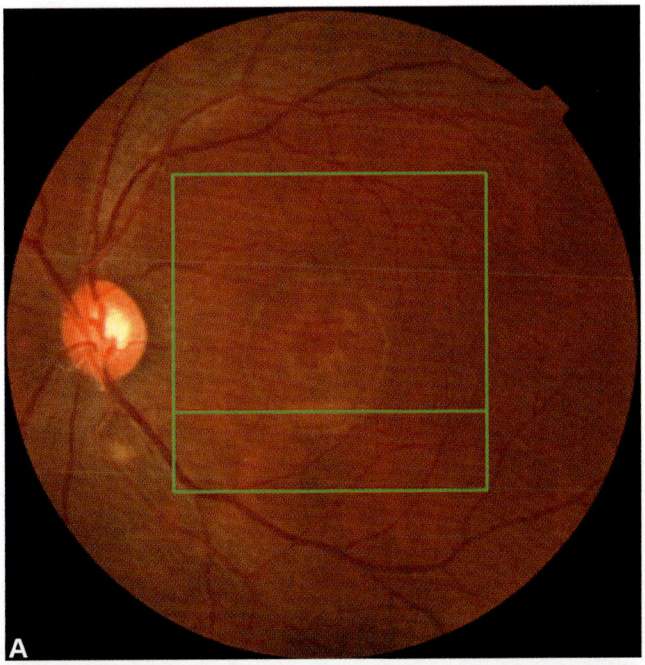

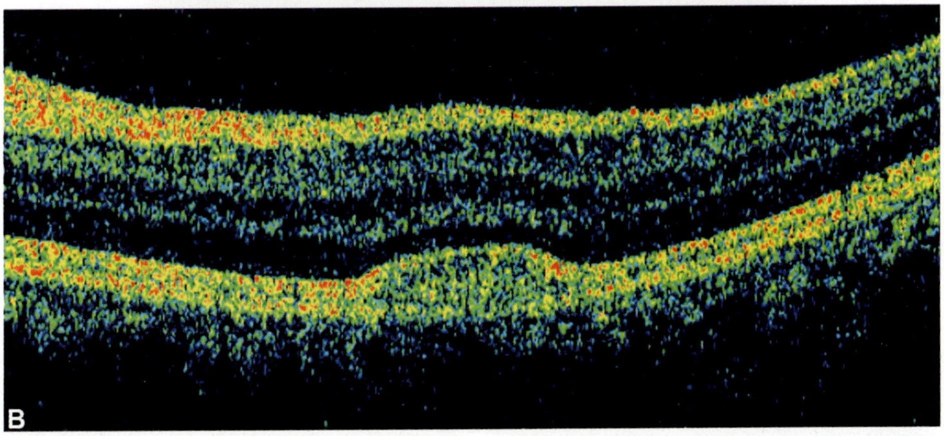

Figures 12.1.9A and B: (A) Color fundus photograph showing the horizontal line scan through the inferior portion of the lesion. (B) Horizontal line scan through the inferior portion of the lesion showing moderate reflectivity between the separated inner and outer RPE layers corresponding to the presence of lipofuschin

Stargardt's Disease

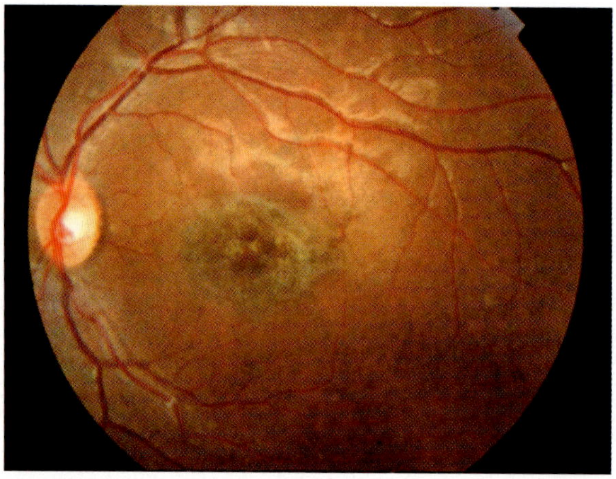

Stargardt's disease is the most prevalent inherited macular dystrophy and accounts for roughly 7 percent of all retinal dystrophies. It is usually inherited as an autosomal recessive trait; however, autosomal dominant inheritance has also been described. The hallmark of this disease is the presence of 'pisciform' flecks which are confined mostly to the posterior pole and macula and are present early in life.Geographic, atrophic RPE patches often coalesce to give the macula a 'beaten bronze' appearance.

Fluorescein Angiography

The most characteristic finding on fluorescein angiography is the phenomenon known as the 'dark' or 'silent' choroid, which appears as a prominent retinal circulation against a hypofluorescent choroid.

CASE 12.2: STARGARDT'S DISEASE

Case Summary

A 13-year-old boy presented with diminished vision in both eyes. His best-corrected visual acuity in the left eye was 6/36. Fluorescein angiography showed 'dark' choroid with a central atrophic area showing hyperfluorescence (Figures 12.2.1 and 12.2.2). The electro-retinogram was normal.

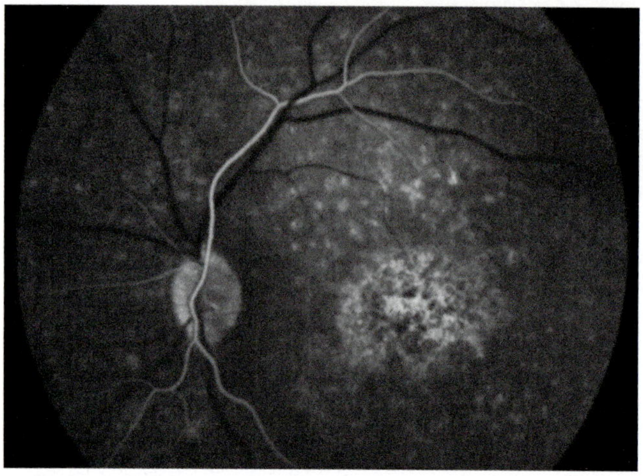

Figure 12.2.1: Early phase angiogram shows 'dark' choroid with a central atrophic area showing hyperfluorescence

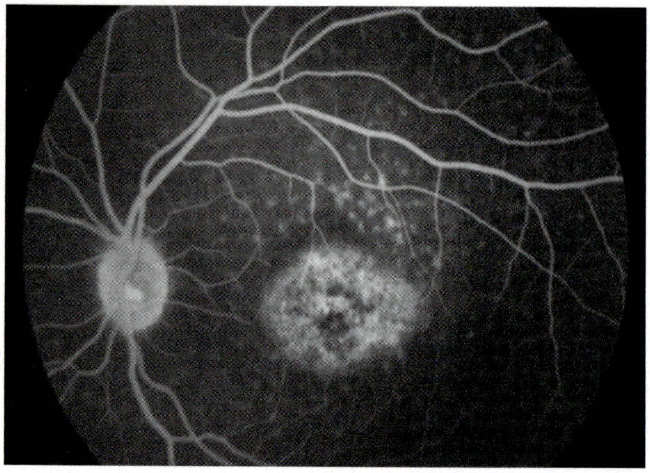

Figure 12.2.2: Late phase angiogram shows increase in the intensity of the hyperfluorescence

Optical Coherence Tomography

Horizontal line scan of the left eye showed foveal atrophy (Figures 12.2.3A to E).

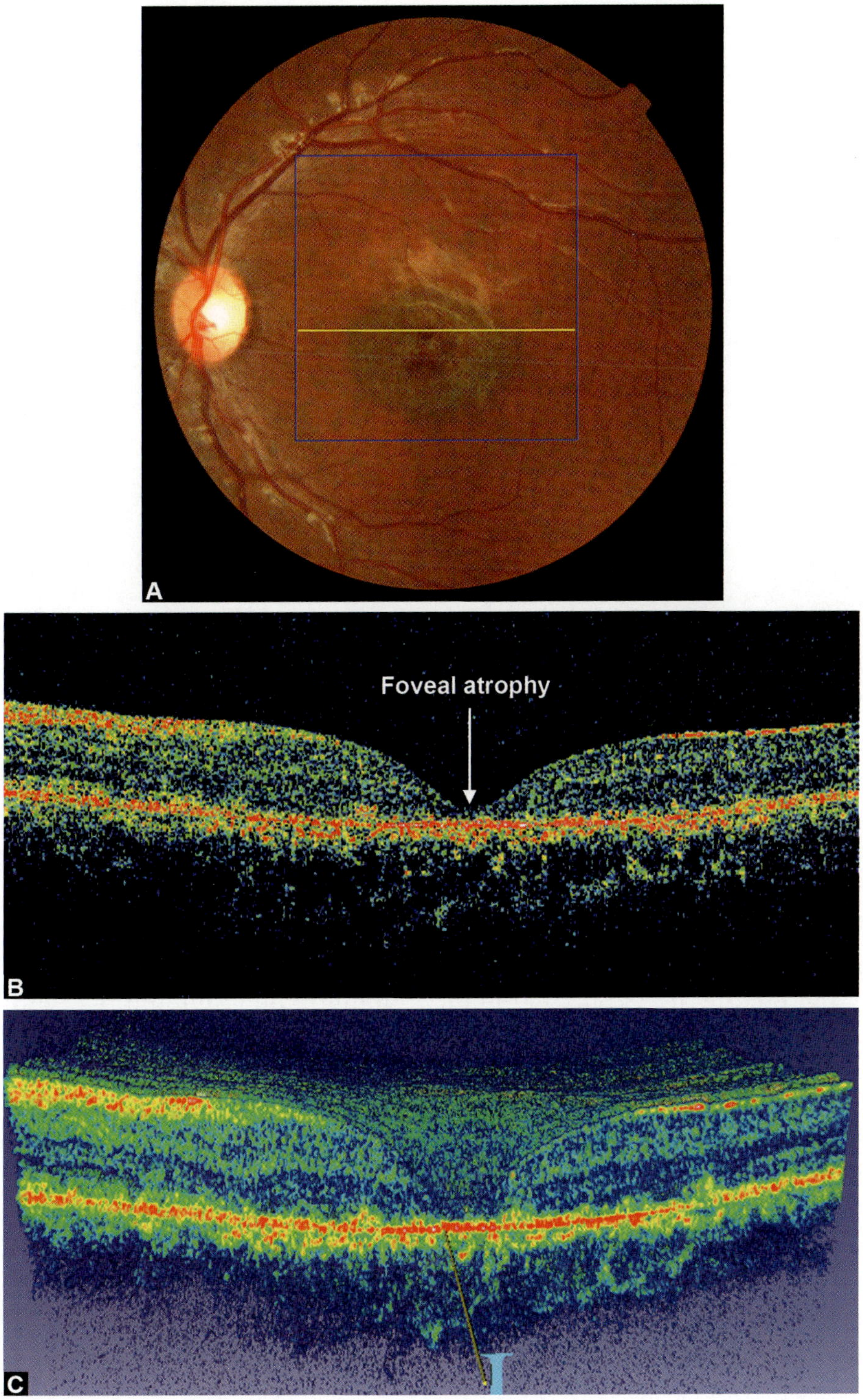

Figures 12.2.3A to C: (A) Color fundus photograph showing the horizontal line scan through the fovea. (B) Horizontal line scan, 2D image showing foveal atrophy. (C) Cropped 3D image showing foveal atrophy

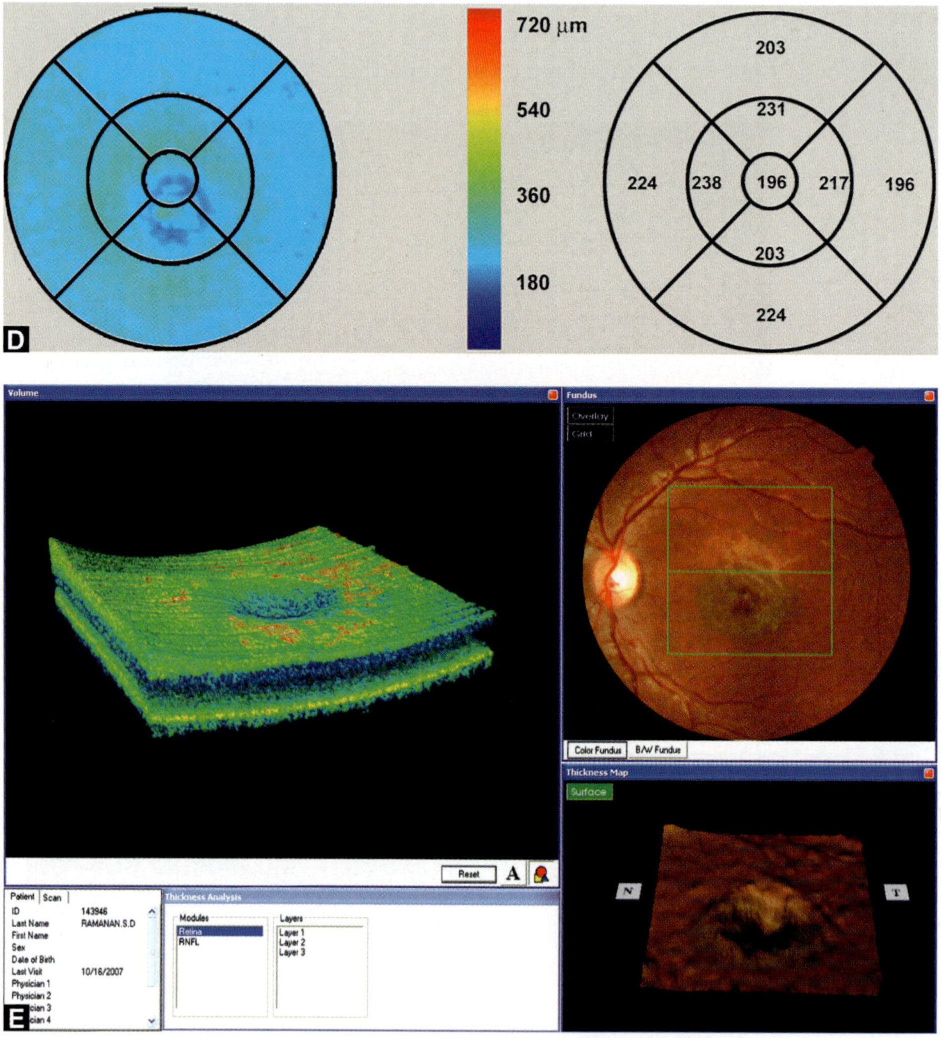

Figures 12.2.3D and E: (D) Macular thickness map showing foveal thickness measuring 196 µm. (E) 3D image of Case 12.2

Central Areolar Choroidal Dystrophy

Central areolar choroidal dystrophy is a rare autosomal dominant macular disease that has been mapped to chromosome 17p. It appears to be a primary dystrophy of either the choroidal vessels or of the pigment epithelium, with secondary involvement of the choroid.

Fluorescein angiography in the early stage of the disease shows background hyperfluorescence from RPE atrophy. When the choriocapillaris is lost, the hyperfluorescence disappears and the choroidal vessels become sharply outlined. The margins of the lesion show hyperfluorescence due to leakage from the choriocapillaris at the edges.

Optical coherence tomography shows retinal thinning with increased backscattering from the choroid.

CASE 12.3: CENTRAL AREOLAR CHOROIDAL DYSTROPHY

Case Summary

A 76-year-old woman with non-proliferative diabetic retinopathy in both eyes presented with difficulty in reading for the past 6 months. Her best-corrected visual acuity was 6/24; N24 in the right eye and 6/60; N24 in the left eye. Fluorescein angiography of the right eye showed prominent choroidal vessels in the early phase with hyperfluorescence at the margins of the lesion towards the late phase (Figures 12.3.1 and 12.3.2).

Optical Coherence Tomography–1

Horizontal line scan showed increased back scattering from under the foveal neurosensory retina with loss of normal retinal architecture. The underlying RPE-choroid complex showed increased hyper-reflectivity probably due to overlying retinal thinning (Figures 12.3.3A to D).

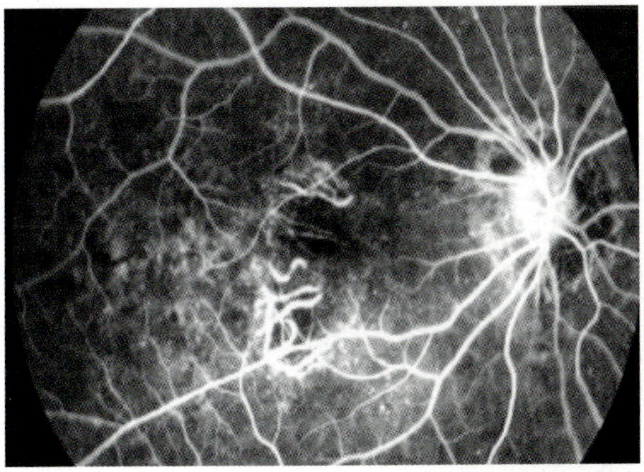

Figure 12.3.1: Early phase angiogram of the right eye shows prominent choroidal vessels

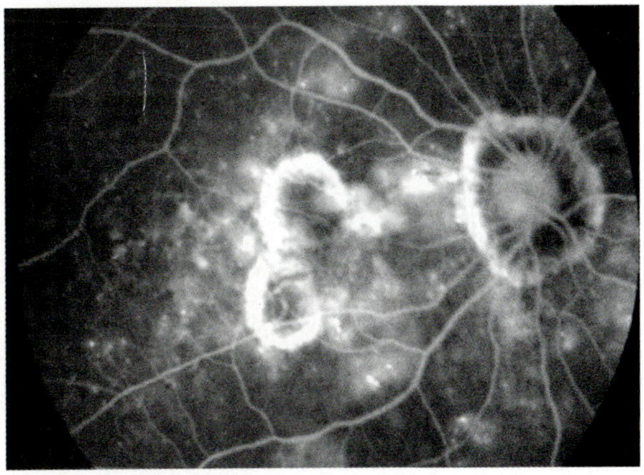

Figure 12.3.2: Late phase angiogram shows hyperfluorescence at the margins of the lesion

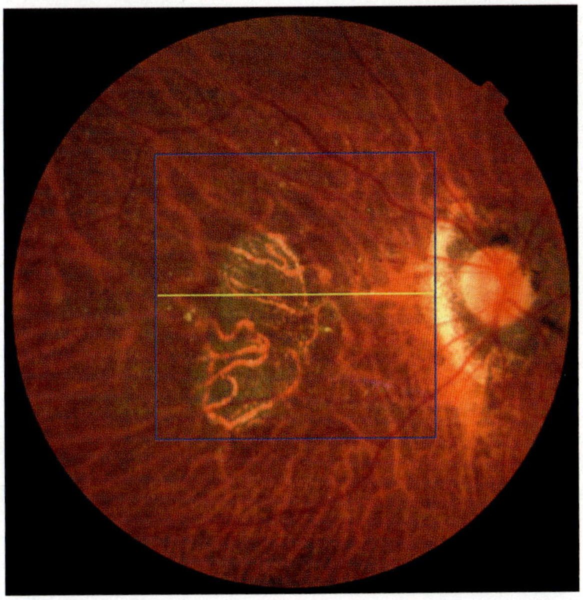

Figure 12.3.3A: Color fundus photograph showing the horizontal line scan through the fovea.

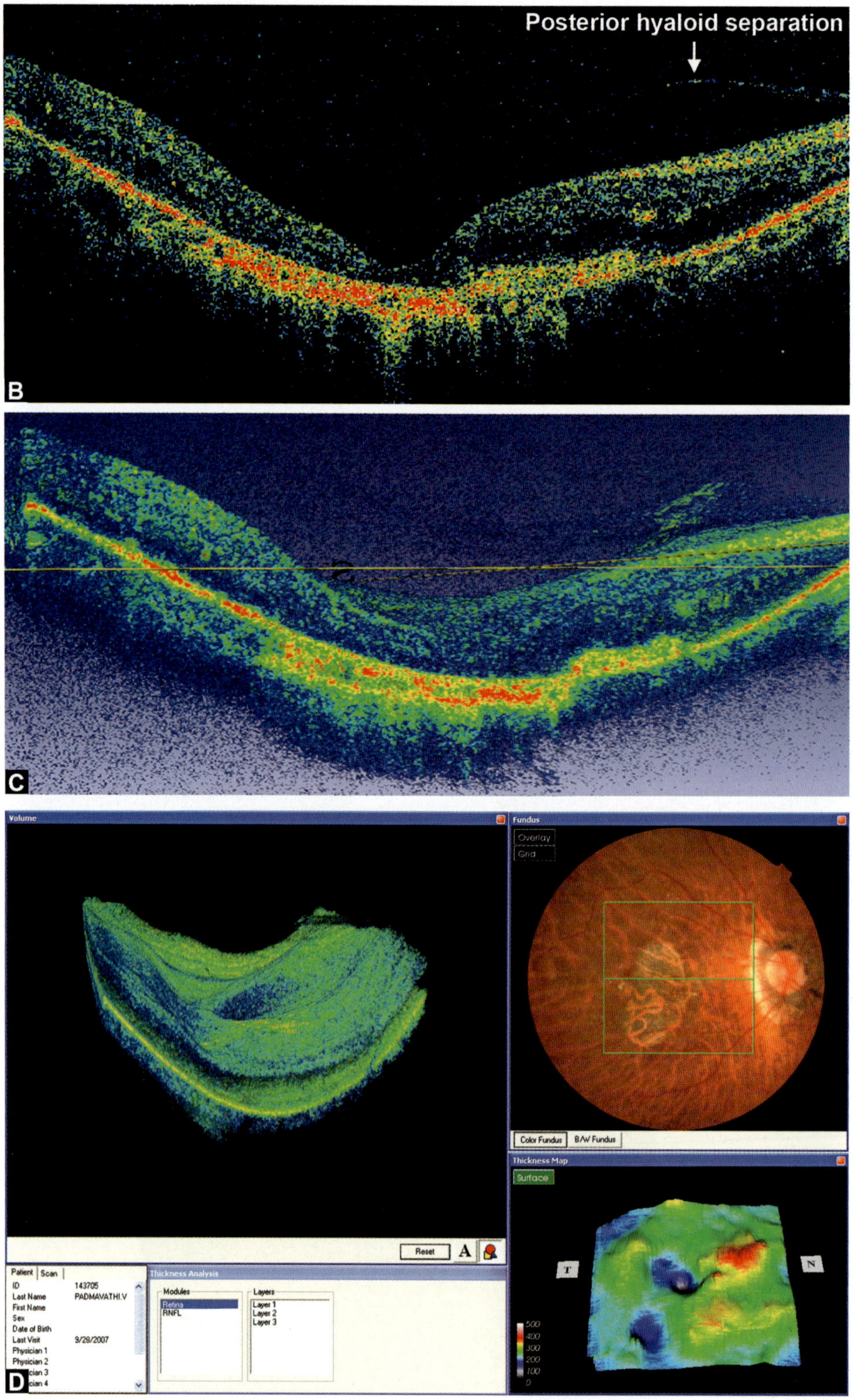

Figures 12.3.3B to D: (B) Horizontal line scan, 2D image showing increased backscattering from under the foveal neurosensory retina with loss of normal retinal architecture. The underlying RPE-choroid complex shows increased hyper-reflectivity probably due to overlying retinal thinning. (C) Cropped 3D image showing increased backscattering from under the foveal neurosensory retina with loss of normal retinal architecture. The underlying RPE-choroid complex shows increased hyper-reflectivity probably due to overlying retinal thinning. (D) 3D image of the right eye of Case 12.3

Fluorescein angiography of the left eye also showed larger choroidal vessels within the area of RPE atrophy with hyperfluorescence at the margins of the lesion in the late phase (Figures 12.3.4 and 12.3.5)

Optical Coherence Tomography–2

Horizontal line scan of the left eye showed retinal thinning with increased back scattering and increased hyper-reflectivity of the underlying RPE-choroid complex (Figures 12.3.6A to D).

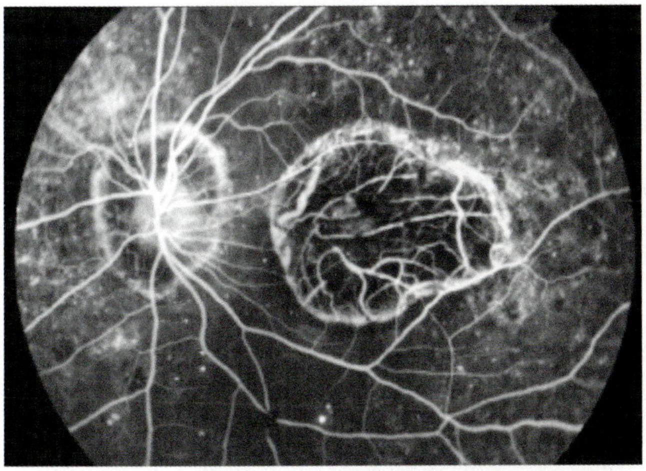

Figure 12.3.4: Early phase angiogram of the left eye shows larger choroidal vessels within the area of RPE atrophy

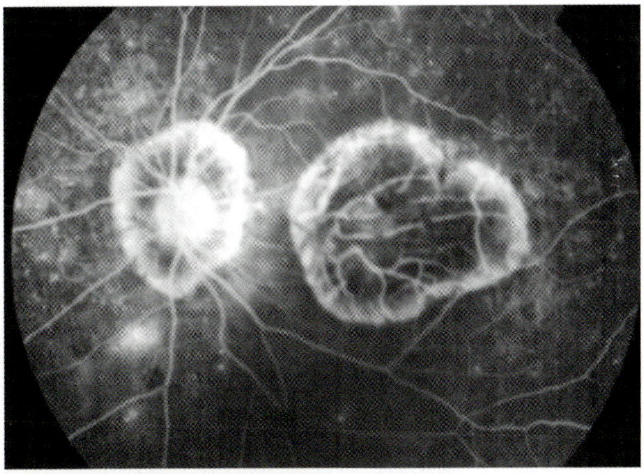

Figure 12.3.5: Late phase angiogram shows hyperfluorescence at the margins of the lesion

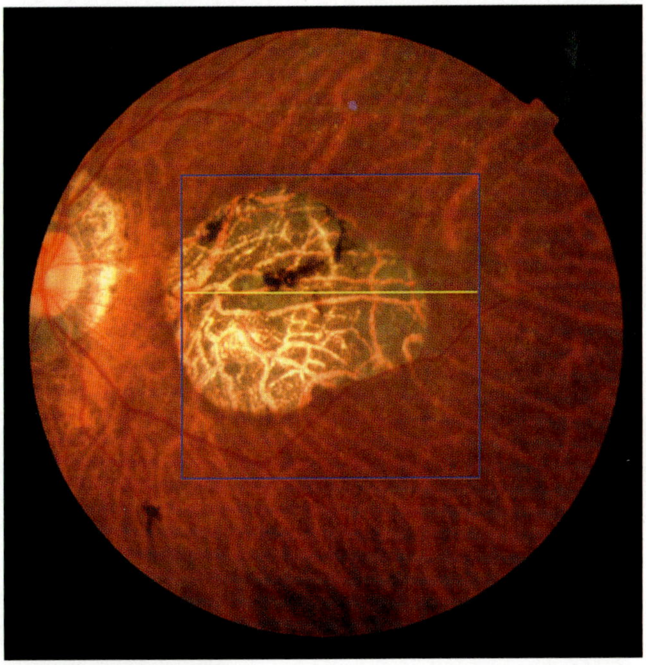

Figure 12.3.6A: Color fundus photograph showing the horizontal line scan through the fovea

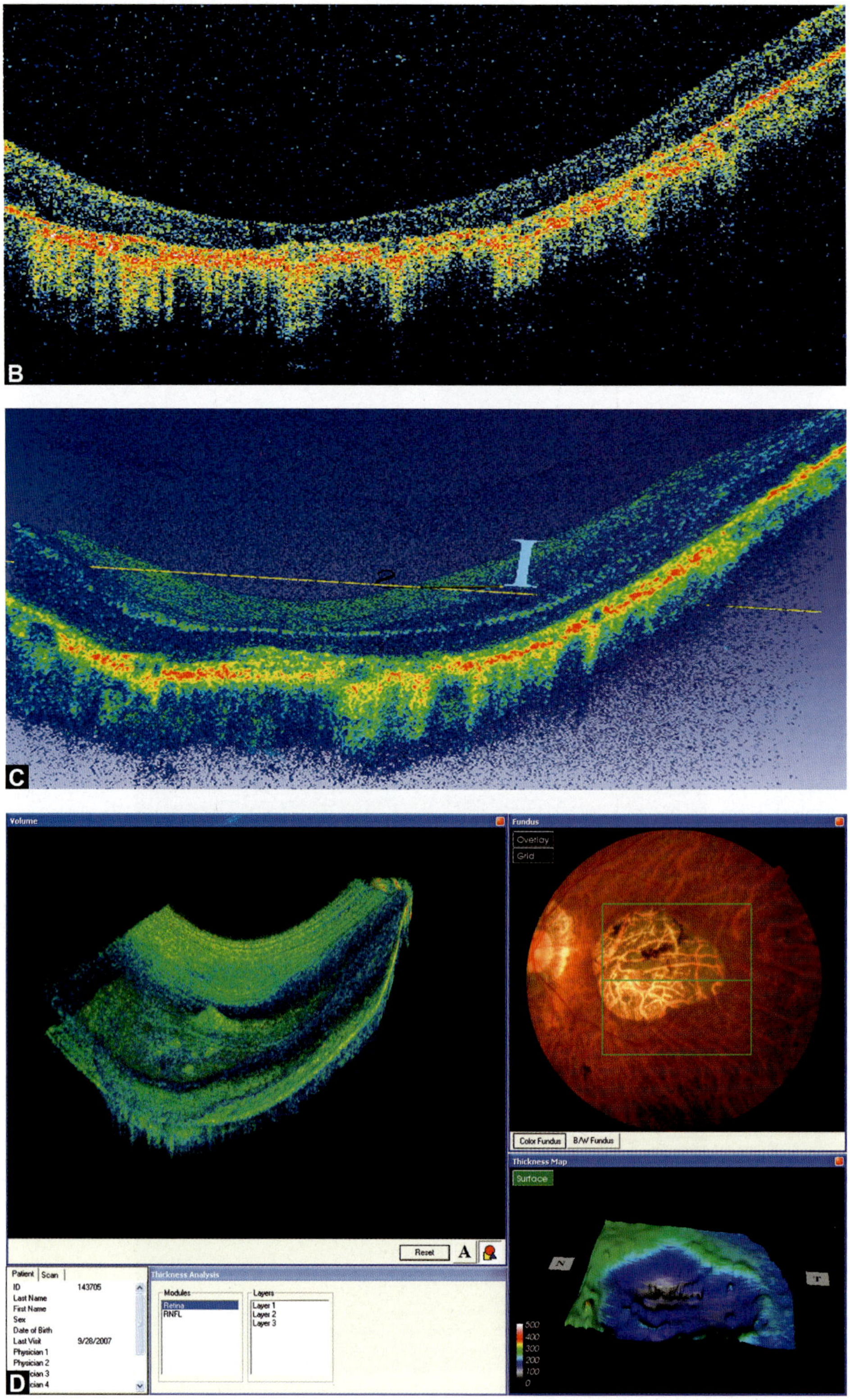

Figures 12.3.6B to D: (B) Horizontal line scan, 2D image showing retinal thinning with increased backscattering and increased hyper-reflectivity of the underlying RPE-choroid complex. (C) Cropped 3D image showing retinal thinning with increased backscattering and increased hyper-reflectivity of the underlying RPE-choroid complex. (D) 3D image of the left eye of Case 12.3

Progressive Cone Dystrophy

Progressive cone dystrophy is inherited either as an autosomal dominant or X- linked disorder, however, sporadic cases can also occur. It usually presents between the first and third decades of life with photoaversion, progressive loss of visual acuity, day blindness and impaired color vision.

CASE 12.4: PROGRESSIVE CONE DYSTROPHY

Case Summary

A 29-year-old male presented with diminished vision in both eyes of one year duration. His best corrected visual acuity in the right eye was 6/18. and left eye was 6/12. There was total loss of color vision in both eyes. The electroretinogram showed reduced cone responses. Fluorescein angiography showed bull's eye pattern of RPE atrophy with ring shaped area of stippled hyperfluorescence (Figures 12.4.1 and 12.4.2).

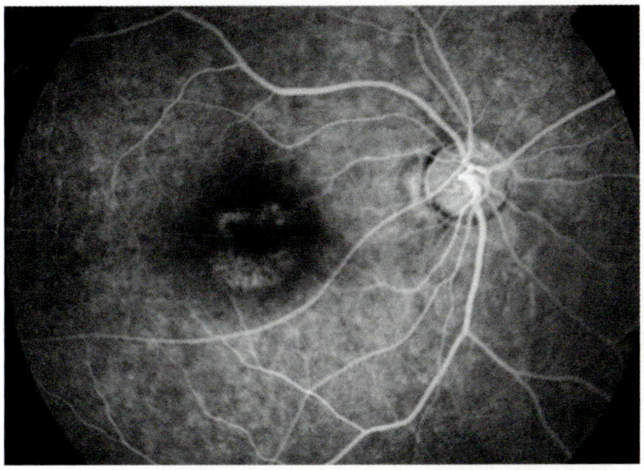

Figure 12.4.1: Early phase angiogram of the right eye shows bull's eye pattern of RPE atrophy with ring shaped area of stippled hyperfluorescence

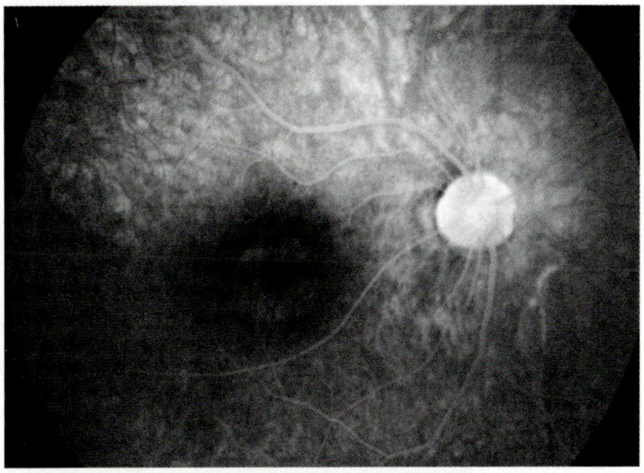

Figure 12.4.2: Late phase angiogram shows bull's eye pattern of RPE atrophy with ring shaped area of stippled hyperfluorescence

Optical Coherence Tomography–1

Horizontal line scan showed retinal thinning. The underlying RPE-choroid complex showed increased hyper-reflectivity probably due to overlying thinning of the retina (Figures 12.4.3A to D).

His best-corrected visual acuity in the left eye was 6/12. Fluorescein angiography showed bull's eye pattern of RPE atrophy with ring shaped area of stippled hyperfluorescence (Figures 12.4.4 and 12.4.5).

Optical Coherence Tomography–2

Horizontal line scan showed retinal thinning with irregularity of the retinal pigment layer. The underlying RPE-choroid complex showed increased hyper-reflectivity probably due to overlying thinning of the retina (Figures 12.4.6A to D).

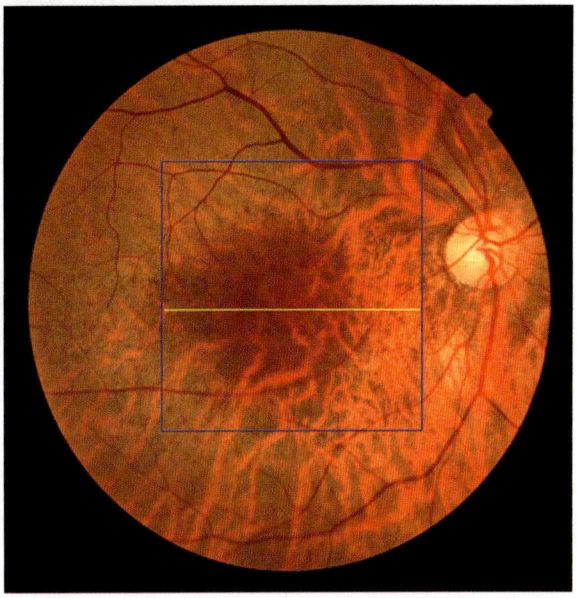

Figure 12.4.3A: Color fundus photograph showing the horizontal line scan through the fovea

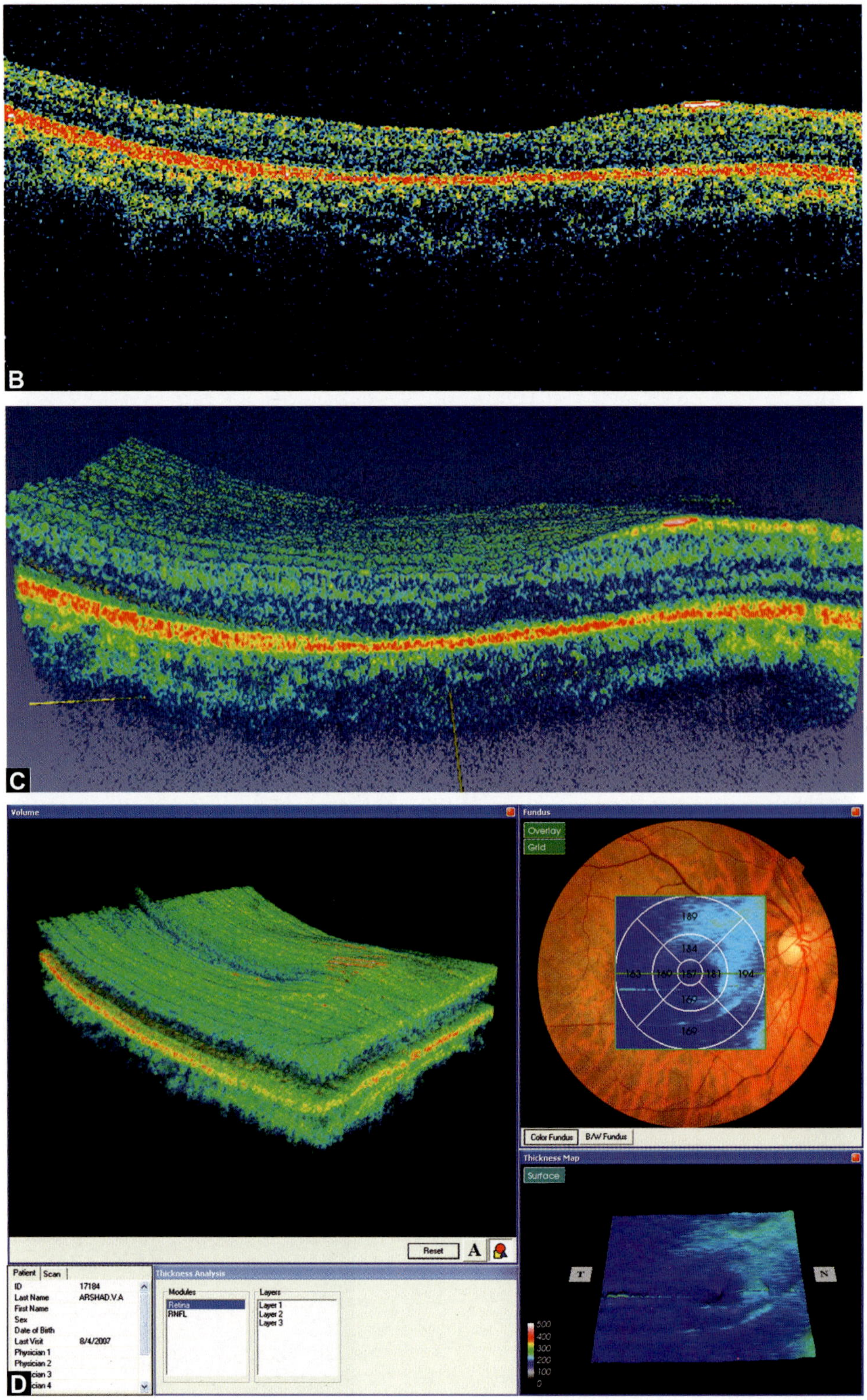

Figures 12.4.3B to D: (B) Horizontal line scan, 2D image showing retinal thinning. The underlying RPE-choroid complex shows increased hyper-reflectivity probably due to overlying thinning of the retina. (C) Cropped 3D image showing retinal thinning. The underlying RPE-choroid complex shows increased hyper-reflectivity probably due to overlying thinning of the retina. (D) 3D image of the right eye of Case 12.4

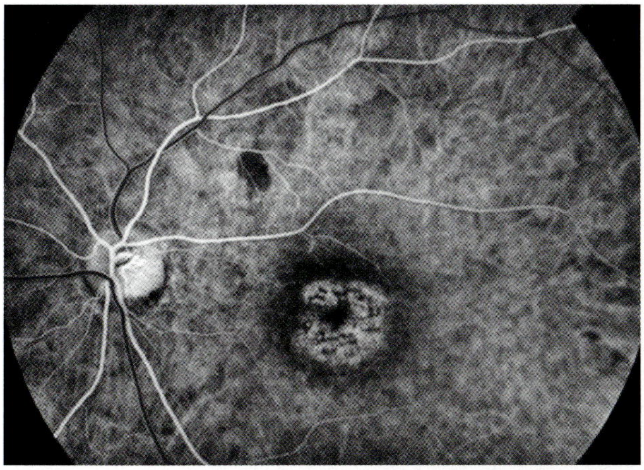

Figure 12.4.4: Early phase angiogram of the left eye shows bull's eye pattern of RPE atrophy with ring shaped area of stippled hyperfluorescence

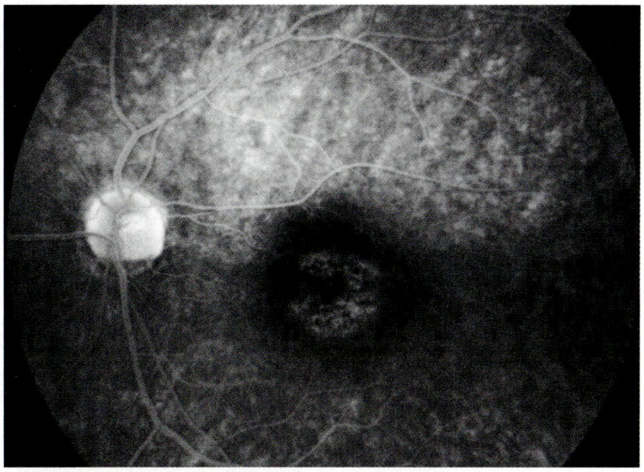

Figure 12.4.5: Late phase angiogram shows bull's eye pattern of RPE atrophy with ring shaped area of stippled hyperfluorescence

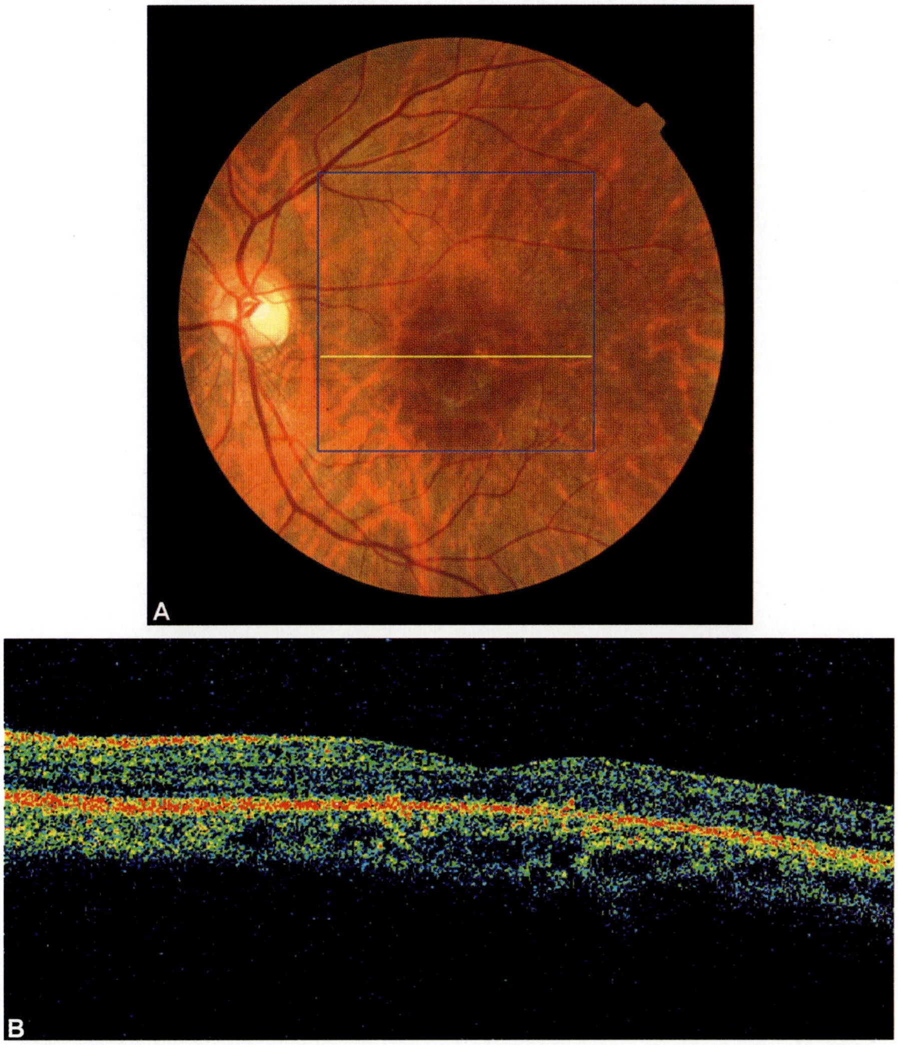

Figures 12 4.6A and B: (A) Color fundus photograph showing the horizontal line scan through the fovea. (B) Horizontal line scan, 2D image showing retinal thinning with irregularity of the retinal pigment layer. The underlying RPE-choroid complex shows increased hyper-reflectivity probably due to overlying thinning of the retina

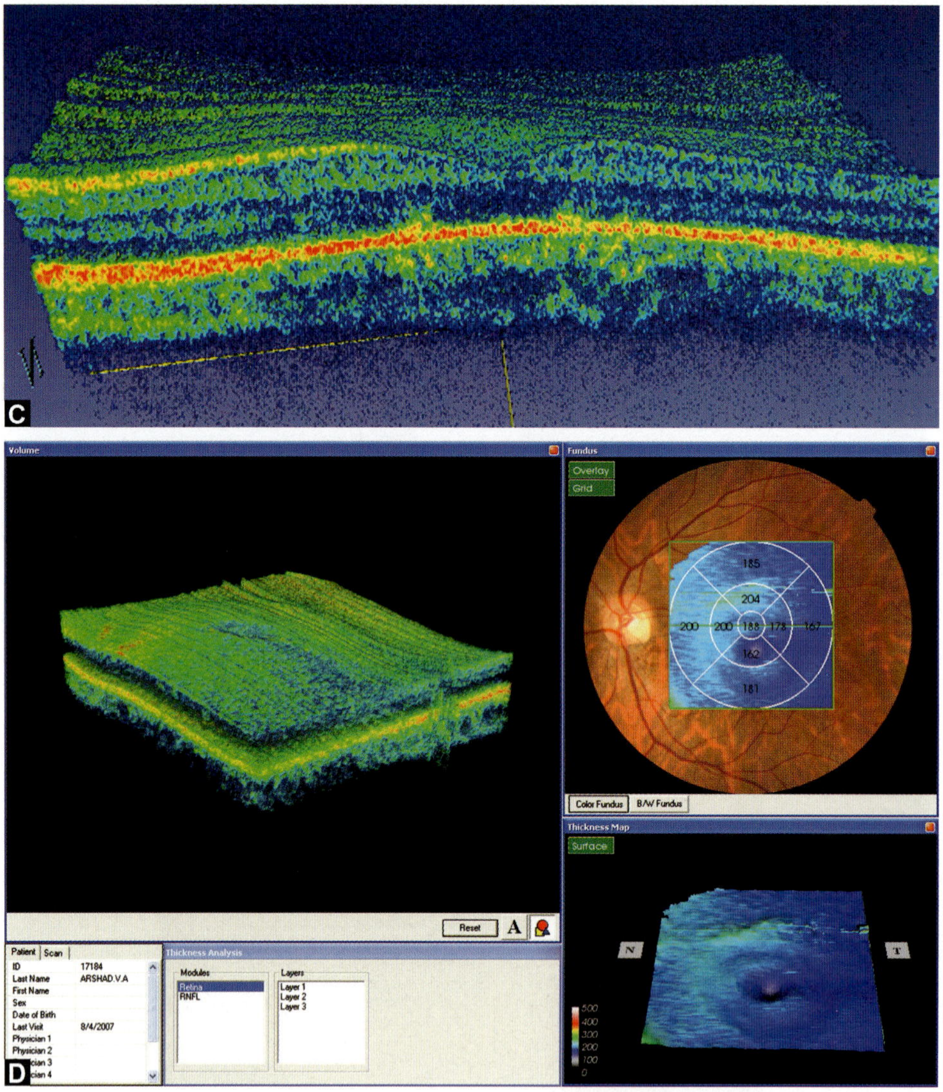

Figures 12 4.6C and D: (C) Cropped 3D image showing retinal thinning with irregularity of the retinal pigment layer. The underlying RPE-choroid complex shows increased hyper-reflectivity probably due to overlying thinning of the retina. (D) 3D image of the left eye of Case 12.4

JUVENILE RETINOSCHISIS

X-linked juvenile retinoschisis is caused by the gene XLRS1 located on band Xp22. XLRS1 encodes a 224 amino acid protein retinoschisin that is expressed in photoreceptor and bipolar cells. Retinoschisin is a secreted protein that is involved in cellular adhesion and cell-cell interactions within the inner nuclear layer as well as synaptic connection between photoreceptors and bipolar cells. Defective or absent retinoschisin may reduce adhesion of the retinal layers, resulting in the creation of schisis cavities

Cystic-like stellate maculopathy or foveal schisis is present almost universally in X-linked juvenile retinoschisis

Fluorescein angiography can help differentiate foveal schisis cavity from cystoid macular edema. In XJR, the angiographic results are normal, whereas in cystoid macular edema, late hyperfluorescence in a petalloid pattern is seen.

Optical coherence tomography reveals cystic spaces primarily in the inner nuclear and outer plexiform layers of the retina arranged in a pallisade fashion. In cystoid macular edema, the cysts are arranged in a petalloid pattern.

CASE 12.5: JUVENILE RETINOSCHISIS

Case Summary

A 9-year-old boy presented with defective vision in both eyes of 3 months duration. His best-corrected visual acuity in the right eye was 6/36;N18

Optical Coherence Tomography–1

Horizontal line scan showed cystic spaces arranged in a pallisade fashion in the inner nuclear layer (Figures 12.5.1A to D)

His best-corrected visual acuity in the left eye was 6/60;N18.

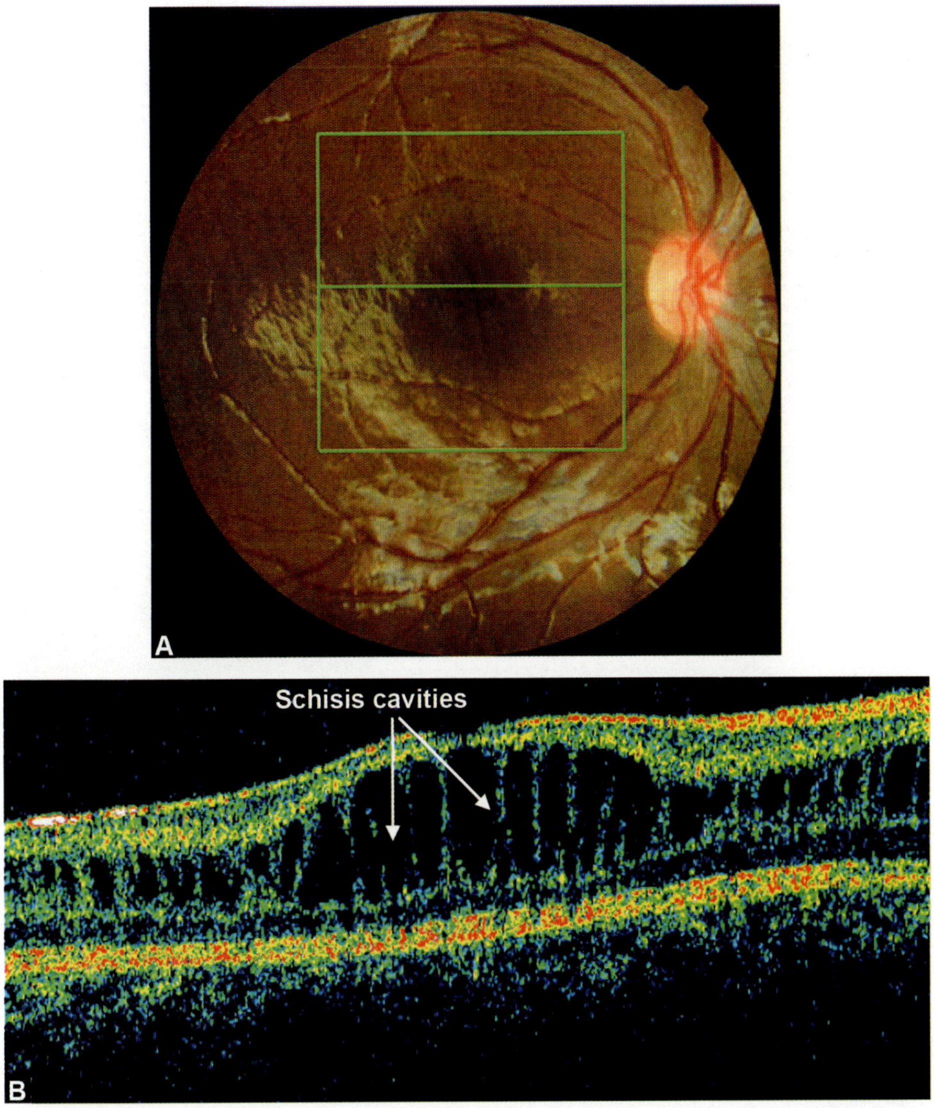

Figures 12.5.1A and B: (A) Color fundus photograph of the right eye showing the horizontal line scan through the fovea. (B) Horizontal line scan, 2D image showing cystic spaces arranged in a pallisade fashion in the inner nuclear layer

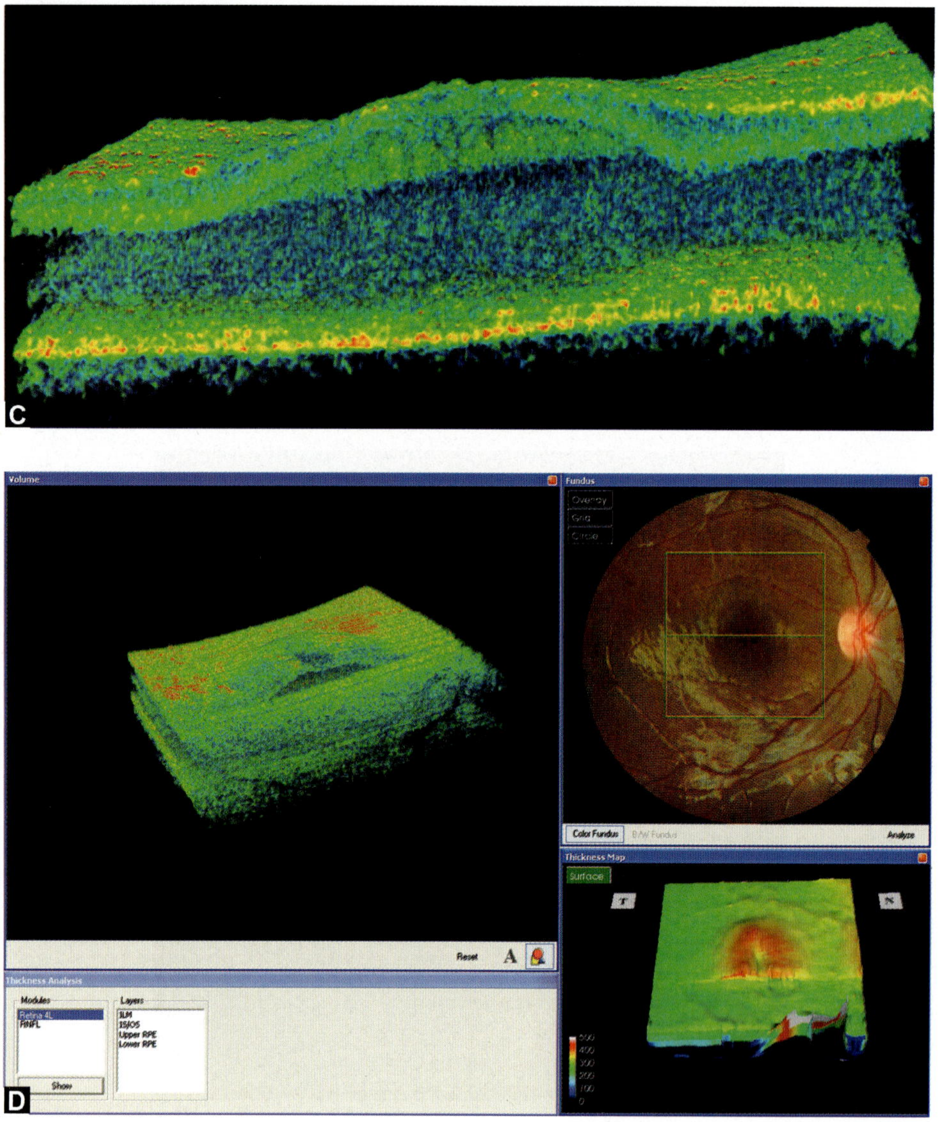

Figures 12.5.1C and D: (C) Cropped 3D image showing cystic spaces arranged in a pallisade fashion in the inner nuclear layer. (D) 3D image of the right eye of Case 12.5

Optical Coherence Tomography–2

Horizontal line scan showed cystic spaces arranged in a pallisade fashion in the inner nuclear layer (Figures 12.5.2A to D)

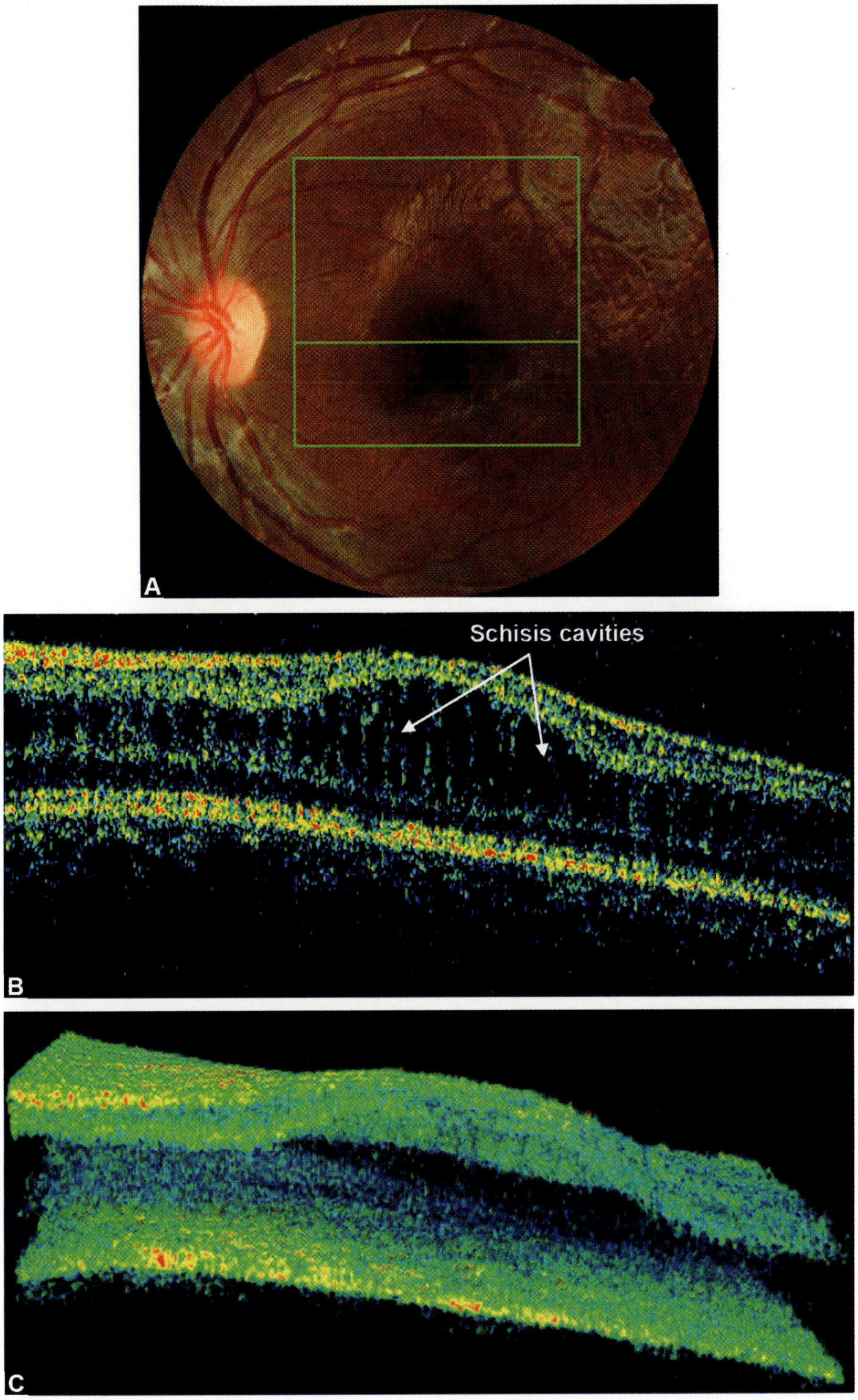

Figures 12.5.2 A to C: (A) Color fundus photograph of the left eye showing the horizontal line scan through the fovea. (B) Horizontal line scan, 2D image showing cystic spaces arranged in a pallisade fashion in the inner nuclear layer. (C) Cropped 3D image showing cystic spaces arranged in a pallisade fashion in the inner nuclear layer

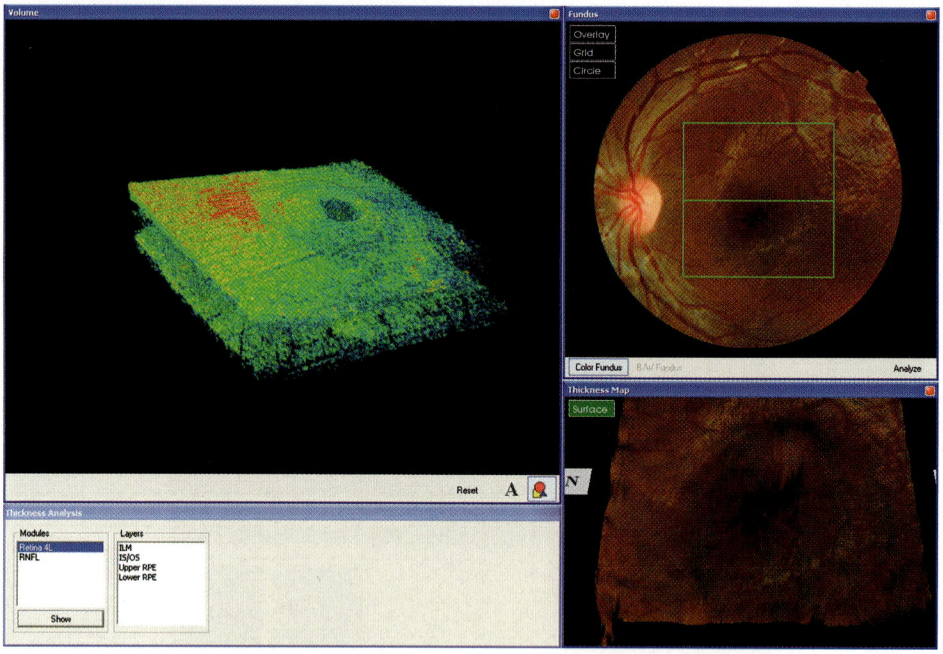

Figure 12.5.2D: 3D image of the left eye of Case 12.5

CONCLUSIONS

1. OCT reveals the location of the cystic spaces which are primarily in the inner nuclear and outer plexiform layers of the retina.
2. It helps to distinguish schisis from retinal detachment.

SUGGESTED READING

1. Chan WM, Choy KW, Wang J, et al. Clin Experiment Ophthalmol. 2004 Aug;32(4):429-32.
2. Gao H, Kusumi R, and Yung C. Optical Coherence Tomography Findings in X-linked Juvenile Retinoschisis. Invest Ophthalmol Vis Sci 2004;45: E-Abstract 3527© 2004 ARVO.

13 Inflammatory Diseases of Retina and Choroid

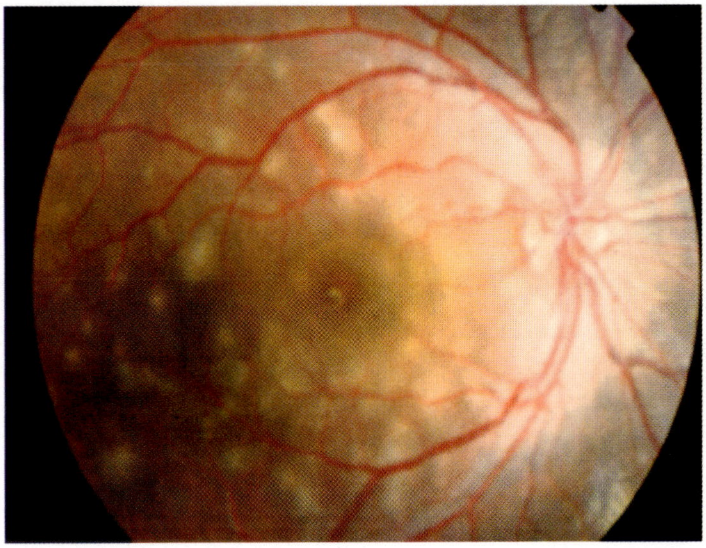

ACUTE POSTERIOR MULTIFOCAL PLACOID PIGMENT EPITHELIOPATHY

Acute posterior multifocal placoid pigment epitheliopathy (APMPPE) is an acquired inflammatory disorder affecting the retina, retinal pigment epithelium, and choroid of otherwise young healthy adults. The disease is self-limiting and is characterized by multiple yellowish white placoid subretinal lesions at the posterior pole. The lesions are frequently bilateral and in various stages of evolution, typically resolving in weeks to months and leaving circumscribed areas of retinal pigment epithelial disturbance.

Fluorescein angiography: The early lesions show a characteristic early hypofluorescence followed by hyperfluorescence in the late phases.The older lesions may show RPE window defects.

Indocyanine green angiography shows numerous round hypofluorescent choroidal defects in which the larger choroidal vessels can be seen.

Optical coherence tomography: In the acute phase, the OCT reveals a mild hyper-reflective area superficial to the RPE and, in the later phases, a nodular hyper-reflective lesion in the plane of the RPE. Rarely a serous retinal detachment is found.

CASE 13.1: ACUTE POSTERIOR MULTIFOCAL PLACOID PIGMENT EPITHELIOPATHY

Case Summary

A 22-year-old male presented with decreased vision in the right eye of two days duration. His best-corrected visual acuity in this eye was 6/18. Fluorescein angiography showed early hypofluorescence with late hyperfluorescence of the lesions (Figures 13.1.1 and 13.1.2).

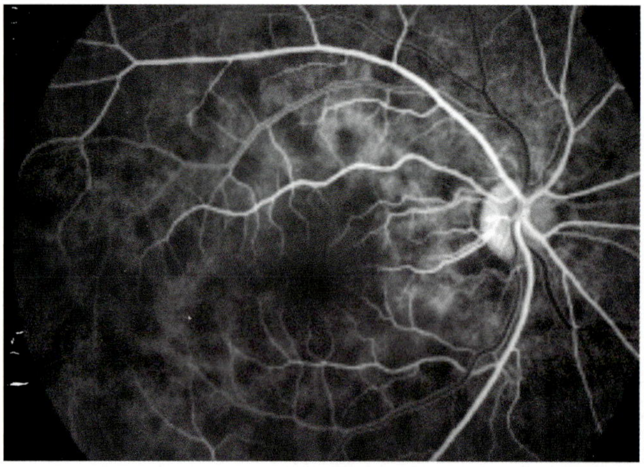

Figure 13.1.1: Early phase angiogram shows hypofluorescence of the lesions

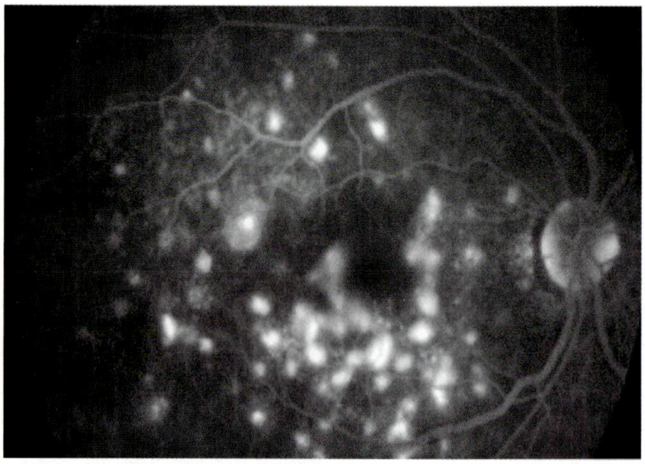

Figure 13.1.2: Late phase angiogram shows hyperfluorescence of the lesions

Optical Coherence Tomography

Horizontal line scan showed loss of foveal contour, central macular thickening and a hypo-reflective space in the subfoveal region consistent with serous retinal detachment (Figures 13.1.3A to E).

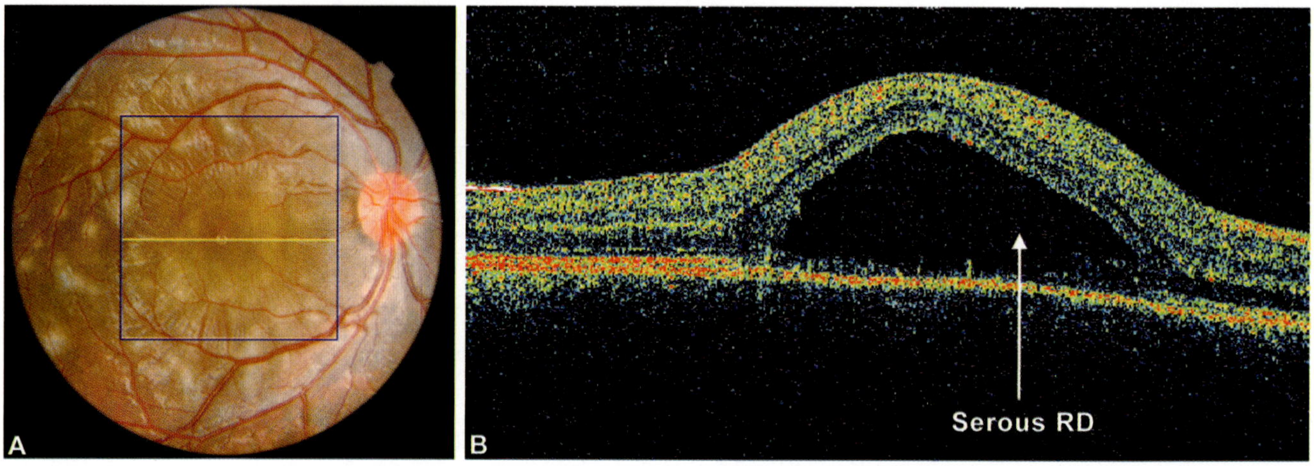

Figures 13.1.3A and B: (A) Color fundus photograph shows horizontal line scan through the fovea. (B) Horizontal line scan through the fovea 2D image showing loss of foveal contour, central macular thickening and a hyporeflective space in the subfoveal region consistent with serous retinal detachment

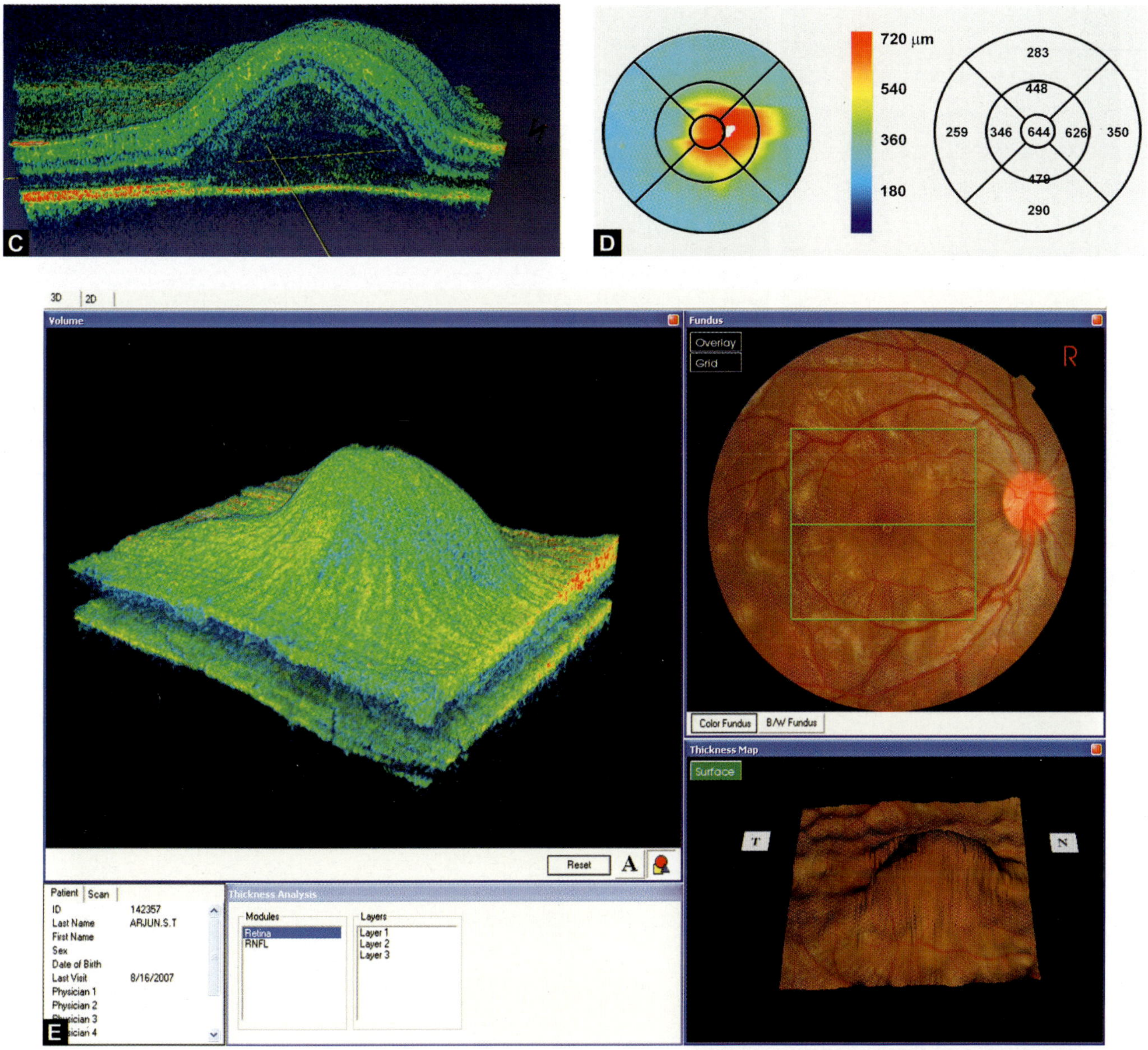

Figures 13.1.3C to E: (C) Cropped 3D image showing loss of foveal contour, central macular thickening and a hyporeflective space in the subfoveal region consistent with serous retinal detachment. (D) Macular thickness map showing foveal thickness measuring 644 µm. (E) 3D image of Case 13.1

The patient was treated with oral steroids and on follow-up 45 days later, the OCT showed resolution of the serous detachment with restoration of the normal foveal contour. The best-corrected visual acuity was 6/6 (Figures 13.1.4A to E).

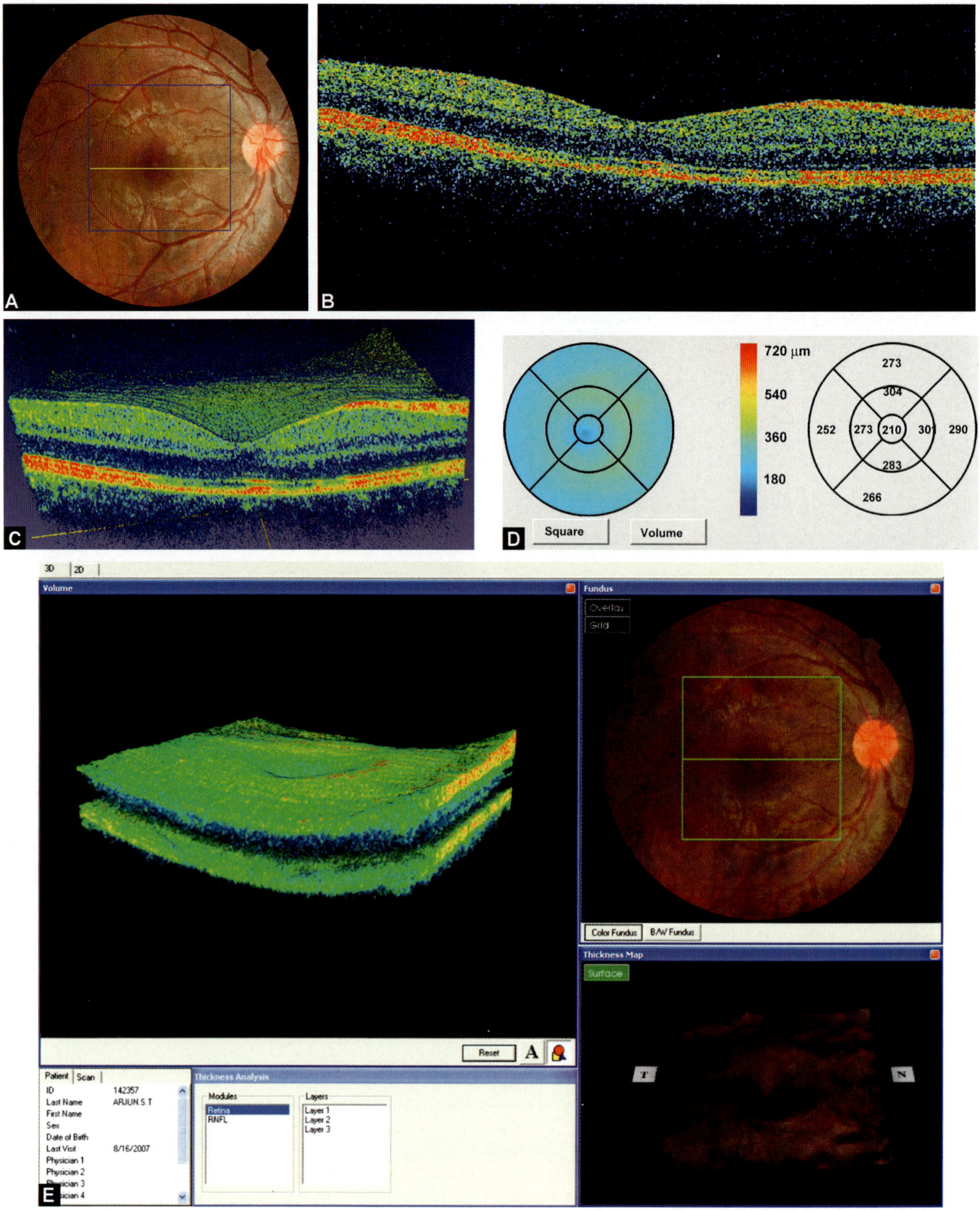

Figures 13.1.4A to E: (A) Color fundus photograph following oral steroids shows horizontal line scan through the fovea. (B) Horizontal line scan through the fovea 2D image showing resolution of the serous detachment with restoration of the normal foveal contour. (C) Cropped 3D image showing resolution of the serous detachment with restoration of the normal foveal contour. (D) Macular thickness map showing foveal thickness measuring 210 μm. (E) 3D image of Case 13.1 following oral steroids

Congenital Toxoplasmosis

Toxoplasmosis is transmitted to the fetus *in utero*. The retinal involvement is part of a generalized infection and is characterized by the presence of a large, atrophic excavated scar in the macula or elsewhere. Most cases are subclinical.

CASE 13.2: CONGENITAL TOXOPLASMOSIS

Case Summary

A 13-year-old boy seen for a routine eye check-up had bilateral healed chorioretinal scars. The scar showed three zones:

1. Outer white zone
2. Intermediate zone with pigmentary hyperplasia
3. Central zone of atrophy

Optical Coherence Tomography–1

Horizontal line scan passing through the superior margin of the scar showed increased hyper-reflectivity from the underlying retinal pigment epithelium and choroid with intact overlying neurosensory retina (Figures 13.2.1A to C).

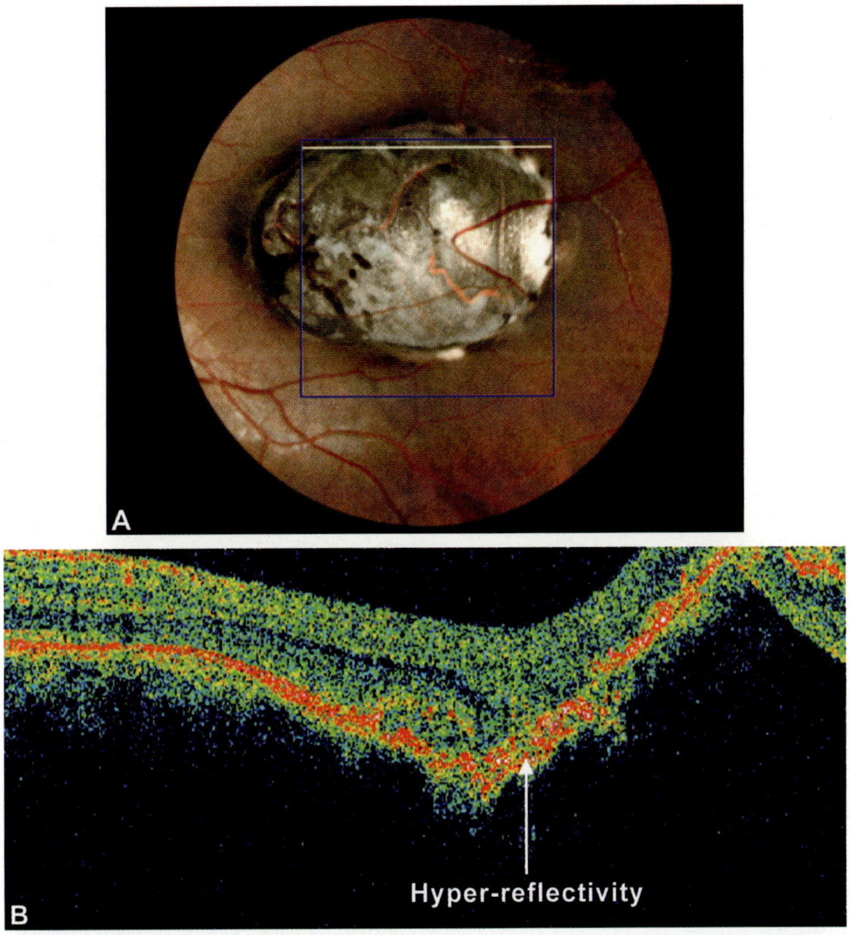

Figures 13.2.1A and B: (A) Color fundus photograph shows horizontal line scan through the superior margin of the scar. (B) Horizontal line scan through the superior margin of the scar 2D image showing increased hyper-reflectivity from the underlying retinal pigment epithelium and choroid with intact overlying neurosensory retina

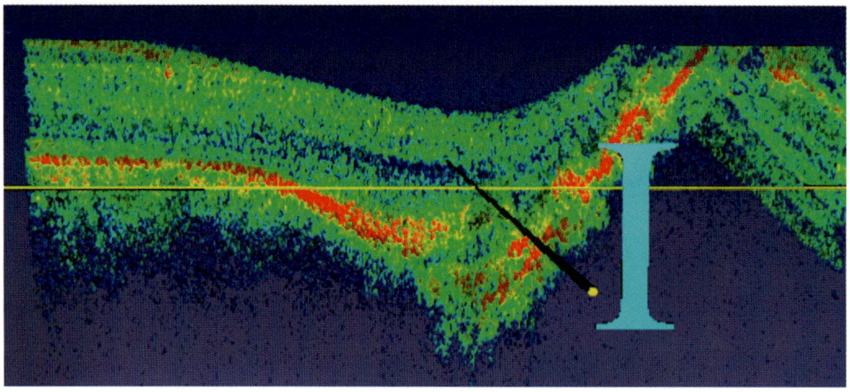

Figure 13.2.1C: Cropped 3D image showing increased hyper-reflectivity from the underlying retinal pigment epithelium and choroid with intact overlying neurosensory retina

Optical Coherence Tomography–2

Horizontal line scan passing through the intermediate zone showed atrophy of the neurosensory retina (Figures 13.2.2A to C).

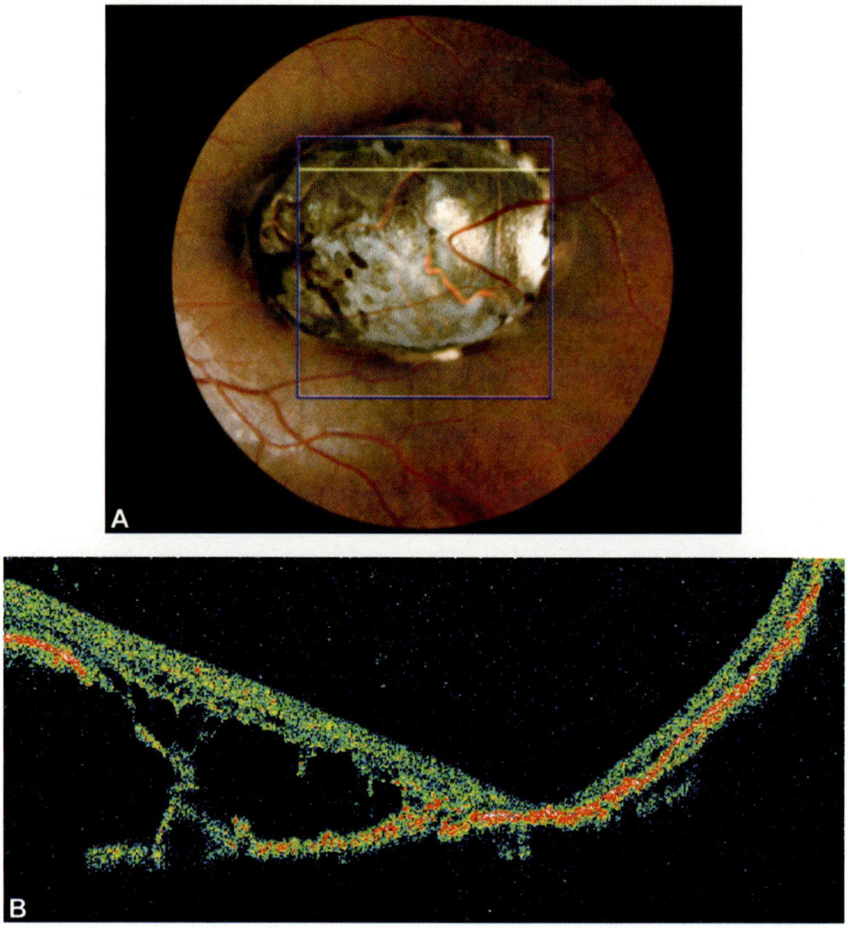

Figures 13.2.2A and B: (A) Color fundus photograph shows horizontal line scan through the intermediate zone. (B) Horizontal line scan through the intermediate zone 2D image showing atrophy of the neurosensory retina

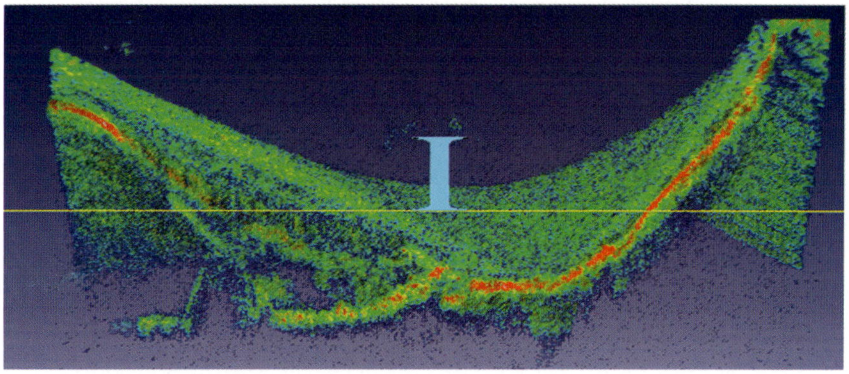

Figure 13.2.2C: Cropped 3D image showing atrophy of the neurosensory retina

Optical Coherence Tomography–3

Horizontal line scan passing through the central zone showed total absence of neurosensory retina over the central area (Figures 13.2.3A to C).

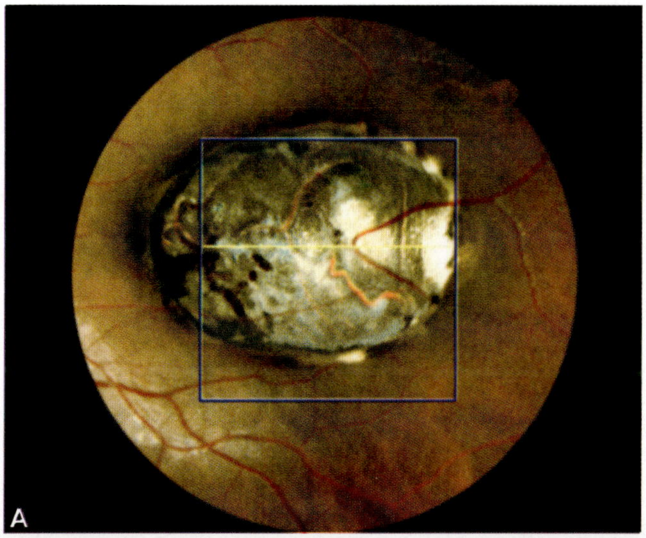

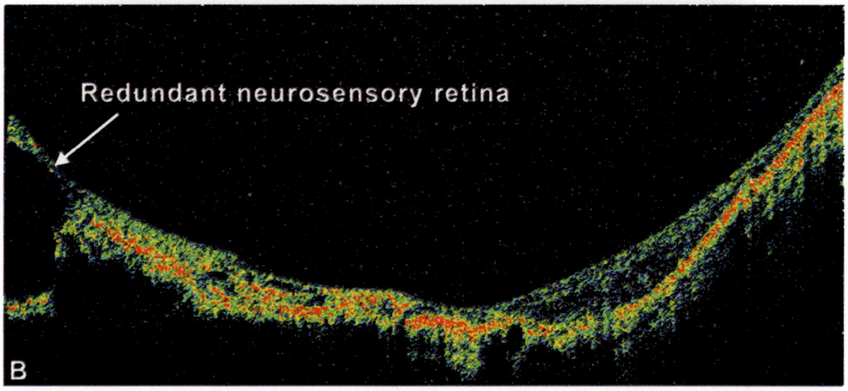

Figures 13.2.3A and B: (A) Color fundus photograph shows horizontal line scan through the central zone. (B) Horizontal line scan through the central zone 2D image showing total absence of neurosensory retina over the central area

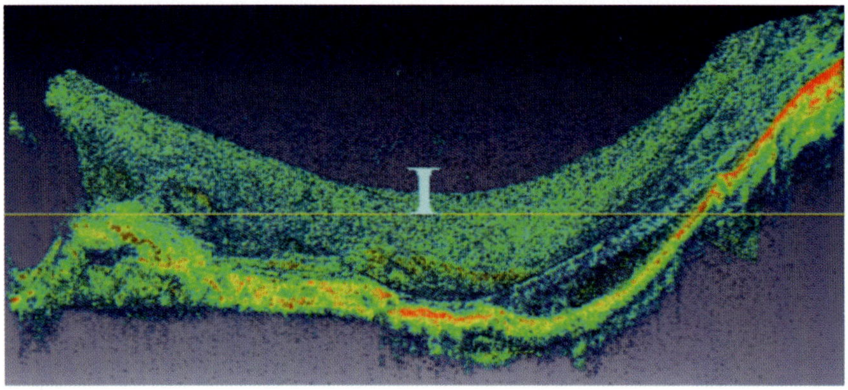

Figure 13.2.3C: Cropped 3D image showing total absence of neurosensory retina over the central area

SUGGESTED READING

1. Chorioretinal inflammatory retinal diseases.In:Puliafito CA, Hee MR, Schuman JS, Fujimoto JG. Optical coherence tomography of ocular diseases. Slack Inc. 1995;249-68.
2. Lim LL, Watzke RC, Lauer AK, Smith JR. Ocular coherence tomography in acute posterior mutifocal pigment epitheliopathy. Clin Experiment Ophthalmol.2006 Nov;34(8):810-2.
3. Lofoco G, Ciucci F, Bardocci A, Quercioli P, Steigerwalt RD Jr, De Gaetano C. Optical coherence tomography findings in a case of acute mutifocal posterior pigment epitheliopathy. Eur J Ophthalmol.2005 Jan-Feb;15(1):143-7.

14 Juxtafoveal Telangiectasia

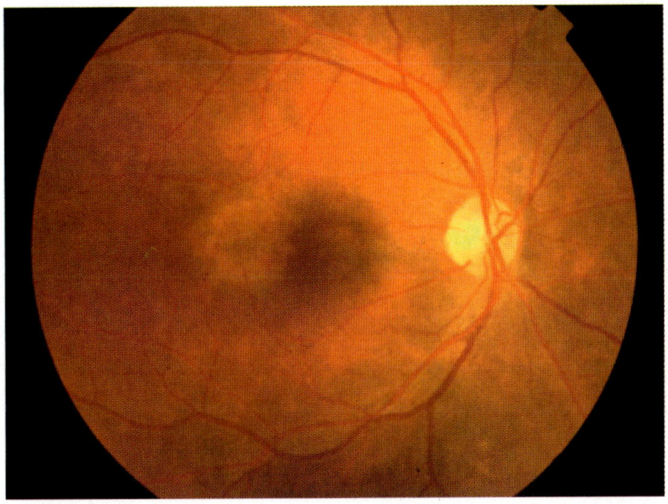

Idiopathic juxtafoveolar retinal telangiectasis (IJT) was first defined in 1982 by Gass and Oyakawa as a unilateral or bilateral disease associated with incompetent retinal capillaries only in the perifoveal or juxtafoveal area. The initial classification, staging, and pathogenesis of IJT were based largely on clinical examination and fluorescein angiography.

Gass defined the following classification:

Group 1A: Unilateral congenital parafoveolar telangiectasis with telangiectatic capillaries temporal to the fovea.

Group 1B: Unilateral, idiopathic, focal juxtafoveolar telangiectasis with a small focal area of incompetent capillaries next to the foveal avascular zone.

Group 2A: Bilateral idiopathic acquired parafoveolar telangiectasis with retinal thickening temporal to the fovea, right-angle venules, retinal pigment epithelial hyperplastic plaques, subretinal neovascularization, and crystalline deposits.

It has 5 stages:

Stage 1: No biomicroscopic abnormality. Fluorescein angiography shows minimal or no capillary dilatation in the early and mild staining in the late phase.

Stage 2: Slight retinal graying with minimal or absent telangiectatic vessels. Fluorescein angiography shows mild capillary telangiectasis.

Stage 3: Clinically shows parafoveolar dilated and blunted retinal venules and refractile deposits. Fluorescein angiography shows capillary dilation with leak in the outer retina.

Stage 4: Stellate foci of black RPE hypertrophy are seen at the posterior end of retinal venules.

Stage 5: Subretinal neovascularization occurs in the parafoveal area. Cystoid edema and yellow exudates are seen only in subretinal neovascularization.

Group 2B: Juvenile occult familial IJT.
Group 3A: Occlusive IJT with visual loss due to obliteration of perifoveal capillaries.
Group 3B: Occlusive IJT associated with central nervous system vasculopathy.

In clinical practice, the most common forms of juxtafoveolar telangiectasis are the unilateral form, which is usually asymptomatic and found typically in men, usually after the age of 40 (type 1B), and the bilateral form, which is found in both men and women, typically between ages 40 and 60 (type 2A). The most common unilateral form of IJT may feature macular edema that affects central visual acuity, whereas the bilateral form presents with parafoveal hemorrhages, retinal pigment epithelium (RPE) hyperplasia, right-angle venules and occasionally choroidal neovascularization, although vision tends to be relatively normal. Group 1B and Group 2A are now referred to as **idiopathic juxtafoveolar retinal telangiectasis**. Recently, photodynamic therapy has been considered in patients with severe disease and choroidal neovascularization.

Optical Coherence Tomography

OCT Features of IJT

1. The earliest finding detected by Spectral domain OCT is a defect in the junction of the inner segment-outer segment photoreceptor layer called IS – OS defect.
2. A unique internal limiting membrane draping across the foveola called ILM drape, related to an underlying loss of tissue.
3. Cystoid spaces within the inner and outer retina.
4. Intensively reflective areas.
5. Retinal pigment epithelial hyperplasia.
6. Absence of retinal thickening despite leakage on fluorescein angiography.
7. Foveal thinning
8. Subretinal neovascularization

CASE 14.1: GROUP 2A IDIOPATHIC JUXTAFOVEOLAR RETINAL TELANGIECTASIS

Case Summary

A 48-year-old woman was seen with decreased vision in both eyes of three years duration. Her best-corrected visual acuity was 6/18 in the right eye. Fluorescein angiography showed telangiectatic vessels temporal to the fovea with staining in the late phase (Figures 14.1.1 and 14.1.2).

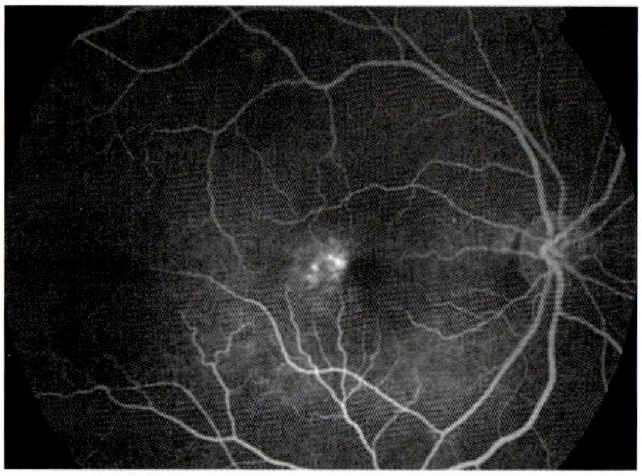

Figure 14.1.1: Early phase angiogram shows telangiectatic vessels temporal to the fovea

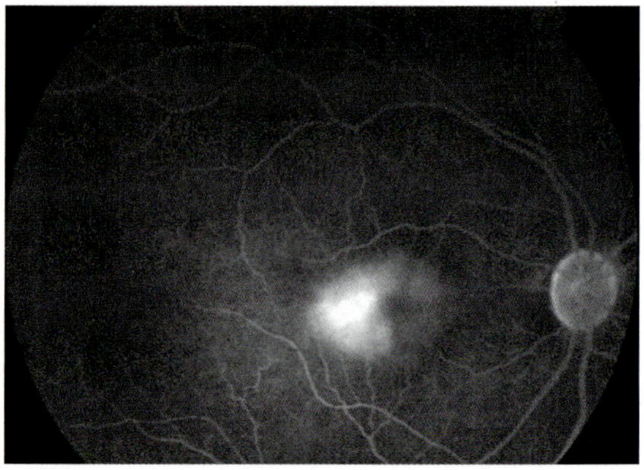

Figure 14.1.2: Late phase angiogram shows parafoveal staining

Optical Coherence Tomography

Horizontal line scan through the fovea showed a small hyporeflective area in the outer retina with an underlying IS-OS defect. Despite the staining seen on fluorescein angiography, there was no increased thickness on OCT, thus showing a lack of correlation between retinal thickening on OCT and leakage on fluorescein angiography (Figures 14.1.3A to E).

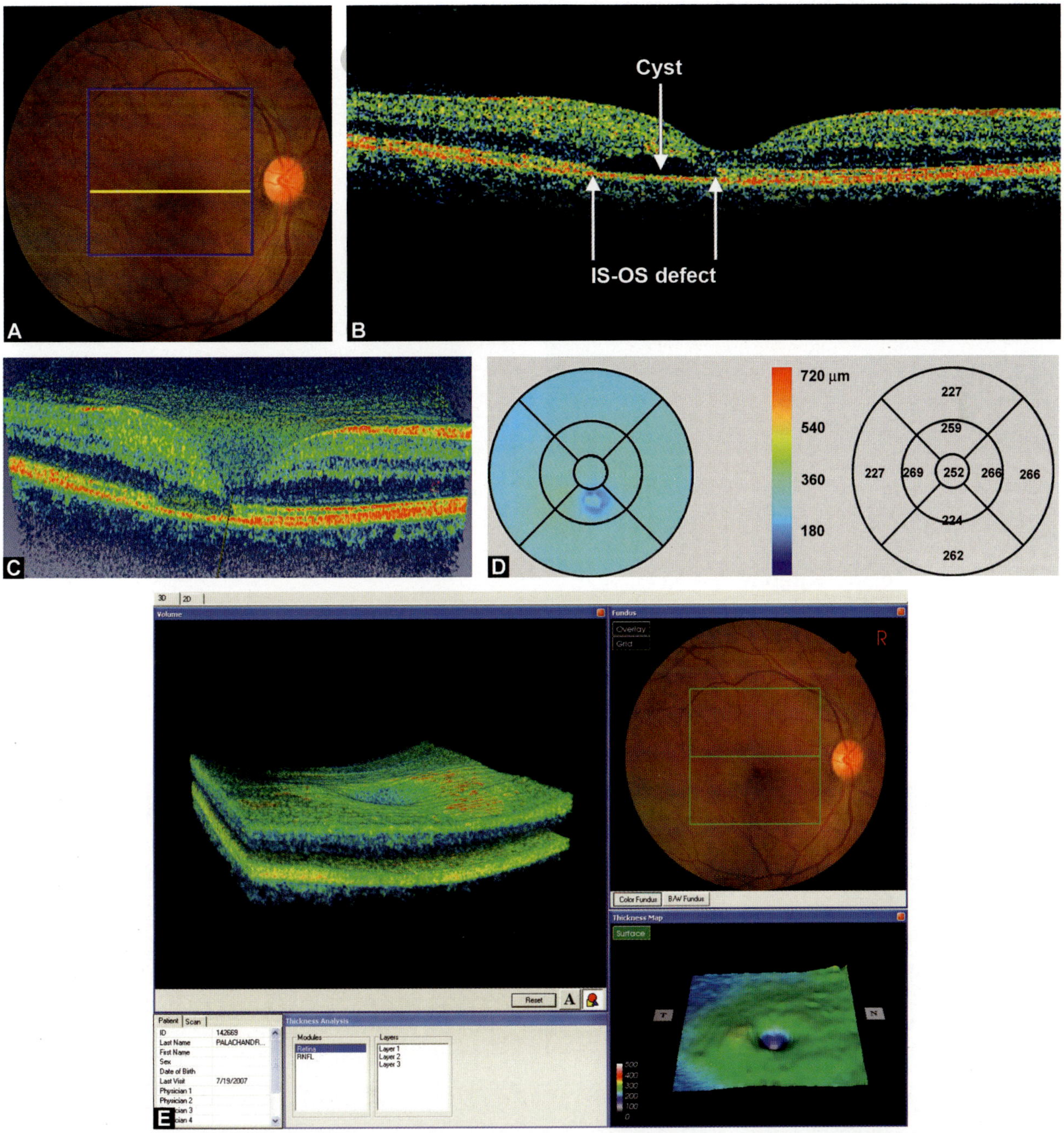

Figures 14.1.3A to E: (A) Color fundus photograph shows horizontal line scan through the fovea. (B) Horizontal line scan through the fovea 2D image showing a small hyporeflective area in the outer retina with an underlying IS-OS defect. (C) Cropped 3D image showing a small hyporeflective area in the outer retina with an underlying IS-OS defect. (D) Macular thickness map showing foveal thickness measuring 252 µm. (E) 3D image of Case 14.1

CASE 14.2: GROUP 2A IDIOPATHIC JUXTAFOVEOLAR RETINAL TELANGIECTASIS

Case Summary

A 69-year-old man with past history of focal photocoagulation was seen for a routine eye check-up. His best-corrected visual acuity in the right eye was 6/24. Fluorescein angiography showed telangiectatic vessels temporal to the fovea with staining in the late phase (Figures 14.2.1 and 14.2.2).

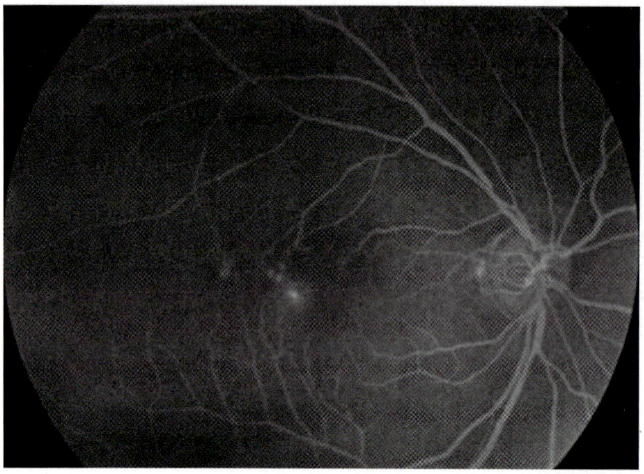

Figure 14.2.1: Early phase angiogram shows telangiectatic vessels temporal to the fovea

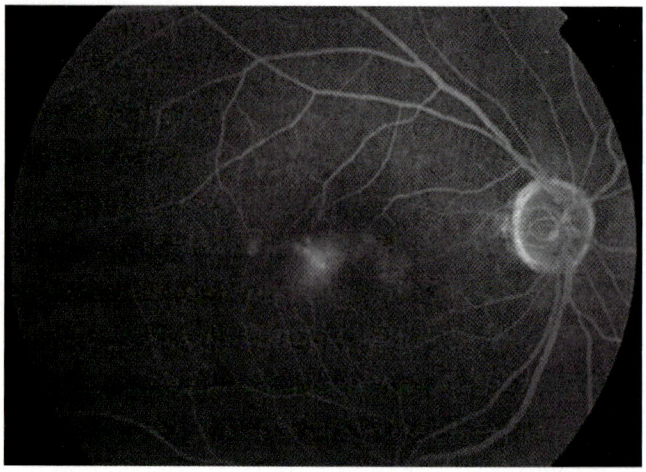

Figure 14.2.2: Late phase angiogram shows parafoveal staining

Optical Coherence Tomography

Horizontal line scan showed the presence of ILM drape and hyporeflective areas under the fovea in the inner and outer retina with an underlying IS-OS defect. There was no increase in retinal thickness despite the leakage seen on fluorescein angiography. There was also evidence of posterior hyaloid separation seen on either side of the fovea (Figures 14.2.3A to E).

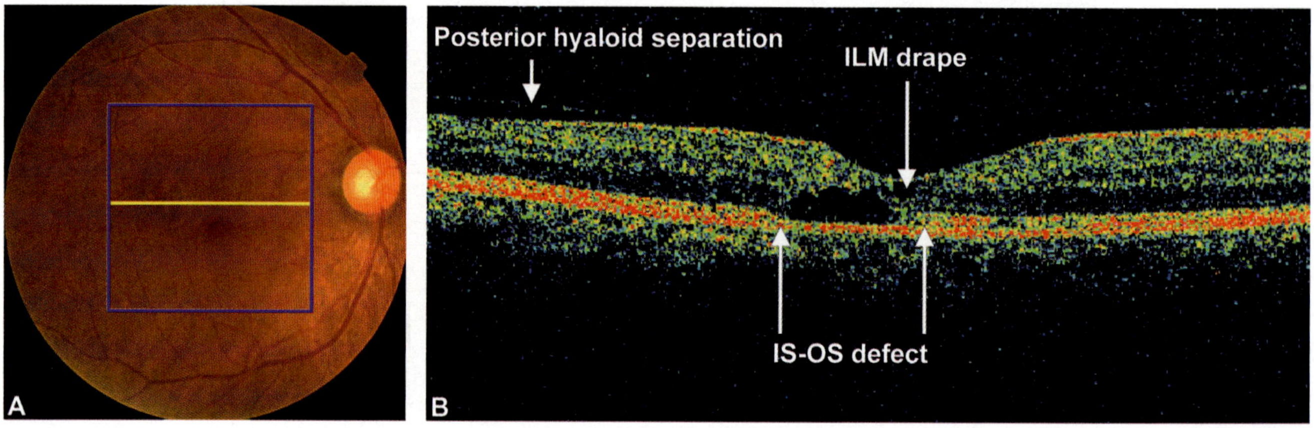

Figures 14.2.3A and B: (A) Color fundus photograph shows horizontal line scan through the fovea. (B) Horizontal line scan through the fovea 2D image showing the presence of ILM drape and hyporeflective areas under the fovea in the inner and outer retina with an underlying IS-OS defect. Perifoveal separation of the posterior hyaloid is evident

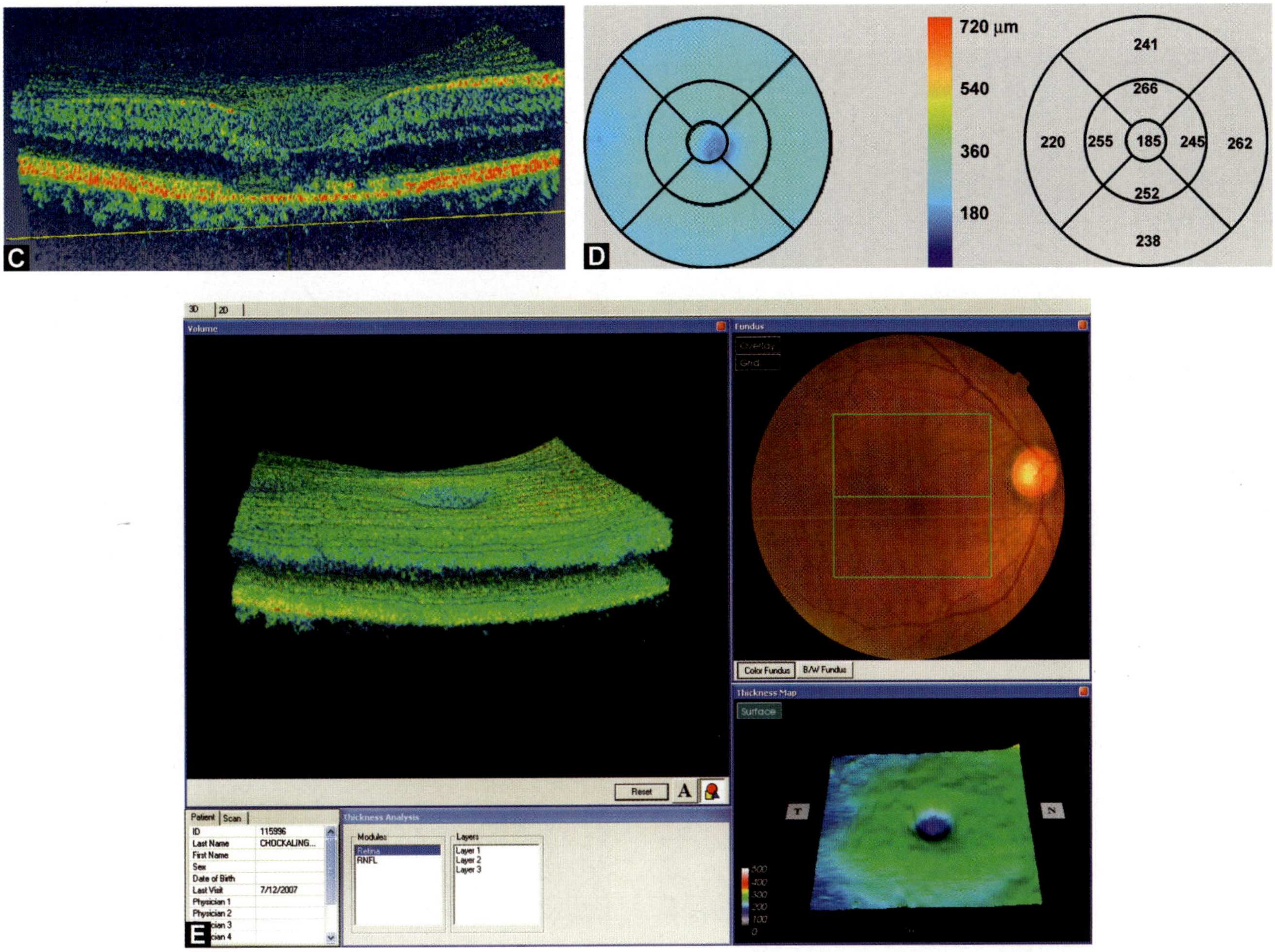

Figures 14.2.3C to E: (C) Cropped 3D image showing the presence of ILM drape and hyporeflective areas under the fovea in the inner and outer retina with an underlying IS-OS defect. Perifoveal separation of the posterior hyaloid is evident. (D) Macular thickness map showing foveal thickness measuring 185 µm. (E) 3D image of Case 14.2

CASE 14.3: GROUP 2A IDIOPATHIC JUXTAFOVEOLAR RETINAL TELANGIECTASIS WITH CHOROIDAL NEOVASCULAR MEMBRANE

Case Summary

A 47-year-old woman was seen with blurring of vision caused by bilateral, acquired, juxtafoveal telangiectasis. Her best-corrected vision in the right eye was 6/9. Fluorescein angiography of the right eye showed mottled hyperfluorescence that increased in the late phase suggesting the presence of underlying classic choroidal neovascular membrane (CNVM) (Figures 14.3.1 and 14.3.2).

Indocyanine green angiography showed the extent of the CNVM (Figures 14.3.3 and 14.3.4).

Optical Coherence Tomography

Horizontal line scan showed IS-OS defect and an area of moderate reflectivity above the RPE, temporal to the fovea with cystic spaces in the overlying retina confirming the presence of a classic CNVM (Figures 14.3.5A to D).The patient was treated with photodynamic therapy and intravitreal Ranibizumab.

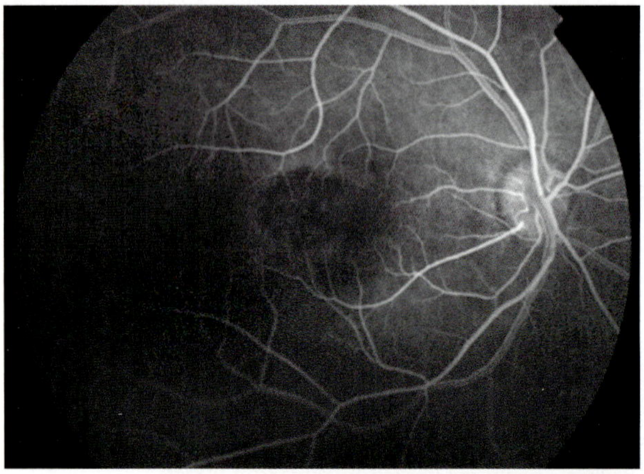

Figure 14.3.1: Early phase angiogram shows mottled hyperfluorescence

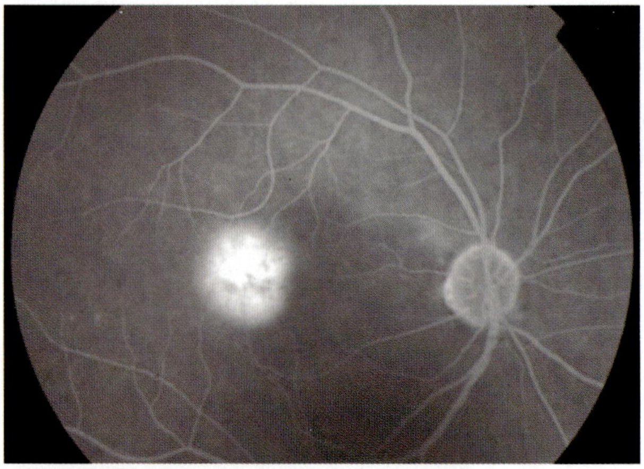

Figure 14.3.2: Late phase angiogram shows CNVM

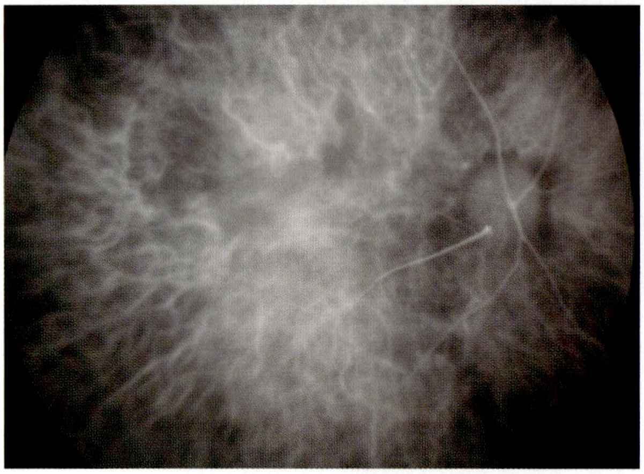

Figure 14.3.3: Early phase ICG shows CNVM

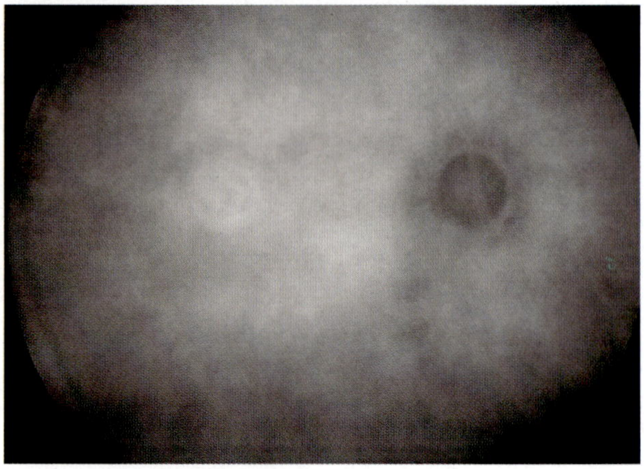

Figure 14.3.4: Late phase ICG shows CNVM

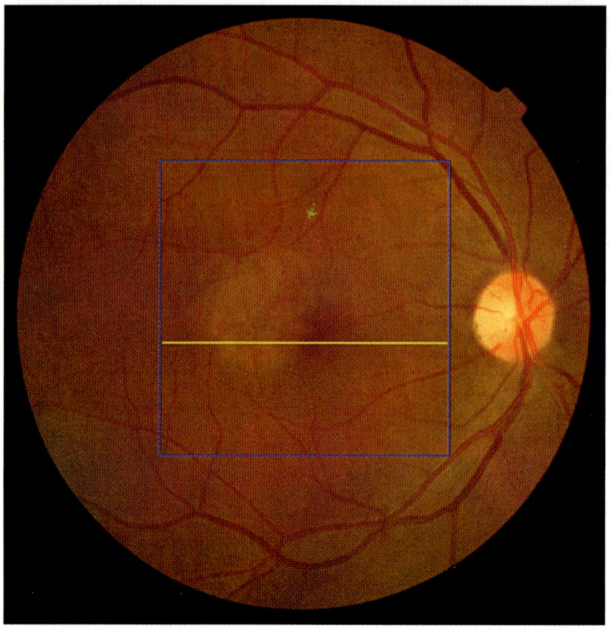

Figure 14.3.5A: Color fundus photograph shows horizontal line scan through the fovea

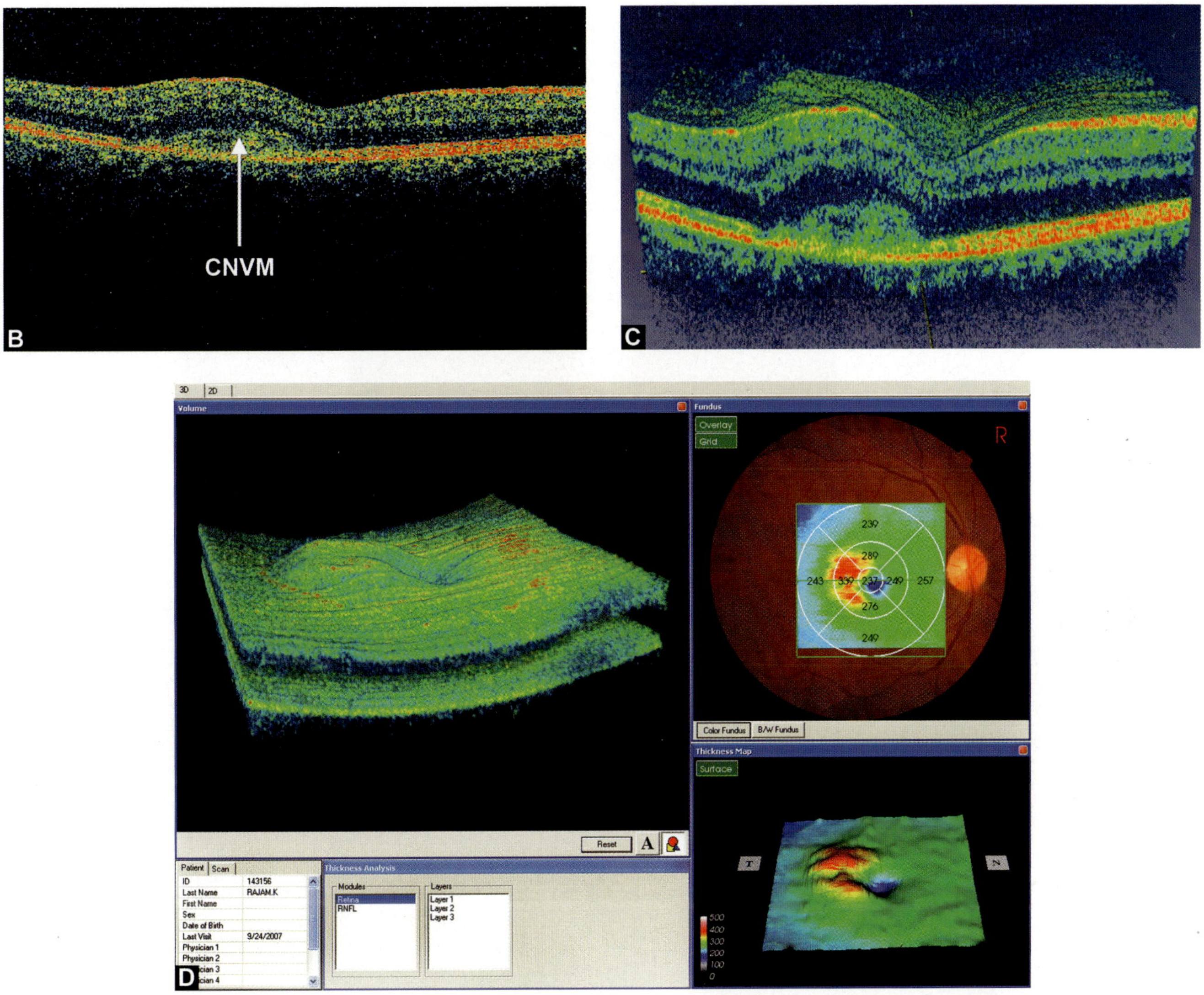

Figures 14.3.5B to D: (B) Horizontal line scan through the fovea 2D image showing IS-OS defect and an area of moderate reflectivity above the RPE, temporal to the fovea with cystic spaces in the overlying retina confirming the presence of a classic CNVM. (C) Cropped 3D image showing IS-OS defect and an area of moderate reflectivity above the RPE, temporal to the fovea with cystic spaces in the overlying retina confirming the presence of a classic CNVM. (D) 3D image of the right eye of Case 14.3

Follow-up

Repeat OCT done one month later, showed regression of the CNVM with formation of scar tissue (Figures 14.3.6A to D). The visual acuity was maintained at 6/9.

Her best-corrected visual acuity in the left eye was 6/6. Fluorescein angiography of the left eye showed telangiectatic vessels temporal to the fovea with staining in the late phase confirming the diagnosis of idiopathic juxtafoveolar retinal telangiectasis (Figures 14.3.7 and 14.3.8).

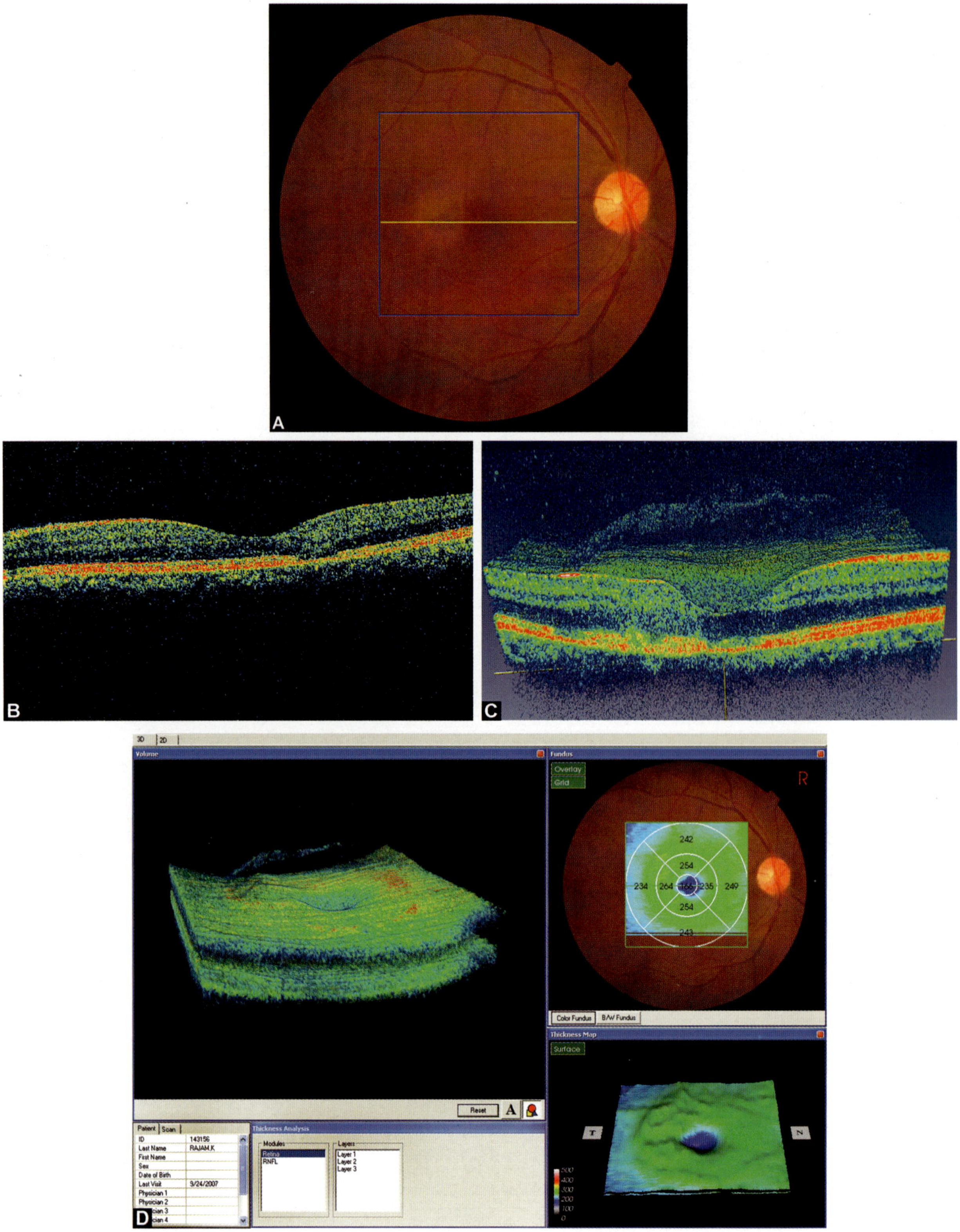

Figures 14.3.6A to D: (A) Color fundus photograph one month following PDT and intravitreal Ranibizumab shows horizontal line scan through the fovea. (B) Horizontal line scan through the fovea 2D image showing regression of the CNVM with formation of scar tissue. (C) Cropped 3D image showing regression of the CNVM with formation of scar tissue. (D) 3D image of the right eye of Case 14. 3, one month following PDT and intravitreal Ranibizumab

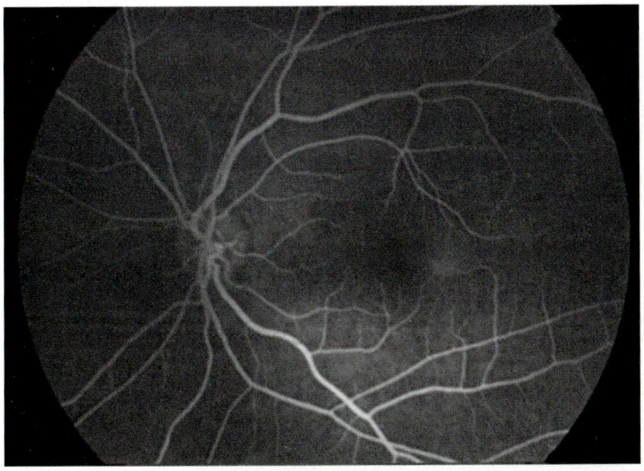

Figure 14.3.7: Early phase angiogram shows telangiectatic vessels temporal to the fovea

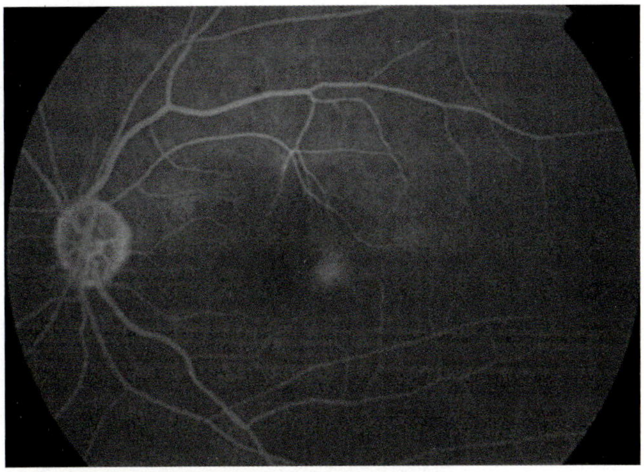

Figure 14.3.8: Late phase angiogram shows temporal parafoveal staining

Optical Coherence Tomography

Horizontal line scan showed IS-OS defect which was the only abnormality evident (Figures 14.3.9A to E).

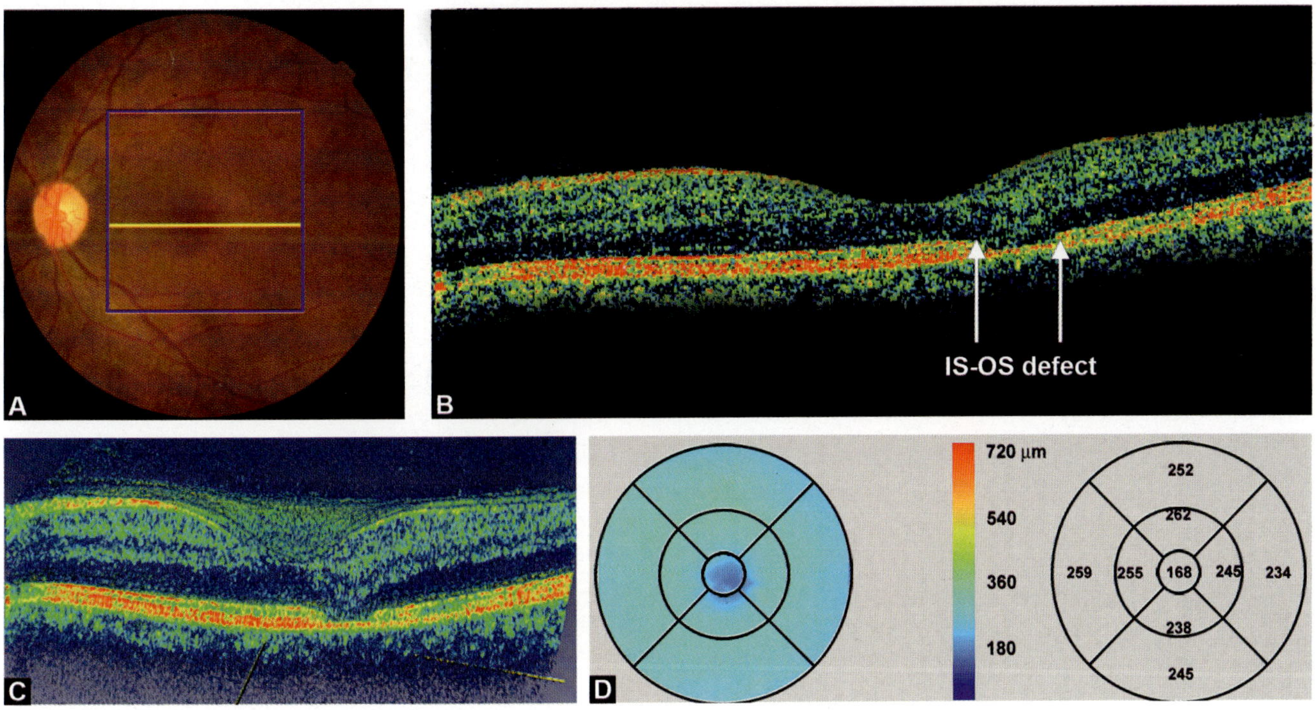

Figures 14.3.9A to D: (A) Color fundus photograph shows horizontal line scan through the fovea. (B) Horizontal line scan through the fovea 2D image showing IS - OS defect. (C) Cropped 3D image showing IS-OS defect. (D) Macular thickness map showing foveal thickness measuring 168 μm

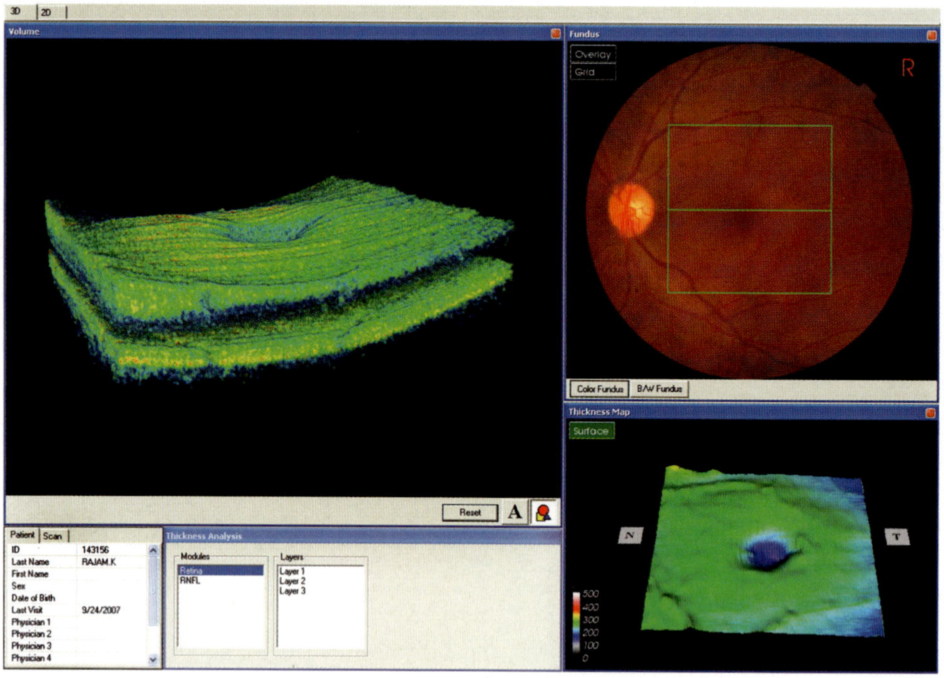

Figure 14.3.9E: 3D image of the left eye of Case 14.3

CONCLUSIONS

1. OCT has made it possible to differentiate whether the pooling seen in fluorescein angiography is due to actual leakage or accumulation of dye in the damaged retinal cells.
2. It helps to establish the cause of visual loss in IJT.
3. The earliest finding detectable on SD OCT is the IS-OS defect.

SUGGESTED READING

1. Gass JD, Oyakawa RT. Idiopathic juxtafoveolar retinal telangiectasis. Arch Ophthalmol 1982;100:769–80. [PubMed]
2. Gass JD, Blodi BA. Idiopathic juxtafoveolar retinal telangiectasis. Update of classification and follow-up study. Ophthalmology. 1993;100:1536–46.
3. Lelia A Paunescu, Tony H Ko, Jay S Duker, Annie Chan, Wolfgang Drexler, Joel S Schuman, et al. Idiopathic Juxtafoveal Retinal Telangiectasis: New Findings by Ultrahigh Resolution Optical Coherence Tomography. Ophthalmol. 2006 Jan;113(1):48-57.

15 Macular Drusen

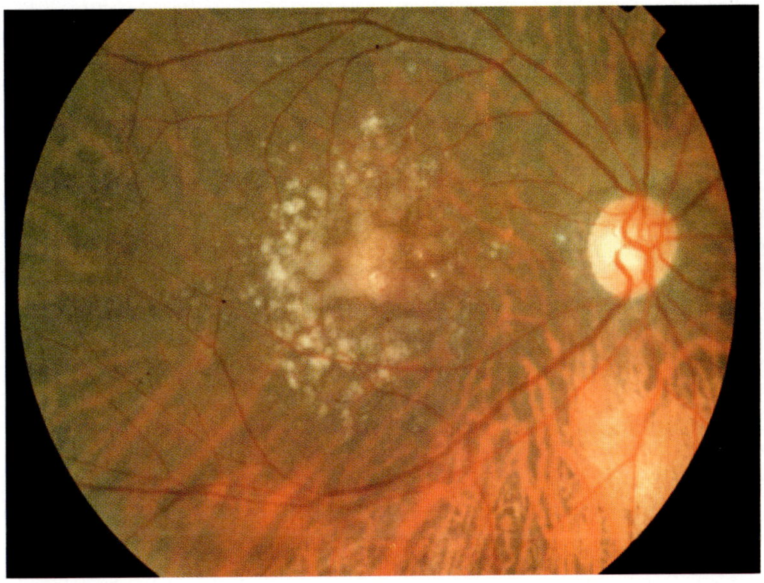

Drusen are rounded, yellowish degenerative formations associated with Bruch's membrane, which are present predominantly at the posterior pole. Progression of the drusen is toward either the atrophic (dry) form or the exudative (wet) form of macular degeneration. Large (>63 μm), amorphous, ill-defined soft drusen and confluent drusen are more likely to progress to advanced age-related macular degeneration, in contrast with discrete, well demarcated, hard drusen.

Fluorescein Angiography

Hard drusen show early hyperfluorescence which increases in the arteriovenous phase and fades in the late phase. Soft drusen on the other hand, do not show hyperfluorescence until the late stages.

Optical Coherence Tomography

Drusen present as undulations or localized increase in the thickness of the retinal pigment epithelium. It is differentiated from pigment epithelial detachment by the absence of optically clear spaces within the undulations.

CASE 15.1: MACULAR DRUSEN

Case Summary

A 78-year-old man was seen for a routine eye check-up. His best-corrected visual acuity in the left eye was 6/6. Fluorescein angiography showed early hyperfluorescence which faded in the late phase confirming the presence of drusens (Figures 15.1.1 and 15.1.2).

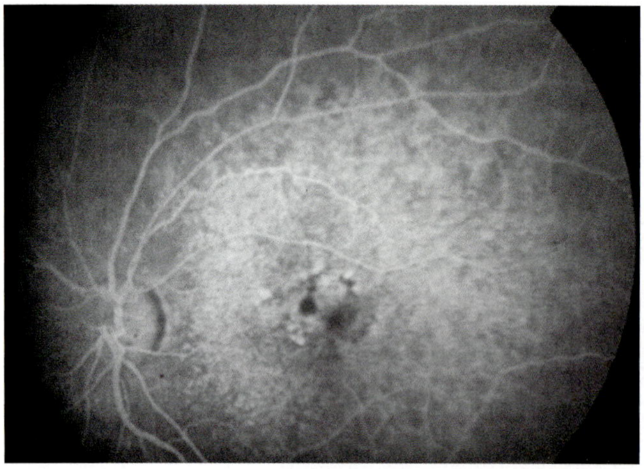

Figure 15.1.1: Early phase of the angiogram showing hyperfluorescence corresponding to the hard drusen

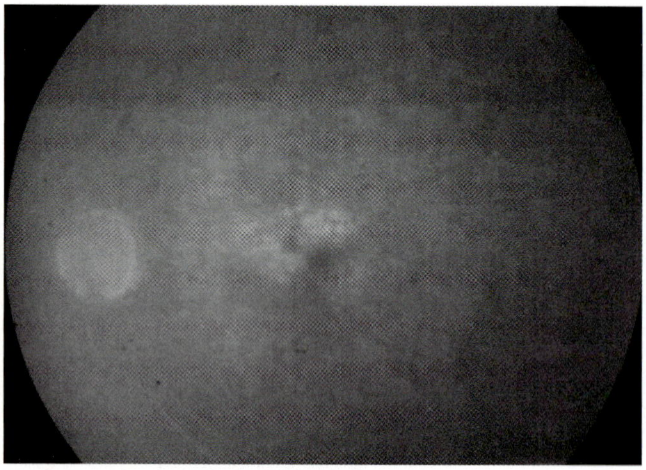

Figure 15.1.2: Late phase of the angiogram showing fading of the hyperfluorescence

Optical Coherence Tomography

Horizontal line scan passing above the fovea through the area of drusens showed irregular elevations of RPE with no shadow from the underlying choroid (Figures 15.1.3A to D).

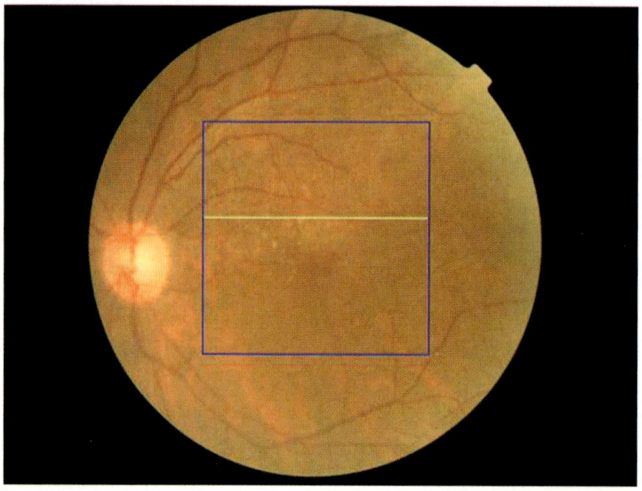

Figure 15.1.3A: Color fundus photograph showing the horizontal line scan above the fovea

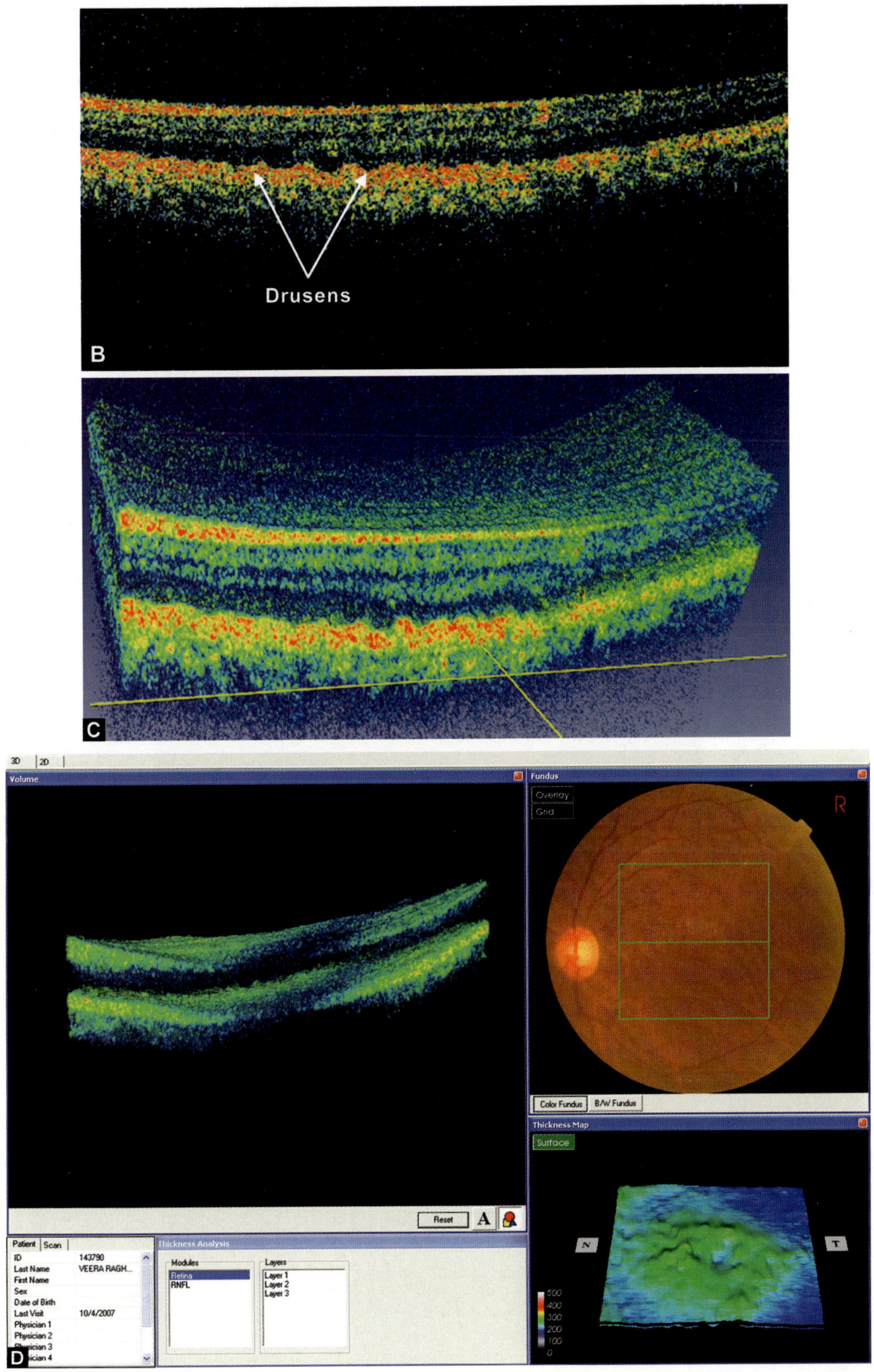

Figures 15.1.3B to D: (B) Horizontal line scan - 2D image showing irregular elevations of RPE with no shadow from the underlying choroid. (C) Cropped 3D image showing irregular elevations of RPE with no shadow from the underlying choroid. (D) 3D image of Case 15.1

CASE 15.2: MACULAR DRUSEN

Case Summary

A 70-year-old man was seen for a routine eye check-up. His best-corrected visual acuity in the right eye was 6/6.

Optical Coherence Tomography

Horizontal line scan through the fovea showed bumps of the RPE with no shadow from the underlying choroid (Figures 15.2.1A to D).

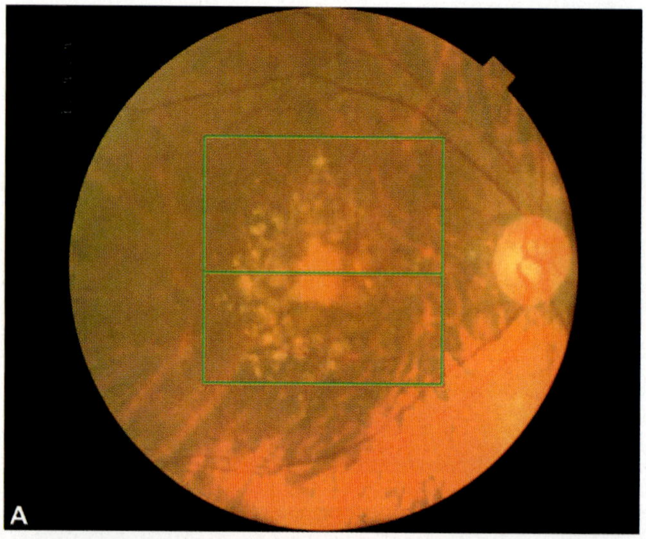

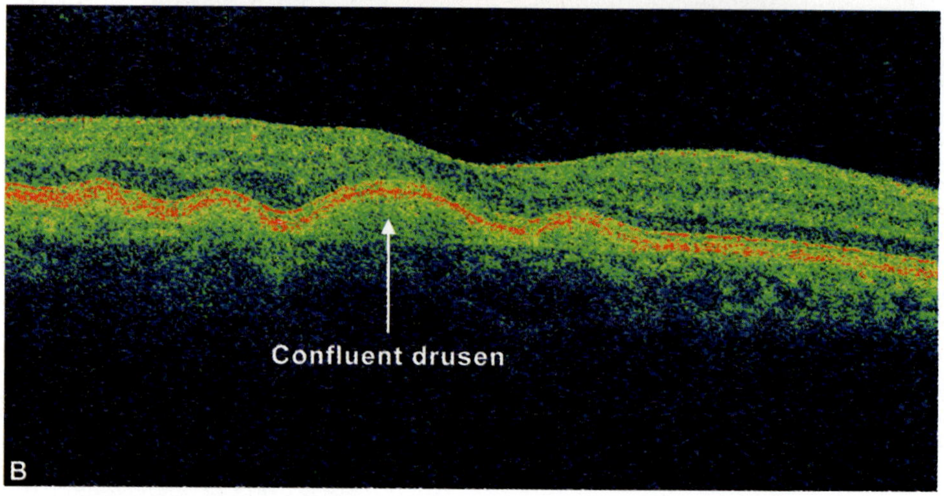

Figures 15.2.1A and B: (A) Color fundus photograph showing the horizontal line scan through the fovea. (B) Horizontal line scan - 2D image showing bumps of the RPE with no shadow from the underlying choroid

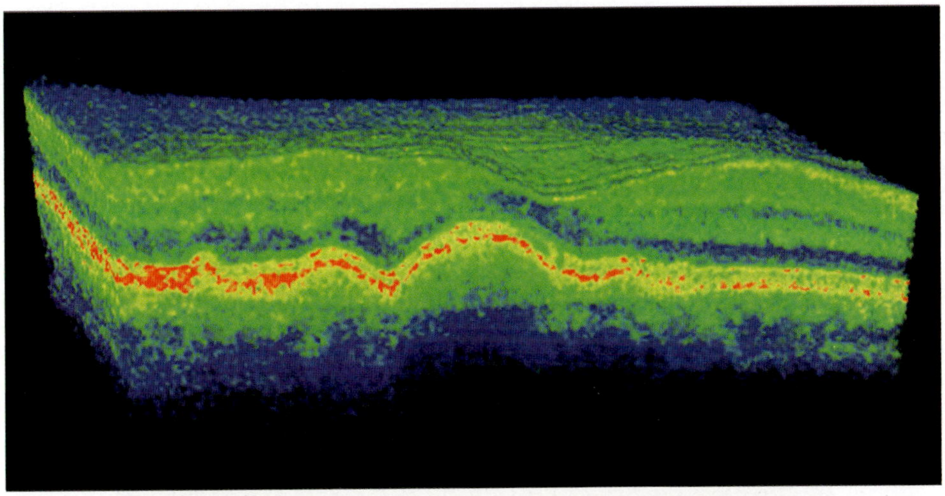

Figure 15.2.1C: Cropped 3D image showing confluent drusen

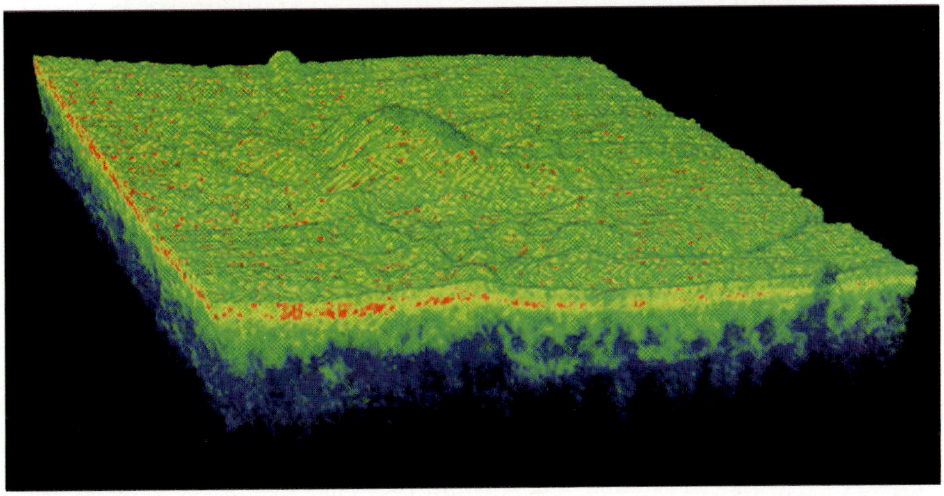

Figure 15.2.1D: Multiple drusen seen after the retinal layers have been peeled upto the RPE (Images with Topcon 3D OCT-2000)

SUGGESTED READING

1. Pieroni C G, Witkin A J, Ko T H, Fujimoto J G, Chan A, Schuman J S, et al.Ultrahigh resolution optical coherence tomography in non-exudative age related macular degeneration. Br J Ophthalmol 2006;90(2):191-7 (PubMed).

16 Macular Hole

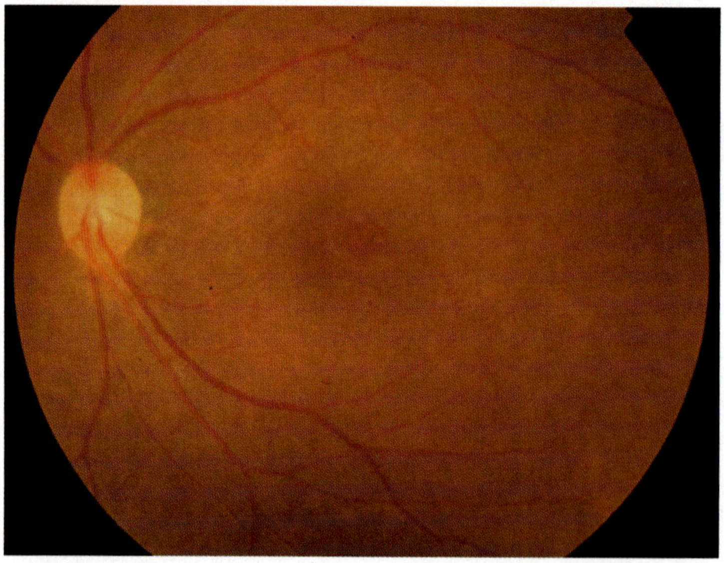

Role of OCT

OCT is a very useful tool in the diagnosis and management of macular holes.

1. It is effective in distinguishing full-thickness macular holes from partial-thickness holes, macular pseudoholes and cysts.
2. It is useful in staging macular holes.
3. It provides a quantitative measure of preoperative hole diameter. This is a prognostic factor to predict postoperative visual outcome and anatomical success rate of macular hole surgery.
4. It is used to evaluate the vitreoretinal interface in patients fellow eyes and thereby predict the chances of a similar occurrence.

OCT Classification of Macular Holes

Stage 1A: Foveal pseudocyst

Stage 1B: Impending macular hole characterized by disruption of outer retina

Stage 2: Lamellar macular hole

Stage 3: Full thickness macular hole without PVD

Stage 4: Full thickness macular hole with PVD

CASE 16.1: STAGE 1 A MACULAR HOLE: FOVEAL PSEUDOCYST

Case Summary

A 73-year-old woman underwent routine check-up of her right eye. Her best-corrected visual acuity was 6/6 in this eye.

Optical Coherence Tomography

Horizontal line scan showed an intraretinal pseudocyst in the inner part of the foveola (Figures 16.1.1A to D). OCT was helpful in detecting the foveal pseudocyst in this patient, which is the first step in the formation of macular hole.

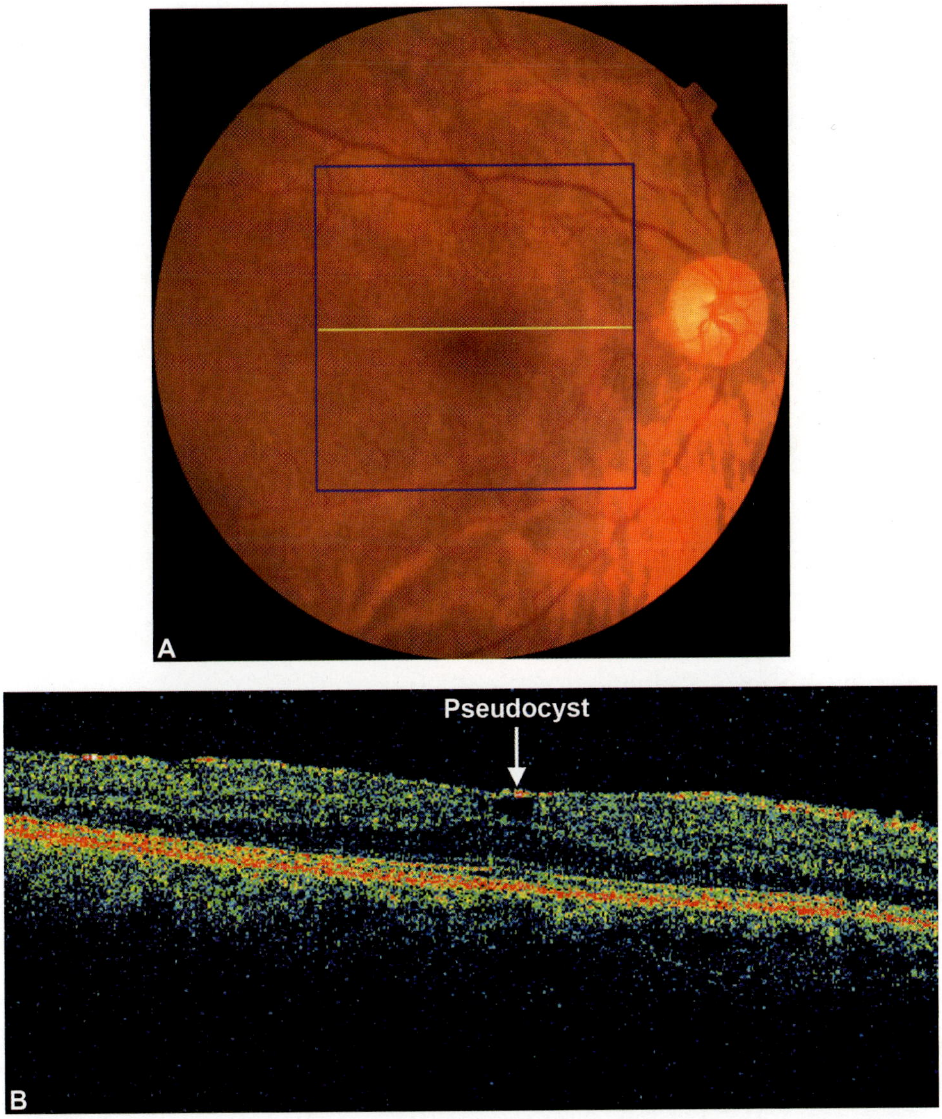

Figures 16.1.1A and B: (A) Color fundus photograph showing the horizontal line scan through the fovea. (B) Horizontal line scan 2D image showing an intraretinal pseudocyst in the inner part of the foveola

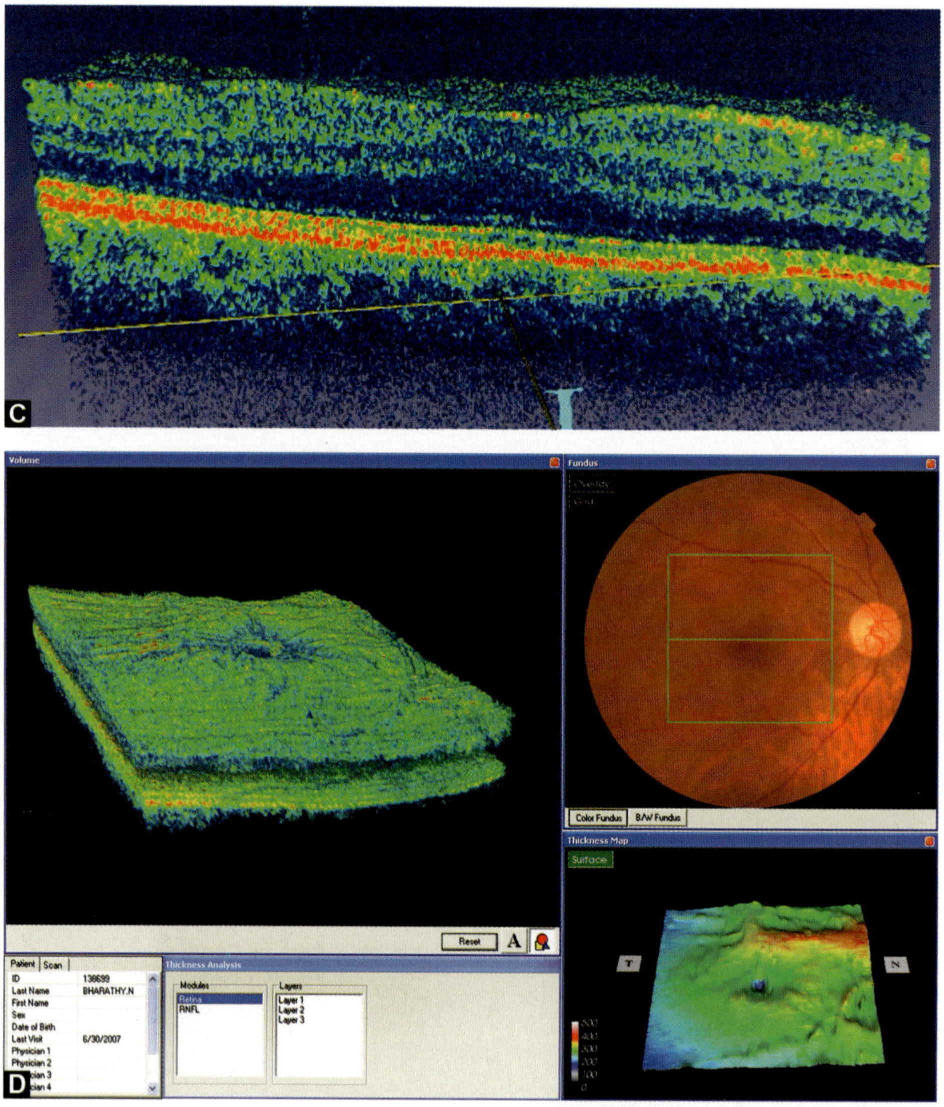

Figures 16.1.1C and D: (C) Cropped 3D image showing an intraretinal pseudocyst in the inner part of the foveola. (D) 3D image of Case 16.1

CASE 16.2: STAGE 2 LAMELLAR MACULAR HOLE

Case Summary

A 60-year-old woman presented with diminished vision in the left eye. Her best-corrected visual acuity was 6/6 in this eye.

Optical Coherence Tomography

Horizontal lines scan showed retinal dehiscence confined to the inner retinal layers suggestive of lamellar macular hole (Figures 16.2.1A to D).

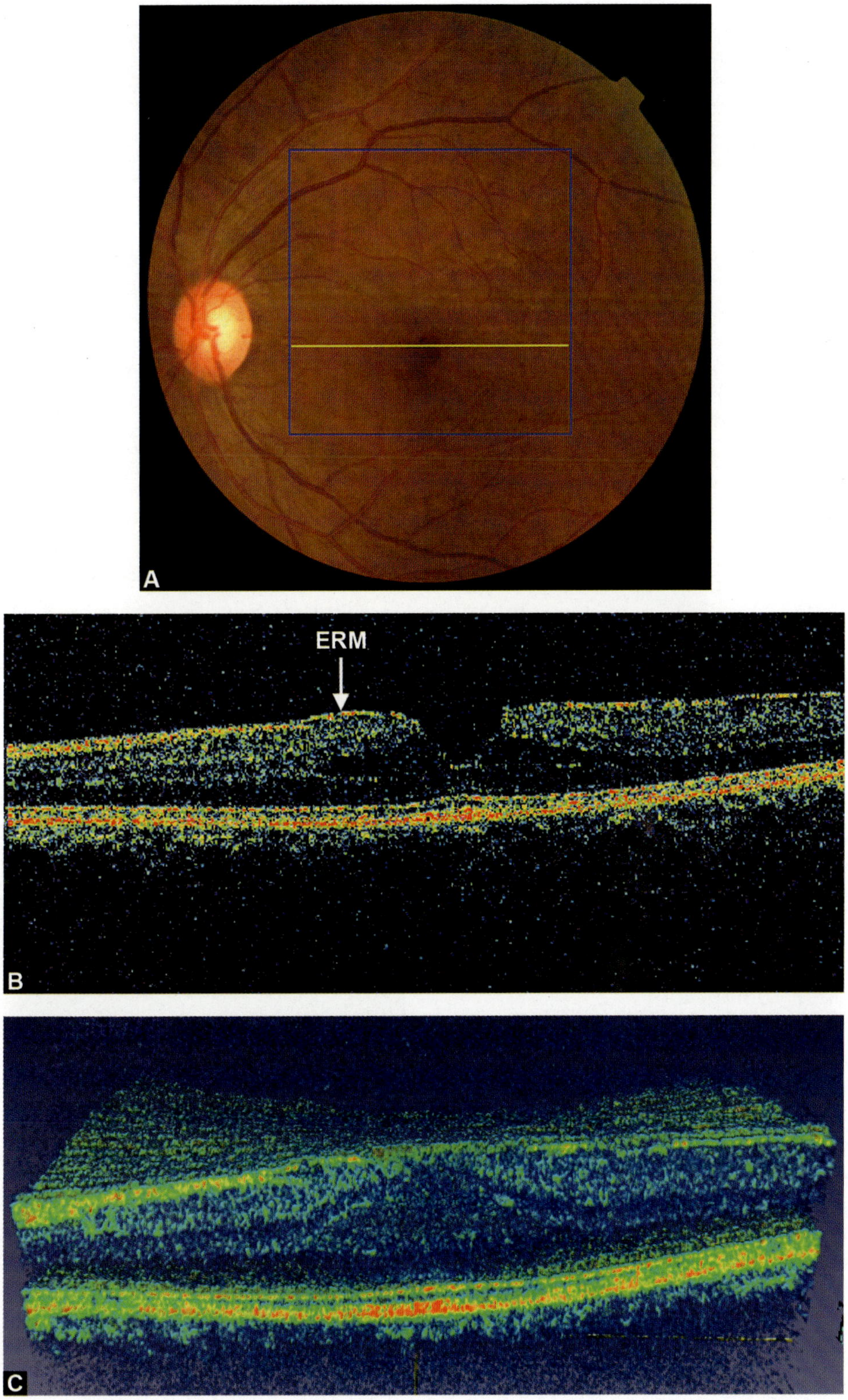

Figures 16.2.1A to C: (A) Color fundus photograph showing the horizontal line scan through the fovea. (B) Horizontal line scan 2D image showing retinal dehiscence confined to the inner retinal layers suggestive of lamellar macular hole. ERM is also evident. (C) Cropped 3D image showing retinal dehiscence confined to the inner retinal layers suggestive of lamellar mac:ular hole. ERM is also evident

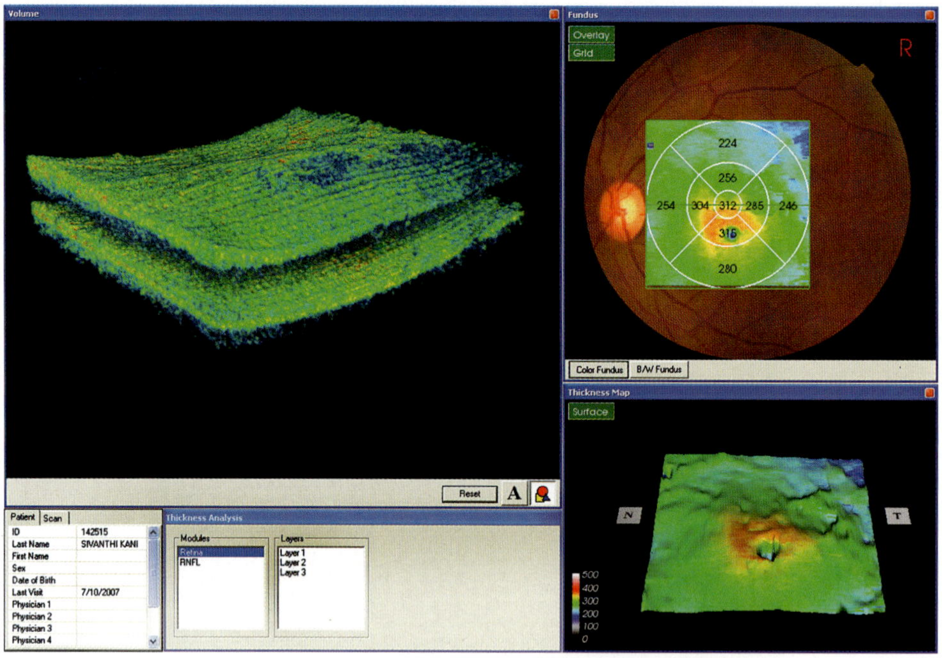

Figure 16.2.1D: 3D image of Case 16.2

CASE 16.3: STAGE 3 MACULAR HOLE

Case Summary

A 73-year-old woman presented with diminished vision in both eyes of one month duration. Her best-corrected visual acuity was 3/60 in the right eye and 4/60 in the left eye.

Optical Coherence Tomography

Horizontal lines scan of the right eye showed the presence of full thickness retinal dehiscence with an overlying operculum (Figures 16.3.1A to D). In spite of the hazy media due to lens changes, the 3D OCT was capable of demonstrating the macular hole.

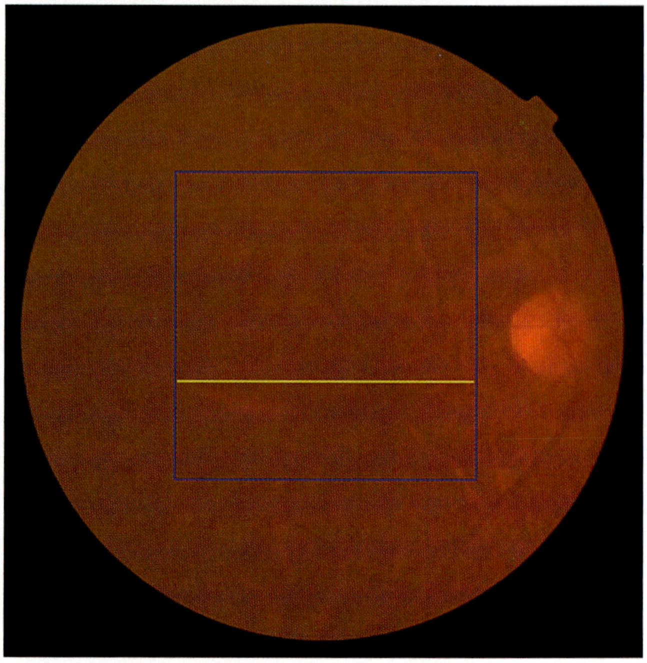

Figure 16.3.1A: Color fundus photograph showing the horizontal line scan through the fovea

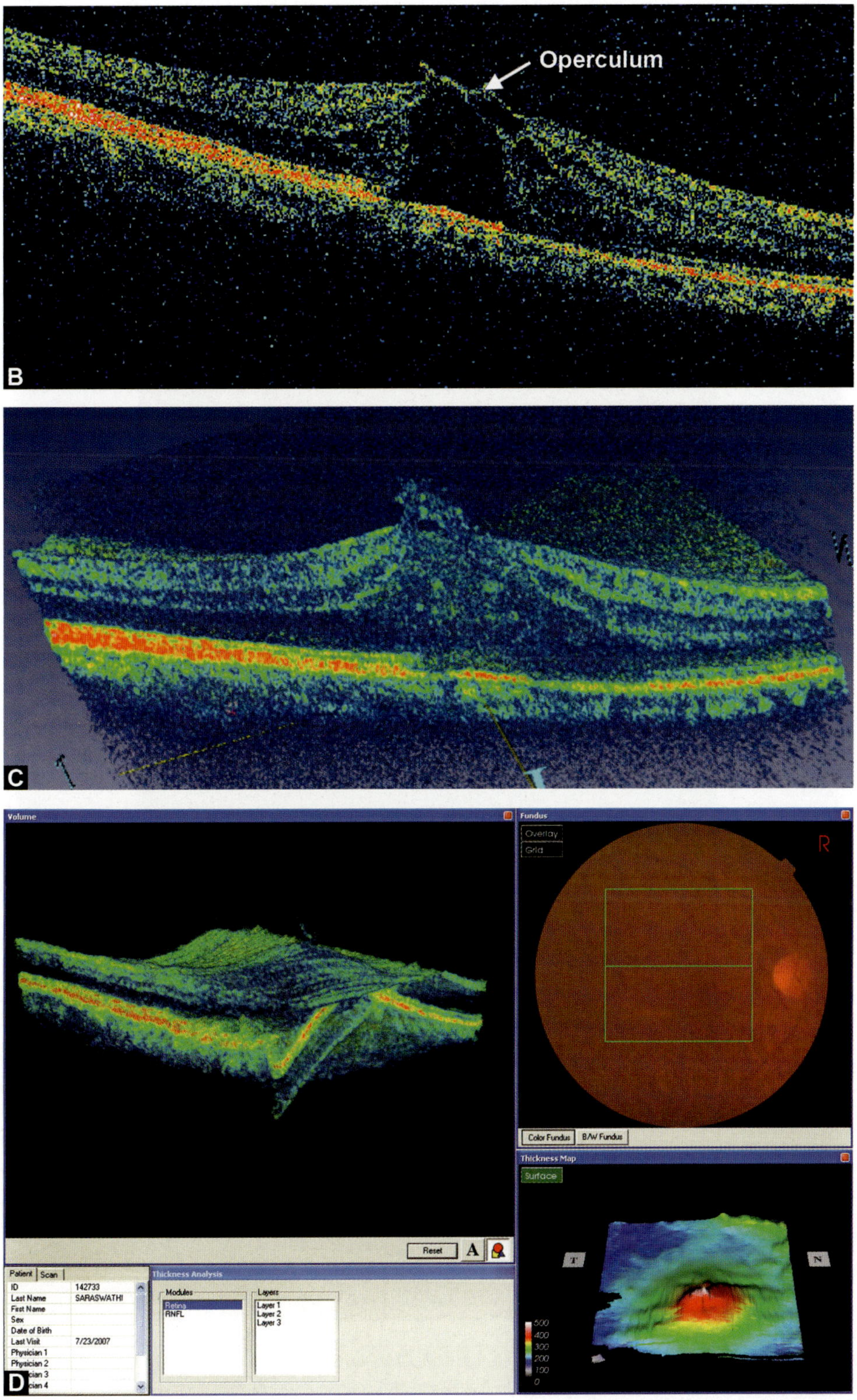

Figures 16.3.1B to D: (B) Horizontal line scan-2D image showing the presence of full thickness retinal dehiscence with an overlying operculum. (C) Cropped 3D image showing the presence of full thickness retinal dehiscence with an overlying operculum. (D) 3D image of Case 16.3

CASE 16.4: STAGE 4 MACULAR HOLE

Optical Coherence Tomography

Horizontal lines scan of the left eye showed the presence of full thickness macular hole with posterior vitreous detachment (Figures 16.4.1A to D). The surrounding retina showed cystic spaces characterized by hyporeflective spaces. In spite of the hazy media due to lens changes, the 3D OCT was capable of demonstrating the macular hole.

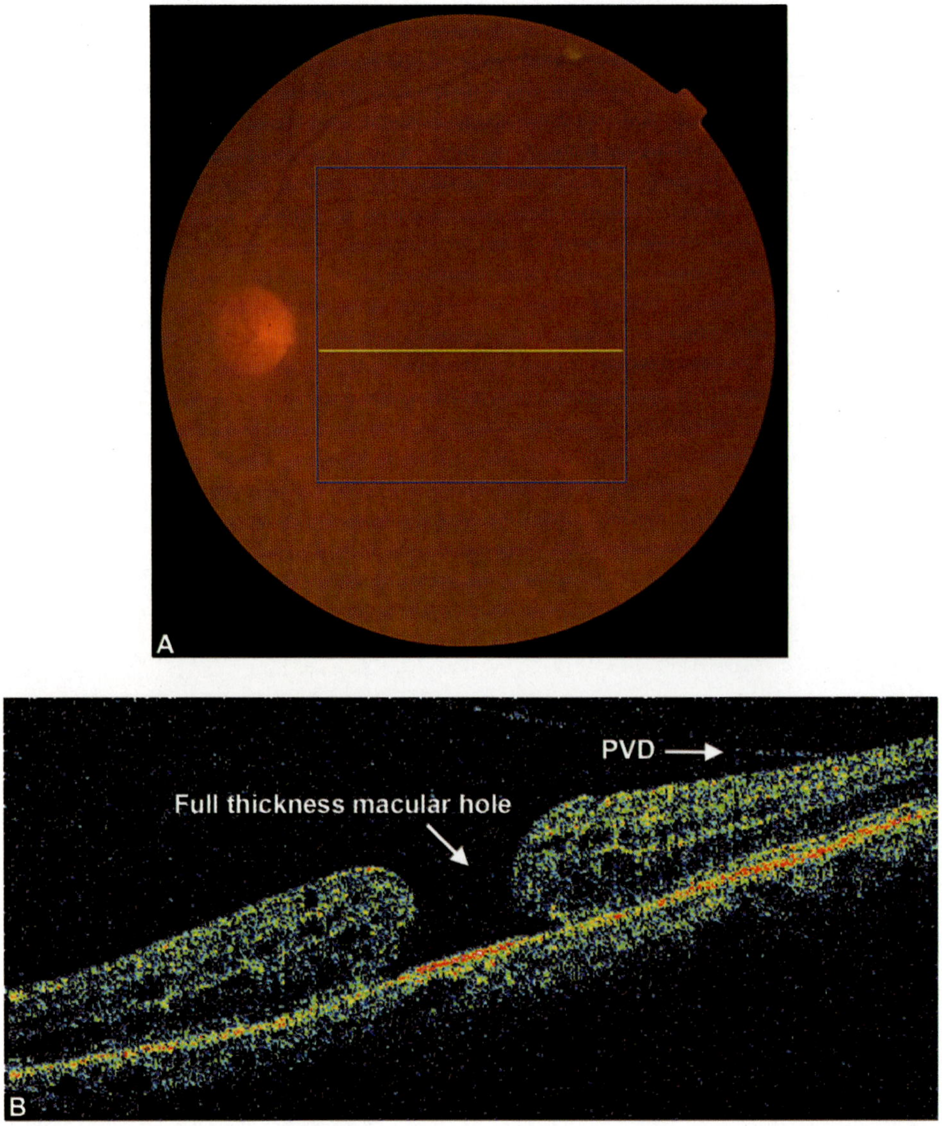

Figures 16.4.1A and B: (A) Color fundus photograph showing the horizontal line scan through the fovea. (B) Horizontal line scan 2D image showing the presence of full thickness macular hole with posterior vitreous detachment. The surrounding retina showed cystic spaces

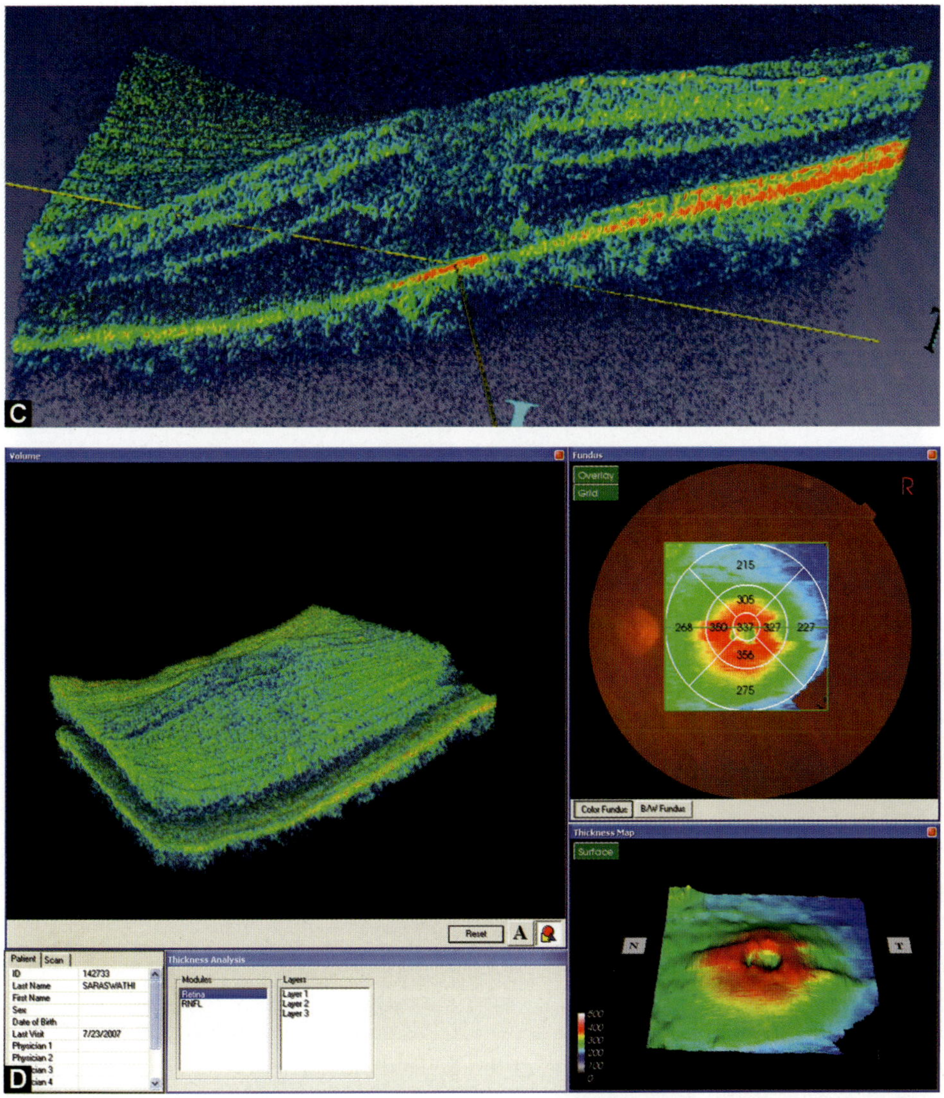

Figures 16.4.1C and D: (C) Cropped 3D image showing the presence of full thickness macular hole with posterior vitreous detachment. The surrounding retina showed cystic spaces. (D) 3D image of Case 16.4

CASE 16.5: STAGE 3 MACULAR HOLE WITH YELLOW DEPOSITS

Case Summary

A 62-year-old woman presented with defective vision in the left eye of 4 months duration. Her best-corrected visual acuity in the left eye was 3/60. Fluorescein angiography in the early phase showed a hyperfluorescent area surrounded by a ring of hypofluorescence which in turn was surrounded by a ring of hyperfluorescence. The late phase showed decreased hyperfluorescence of the lesion (Figures 16.5.1 and 16.5.2).

Optical Coherence Tomography

Horizontal lines scan of the left eye showed the presence of full thickness macular hole. The surrounding retina showed cystic spaces characterized by hyporeflective areas. Hyper-reflective irregularities corresponding to the yellow deposits were evident at the base of the hole (Figures 16.5.3A to F).

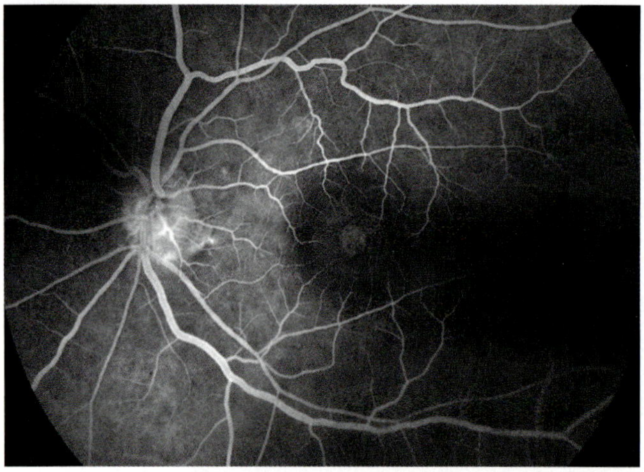

Figure 16.5.1: Early phase fluorescein angiogram showing hyperfluorescence surrounded by a rim of hypofluorescence

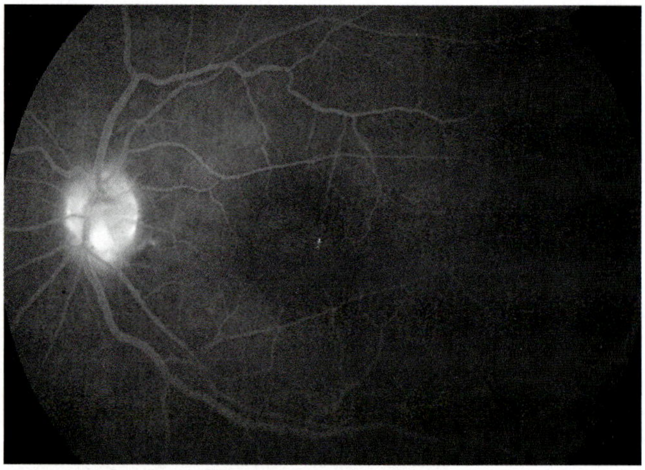

Figure 16.5.2: Late phase fluorescein angiogram showing decrease in hyperfluorescence

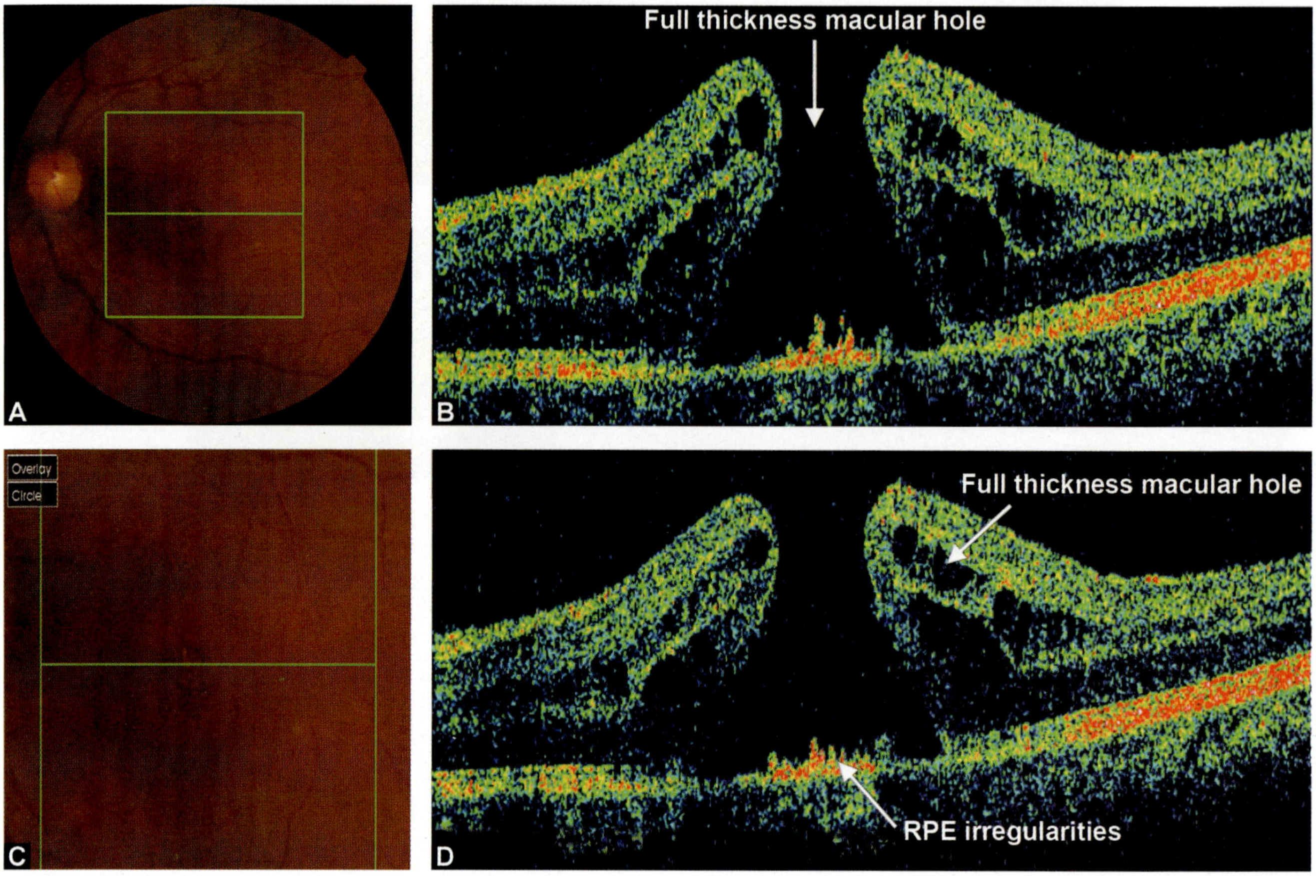

Figures 16.5.3A to D: (A) Color fundus photograph showing the horizontal line scan through the fovea. (B) Horizontal line scan 2D image showing the presence of full thickness macular hole with cystic spaces in the surrounding retina. Hyper-reflective irregularities are evident at the base of the hole. (C) Color fundus photograph (zoomed image) showing the horizontal line scan through the fovea. (D) Horizontal line scan 2D image showing the presence of full thickness macular hole with cystic spaces in the surrounding retina. Hyper-reflective irregularities corresponding to the yellow deposits are evident at the base of the hole

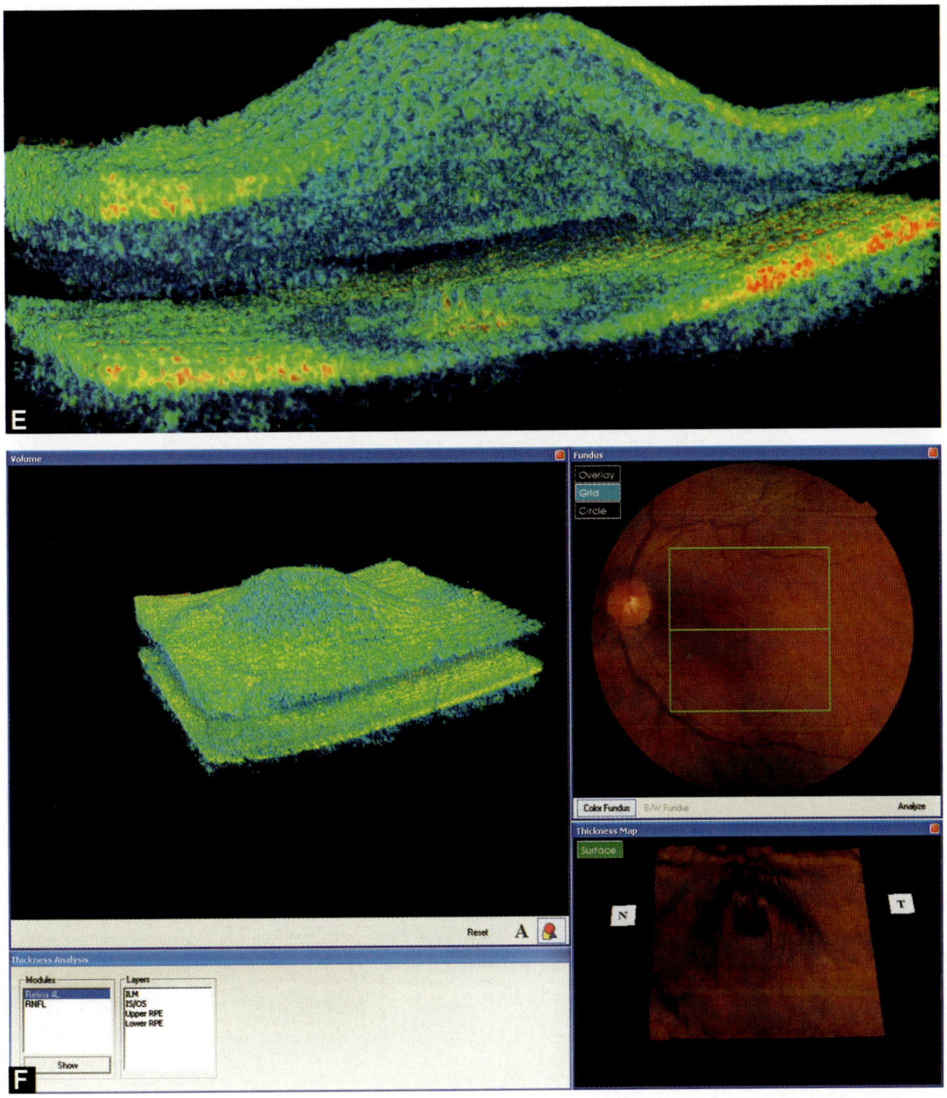

Figures 16.5.3E and F: (E) Cropped 3D image showing the presence of full thickness macular hole with cystic spaces in the surrounding retina. Hyper-reflective irregularities are evident at the base of the hole. (F) 3D image of case 16.5

CASE 16.6: STAGE 4 MACULAR HOLE WITH YELLOW DEPOSITS

Case Summary

A 61-year-old woman presented with defective vision in the left eye of 4 months duration. Her best-corrected visual acuity in the left eye was 6/60; N36

Optical Coherence Tomography

Horizontal lines scan of the left eye showed the presence of full thickness macular hole with cystic spaces in the surrounding retina. In addition, there were hyper-reflective RPE protrusions which corresponded to the yellow deposits seen at the base of the hole. Posterior vitreous detachment was also evident (Figures 16.6.1A to D).

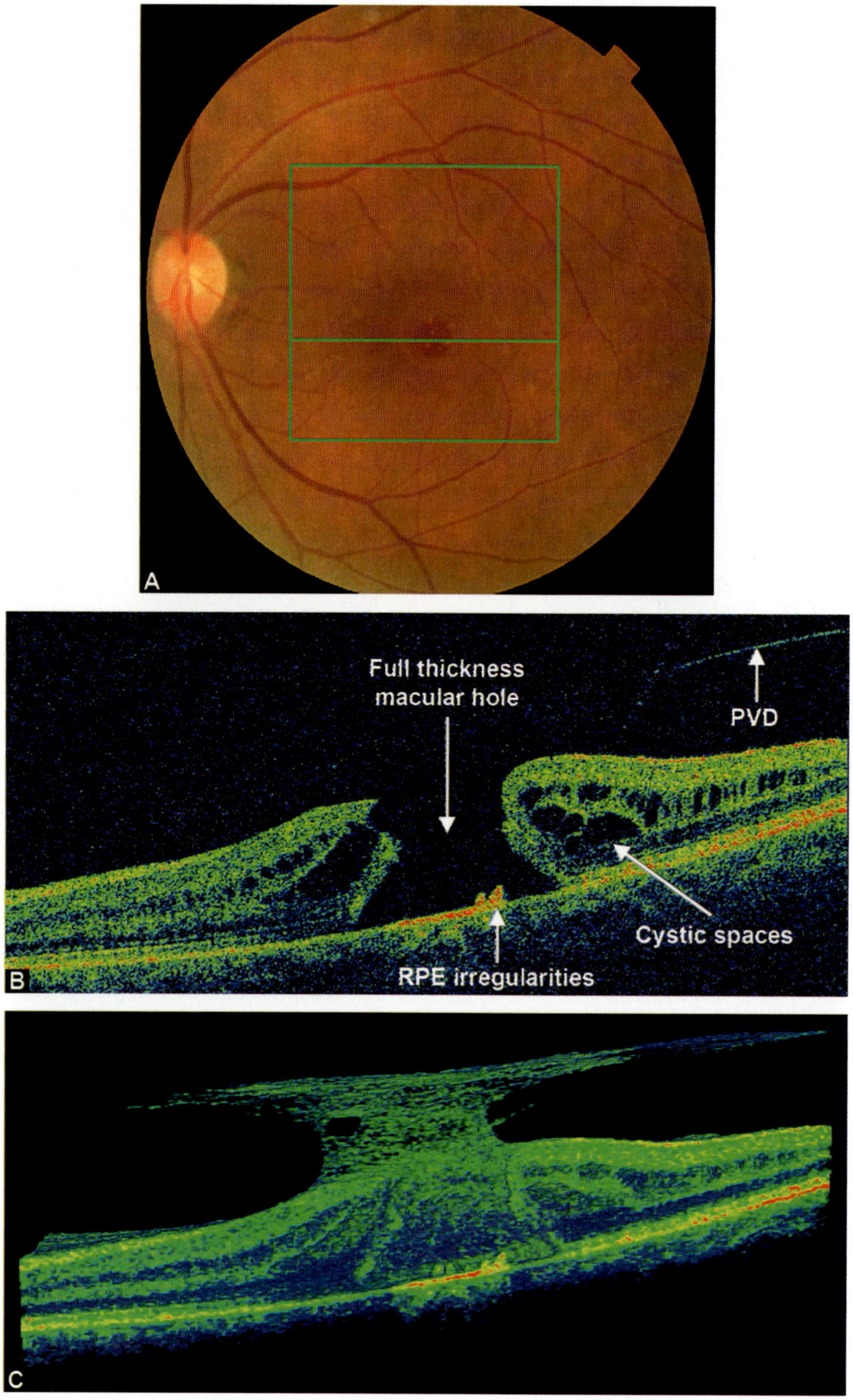

Figures 16.6.1A to C: (A) Color fundus photograph showing the horizontal line scan through the fovea. (B) Horizontal line scan 2D image showing the presence of full thickness macular hole with cystic spaces in the surrounding retina. Hyper-reflective RPE protrusions which correspond to the yellow deposits are seen at the base of the hole. Posterior vitreous detachment is evident. (C) Cropped 3D image showing the presence of full thickness macular hole with cystic spaces in the surrounding retina. Hyper-reflective RPE protrusions which correspond to the yellow deposits are seen at the base of the hole. Posterior vitreous detachment with vitreomacular traction is evident

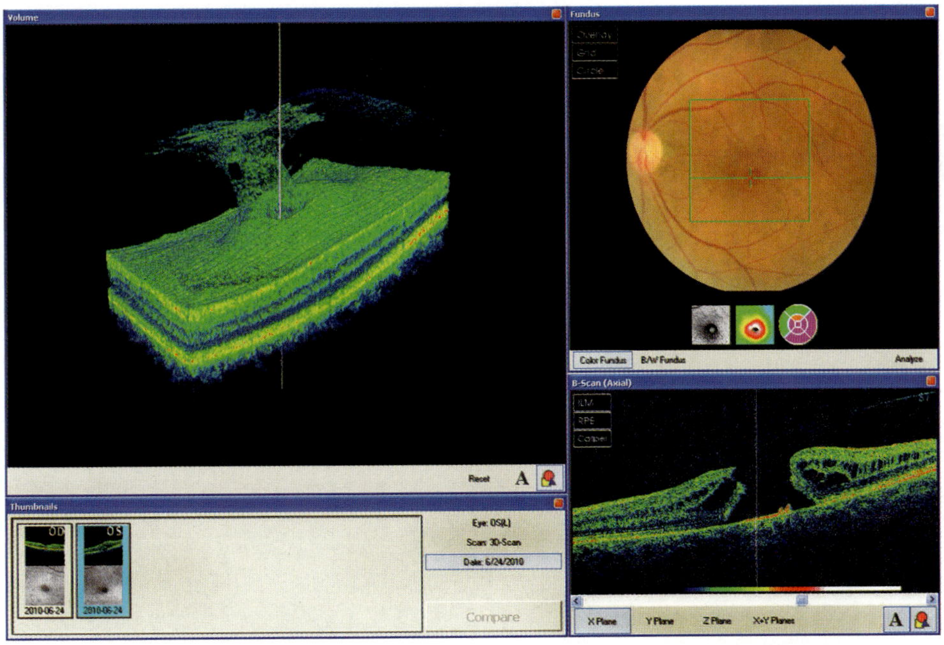

Figure 16.6.1D: 3D image of Case 16.6 **(Images with Topcon 3D OCT-2000)**

SUGGESTED READING

1. Haouchine B, Massin P, Tadayoni R, Erqinay A, Gaudric A. Am J Ophthalmol 2004;138(5):732-9.
2. Hee MR, Puliafito CA, Wong C, Duker JS, Reichel E, Schuman JS, et al. Optical coherence tomography of macular holes. Ophthalmol 1995;102(5):748-56.
3. Ullrich S, Haritoglou C, Gass C, Schaumberger M, Ulbig MW, Kampik A. Macular hole size as a prognostic factor in macular hole surgery. Br J Ophthalmol 2002;86(4):390-3.
4. Witkin AJ, Ko TH, Fujimoto JG, Schuman JS, Baumal CR, Rogers AH, et al. Redefining lamellar holes and the vitreomacular interface: an ultrahigh-resolution optical coherence tomography study. Ophthalmol 2006;113(3):388-97.

17 Medullated Nerve Fibers

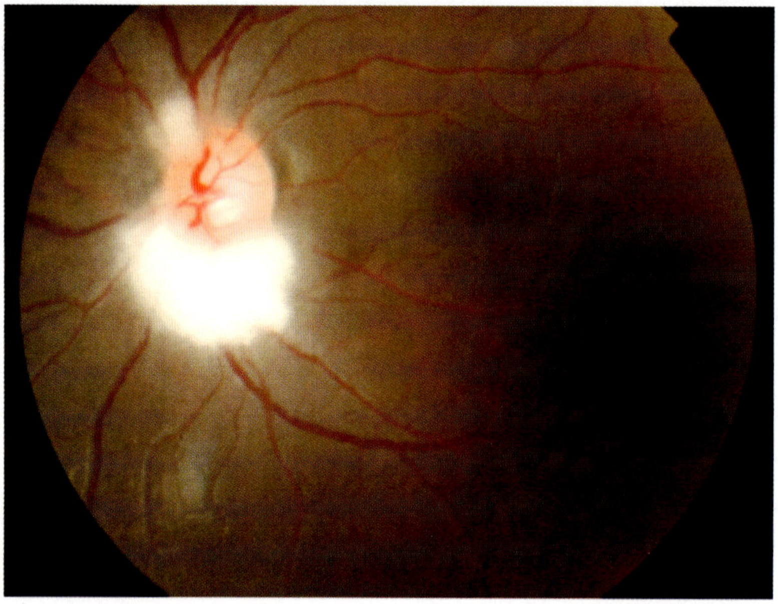

Medullated nerve fiber is a congenital abnormality in which the superficial layer of the nerve fibers fail to demyelinate during the later part of intrauterine life.

Fluorescein angiography shows masking of the retinal vessels without any evidence of leakage.

Optical coherence tomography shows increased reflectivity in the superficial layers.

CASE 17.1: MEDULLATED NERVE FIBERS

Case Summary

A 23- year-old female was seen for a routine eye examination. Her best-corrected visual acuity in the left eye was 6/12. Fluorescein angiography showed fuzziness overlying the vessels at the superior and inferior portions of the disc (Figures 17.1.1 and 17.1.2).

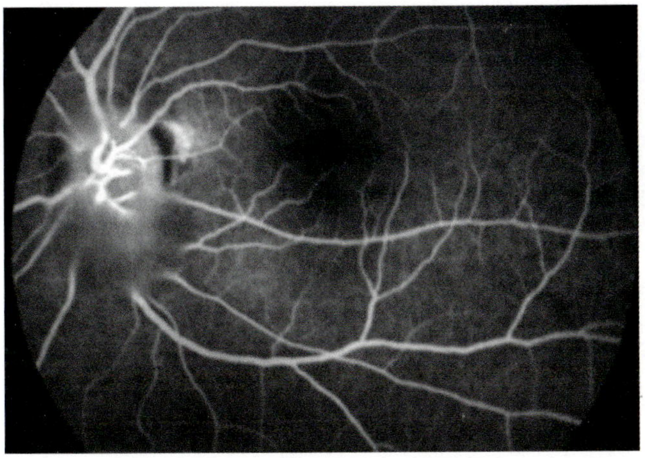

Figure 17.1.1: Early phase angiogram showing fuzziness overlying the vessels adjacent to the disc

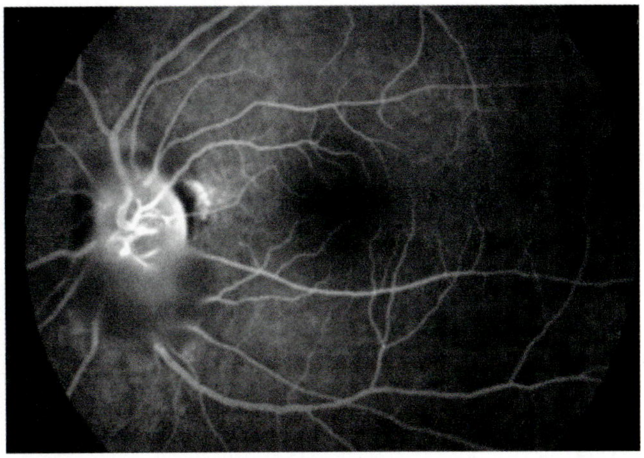

Figure 17.1.2: Late phase angiogram showing fuzziness overlying the vessels adjacent to the disc

Optical Coherence Tomography

Horizontal line scan through the medullated nerve fibers showed hyper-reflectivity (Figures 17.1.3A to D).

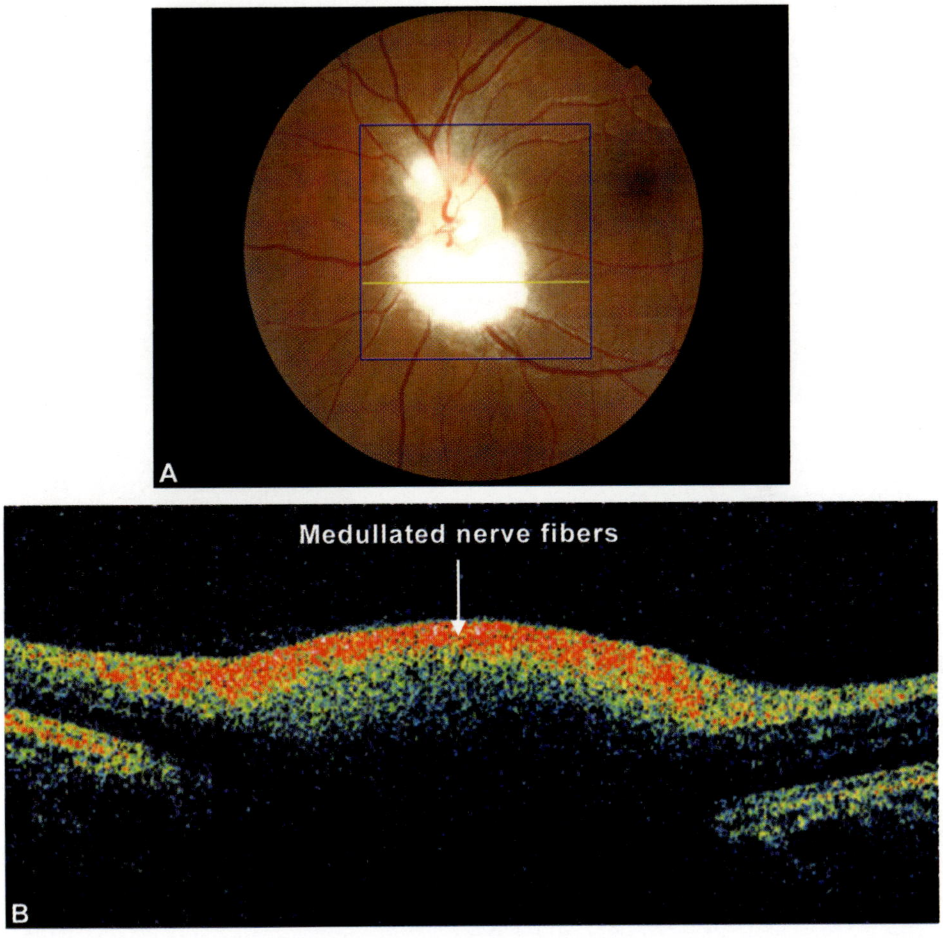

Figures 17.1.3A and B: (A) Color fundus photograph showing the horizontal line scan passing through the medullated nerve fibers. (B) Horizontal line scan through the medullated nerve fibers 2D image showing hyper-reflectivity

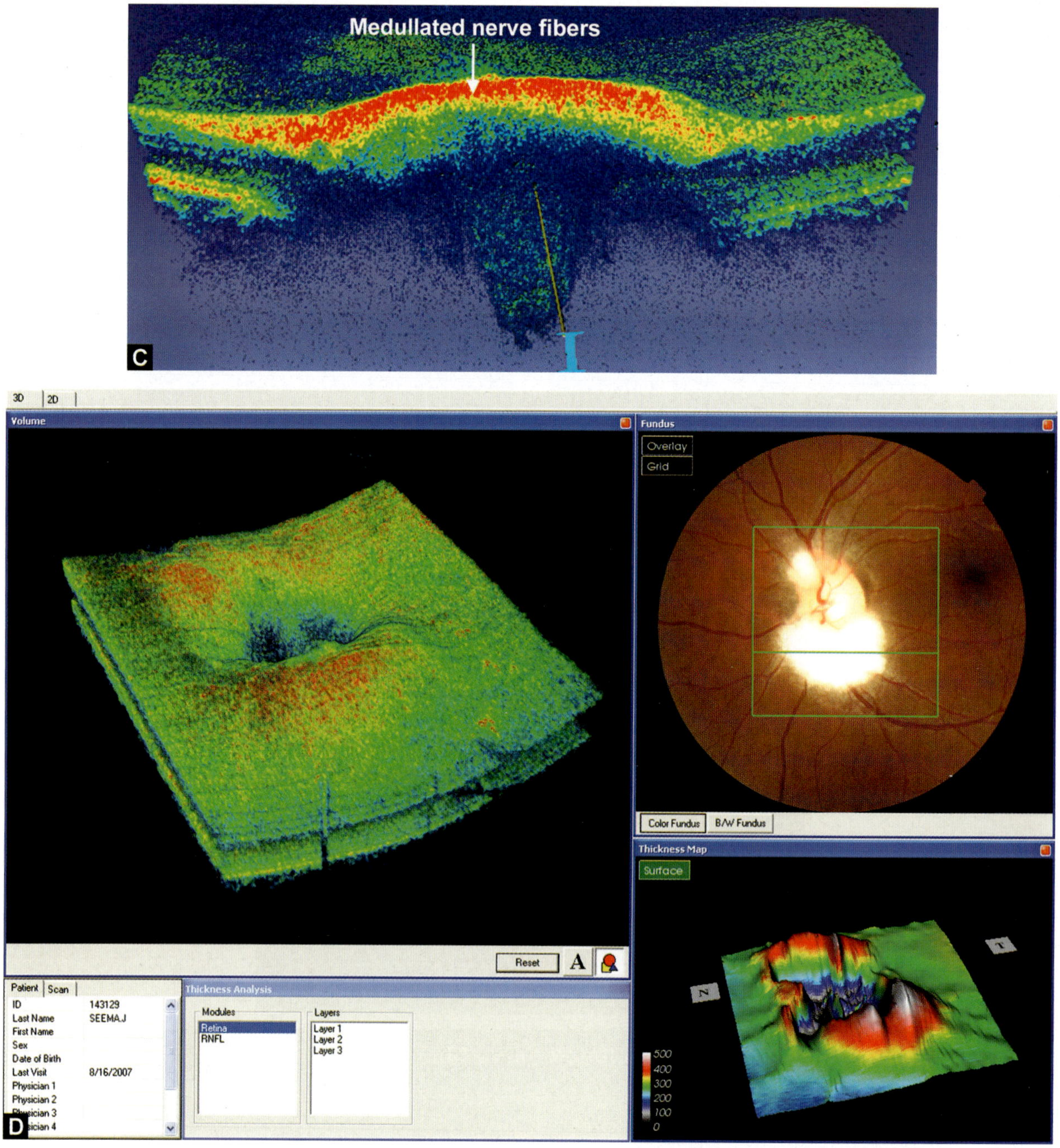

Figures 17.1.3C and D: (C) Cropped 3D image showing hyper-reflectivity. (D) 3D image of Case 17.1

18 Neovascular Age-related Macular Degeneration

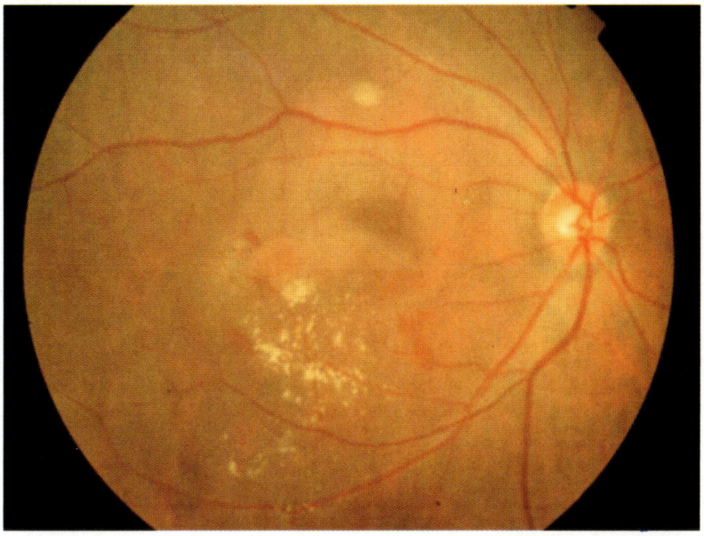

Age-related macular degeneration (ARMD) is the leading cause of irreversible visual loss. It is a bilateral disorder with CNV membranes developing in 26 percent of eyes that were initially free of neovascular ARMD. Neovascular ARMD is characterized by the formation of choroidal neovascularization initially under the RPE resulting in clinical findings such as subretinal hemorrhage, subretinal fluid, retinal edema, RPE detachments, and, eventually, disciform scarring.

Macular photocoagulation study investigators defined two rapid sequence fluorescein angiography (RSFA) leakage patterns for choroidal neovascularization:

1. Classic, which results in discrete and early hyperfluorescence with late leakage into the overlying neurosensory retinal detachment.
2. Occult, which in turn is categorized into two basic forms:
   i. Late leakage of undetermined source manifests as regions of stippled or ill-defined leakage into an overlying neurosensory retinal detachment, without a distinct source identified on the early frames of the angiogram.
   ii. Fibrovascular PEDs appear as irregular elevation of the RPE associated with stippled leakage into an overlying neurosensory retinal detachment in the early and late frames of the angiogram.

Depending on the distance from the foveal avascular zone, the leakage is classified as subfoveal, juxtafoveal (1-199 μm) or extrafoveal (200-250 μm).

Role of OCT

1. OCT makes it possible to image all of the components of neovascular age-related macular degeneration. The typical components include serous elevation of the retinal pigment epithelium, serous elevation of the retina, and subretinal pigment epithelial and subretinal hemorrhages. Hard exudates can be found at the peripheral borders of the serous detachments. Choroidal neovascular membranes result in these serous elevations and hemorrhages.
2. OCT is useful in the detection of occult CNV, which are difficult to identify clinically and with fluorescein angiography.
3. OCT is particularly useful in the evaluation of the results of photodynamic therapy (PDT), indocyanine green mediated photothrombosis (i-MP), transpupillary thermotherapy (TTT) and the new antiangiogenic therapies.

Following PDT, 5 stages have been described:

Stage 1: Seen within one week of therapy and characterized by acute inflammatory response with increase in subrertinal fluid.

Stage 2: Seen within 1-4 weeks of treatment and characterized by resolution of serous fluid with restoration of the foveal contour.

Stage 3: Seen between 4-12 weeks and is characterized by the presence of either greater subretinal fluid relative to fibrous tissue suggestive of active CNV Stage 3a or more fibrous tissue with minimal subretinal fluid suggesting inactivity Stage 3b.

Stage 4: Characterized by the presence of cystoid spaces.

Stage 5: Resolution of subretinal fluid with thinning of the retina and merging of fibrous tissue with it.

CASE 18.1: NEOVASCULAR ARMD

Case Summary

A 58-year-old woman presented with metamorphopsia in the right eye. Her best-corrected visual acuity was 6/24 in this eye. Fluorescein angiography showed a large subfoveal predominantly classic CNVM with a surrounding rim of subretinal hemorrhage (Figures 18.1.1 and 18.1.2).

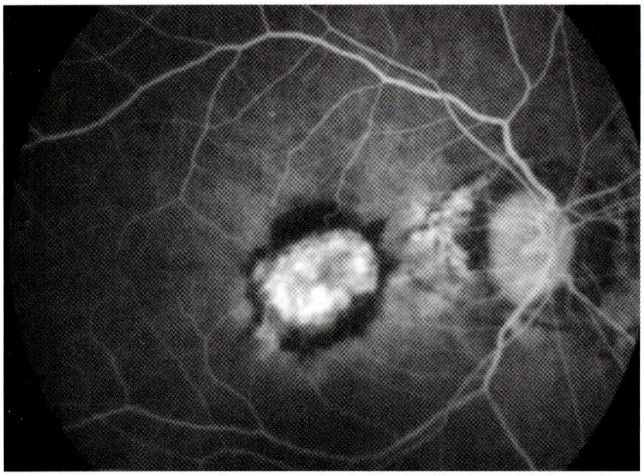

Figure 18.1.1: Early phase angiogram showing classic CNVM

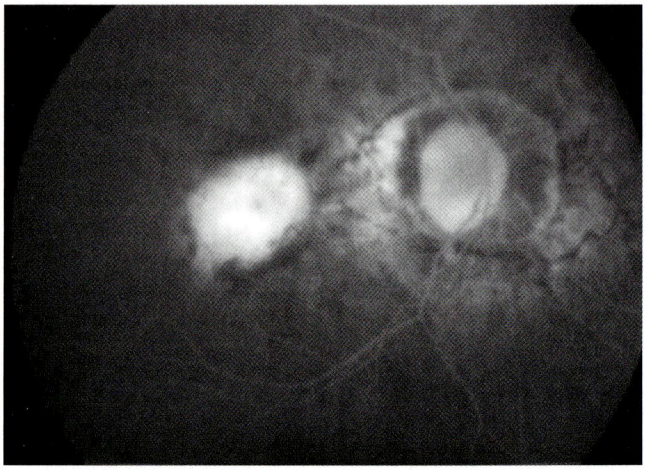

Figure 18.1.2: Late phase angiogram showing classic CNVM

Optical Coherence Tomography

Horizontal line scan showed an area of moderate reflectivity with overlying retinal edema and minimal subretinal fluid indicating an active CNVM (Figures 18.1.3A to D).

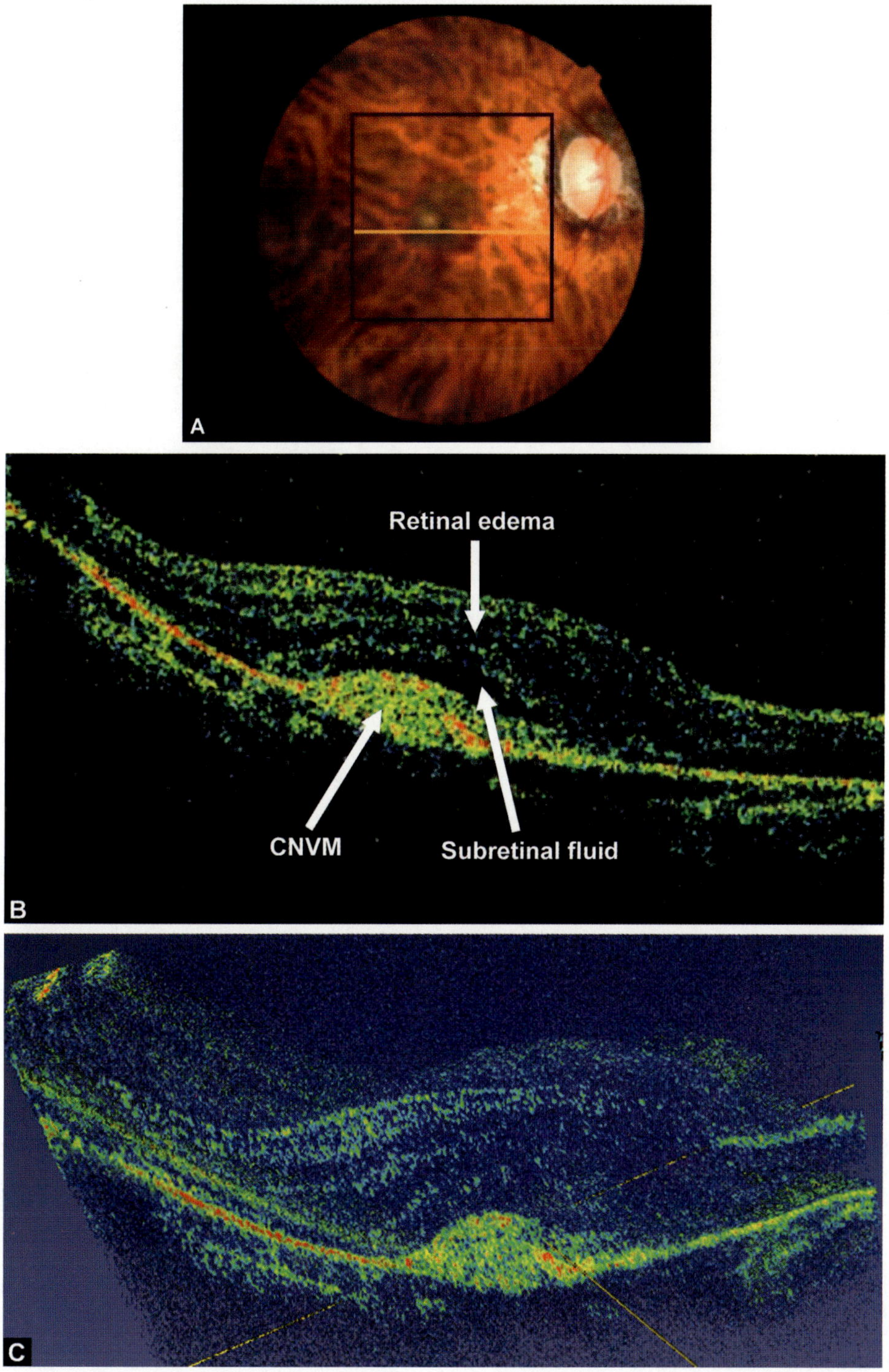

Figures 18.1.3A to C: (A) Color fundus photograph showing the horizontal line scan through the fovea. (B) Horizontal line scan 2D image showing an area of moderate reflectivity with overlying retinal edema and minimal subretinal fluid indicating an active CNVM. (C) Cropped 3D image showing the an area of moderate reflectivity with overlying retinal edema and minimal subretinal fluid indicating an active CNVM

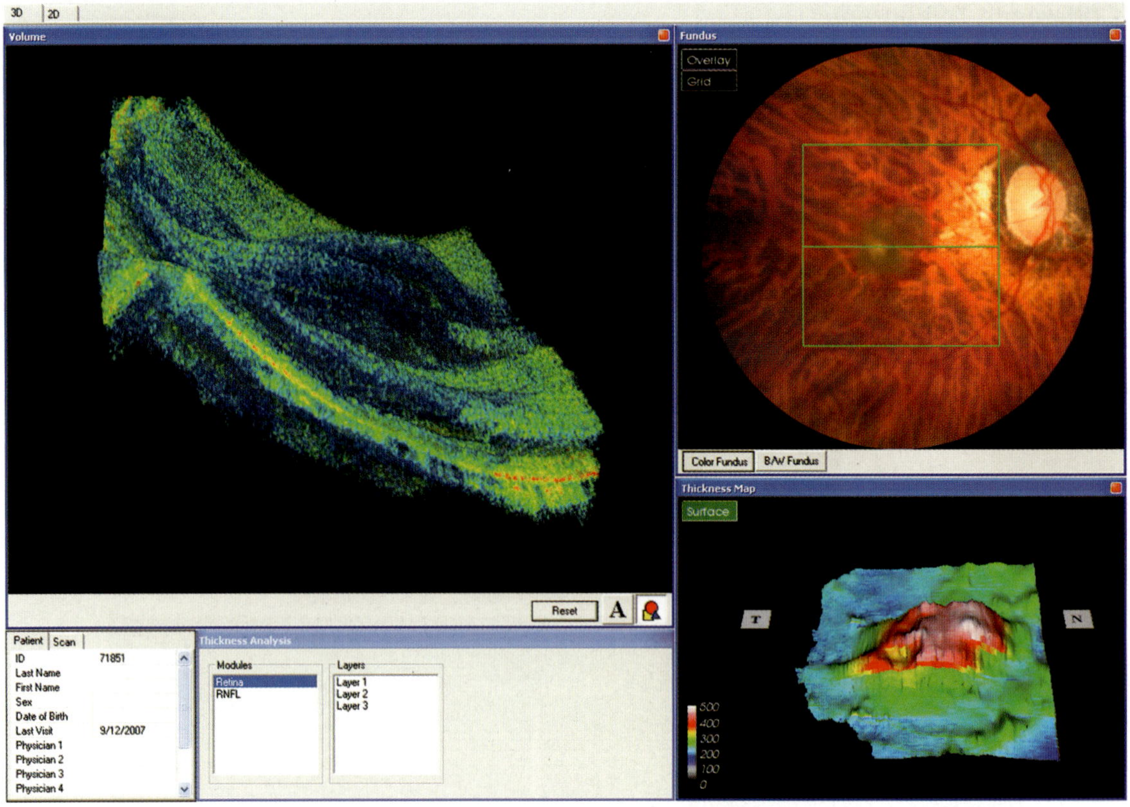

Figure 18.1.3D: 3D image of Case 18.1

CASE 18.2: NEOVASCULAR ARMD

Case Summary

A 72-year-old man presented with difficulty in reading and metamorphopsia in the right eye of five months duration. His best-corected visual acuity was 6/18 in this eye. Fluorescein angiography showed a hemorrhagic pigment epithelial detachment with evidence of occult CNVM (Figures 18.2.1 and 18.2.2).

Indocyanine green angiography showed the extent of the CNVM (Figures 18.2.3 and 18.2.4).

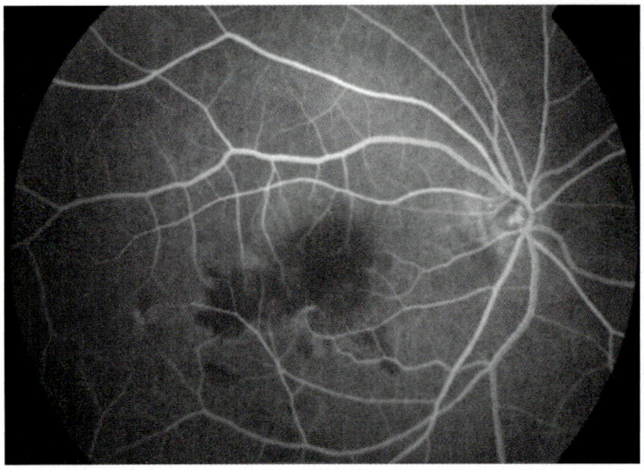

Figure 18.2.1: Early phase angiogram showing blocked fluorescence due to hemorrhage

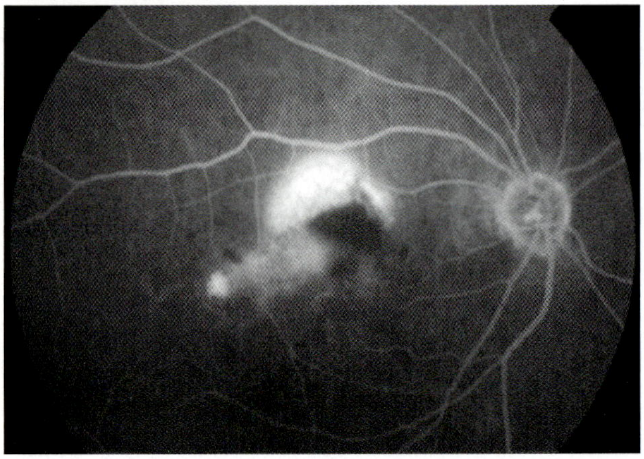

Figure 18.2.2: Late phase angiogram showing hemorrhagic PED and occult CNVM

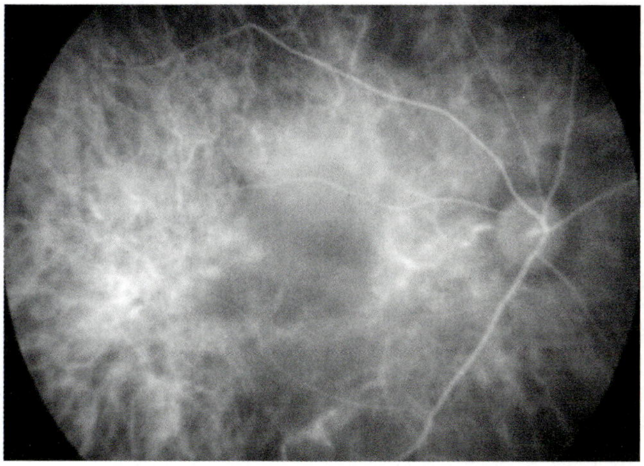

Figure 18.2.3: Early phase ICG showing CNVM

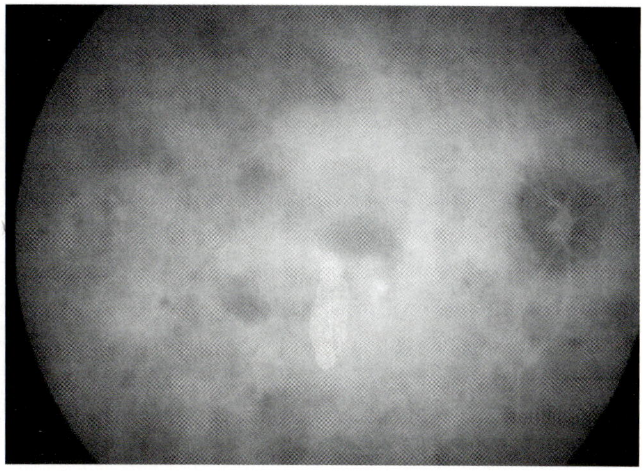

Figure 18.2.4: Late phase ICG showing CNVM

Optical Coherence Tomography–1

Horizontal line scan showed a large elevation of the RPE consistent with RPE detachment. The blood cells contained within the detachment induce a shadow effect that prevents the choriocapillaris from being seen. Serous elevation of the retinal can be seen on either side of the RPE detachment (Figures 18.2.5A to D).

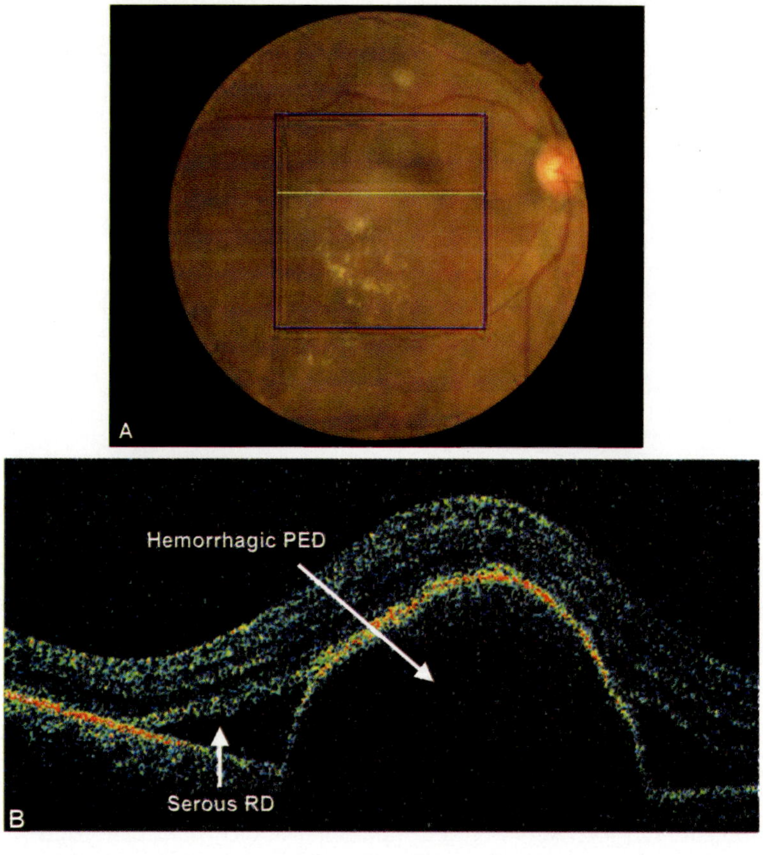

Figures 18.2.5A and B: (A) Color fundus photograph showing the horizontal line scan passing through the hemorrhagic PED. (B) Horizontal line scan 2D image showing a large elevation of the RPE consistent with RPE detachment. The blood cells contained within the detachment induce a shadow effect that prevents the choriocapillaris from being seen. Serous elevation of the retinal can be seen on either side of the RPE detachment

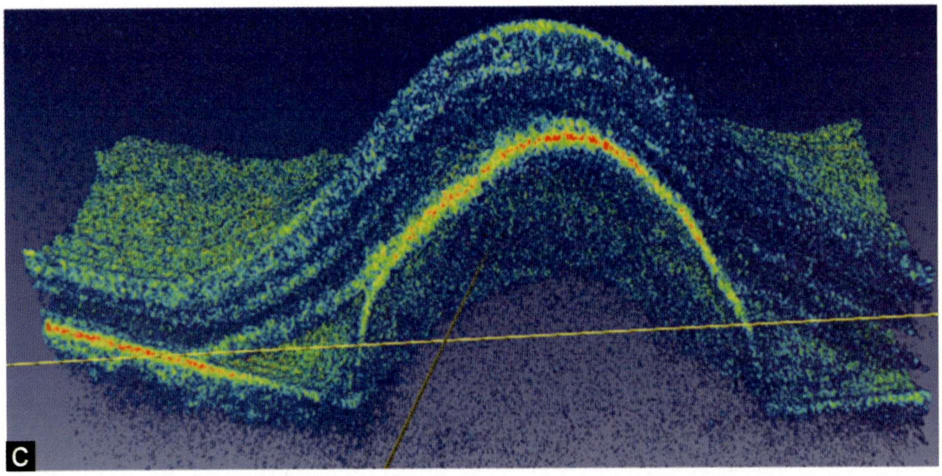

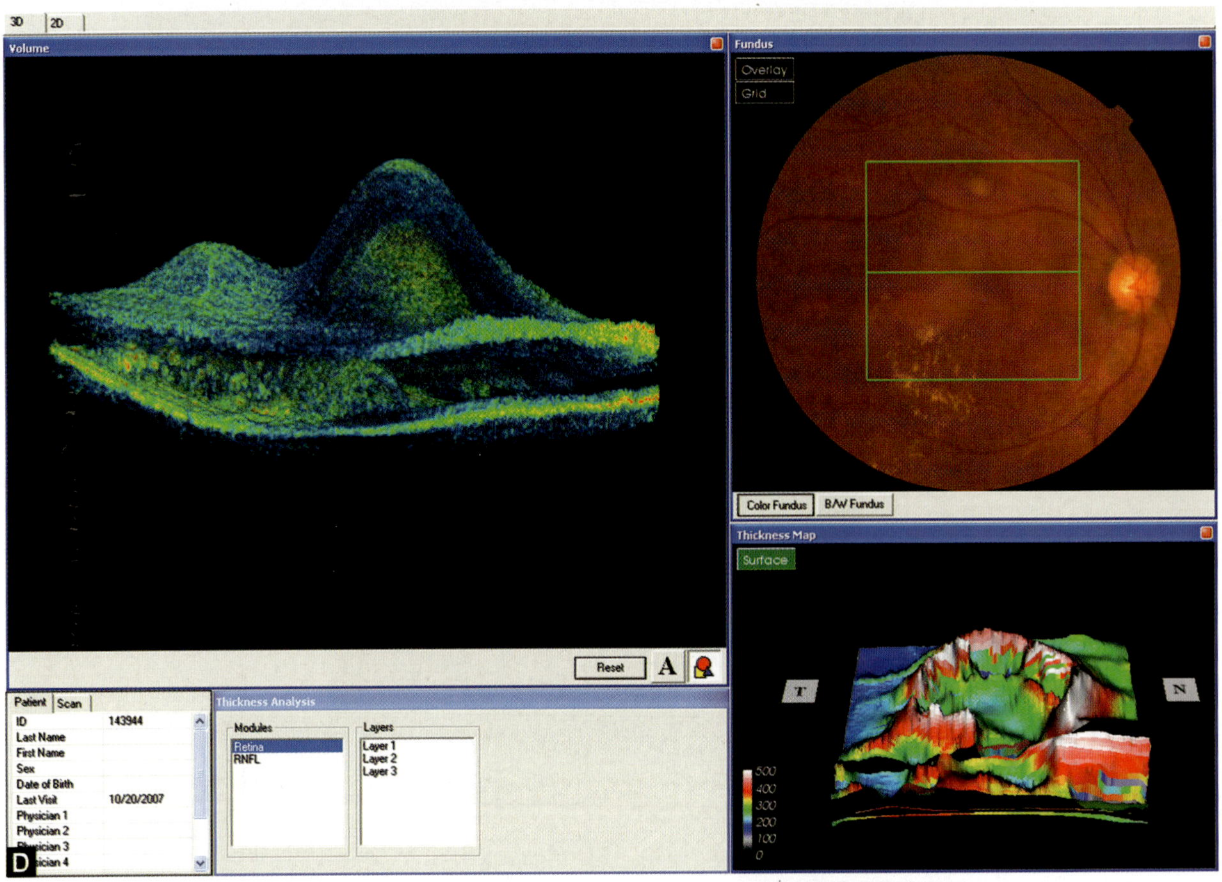

Figures 18.2.5C and D: (C) Cropped 3D image showing a large elevation of the RPE consistent with RPE detachment. The blood cells contained within the detachment induce a shadow effect that prevents the choriocapillaris from being seen. Serous elevation of the retinal can be seen on either side of the RPE detachment. (D) 3D image of Case 18.2

Optical Coherence Tomography–2

Horizontal line scan showed a hemorrhagic pigment epithelial detachment. On the right side of the detachment, the retinal pigment epithelium is disrupted due to the presence of a choroidal neovascular membrane (Figures 18.2.5E to G).

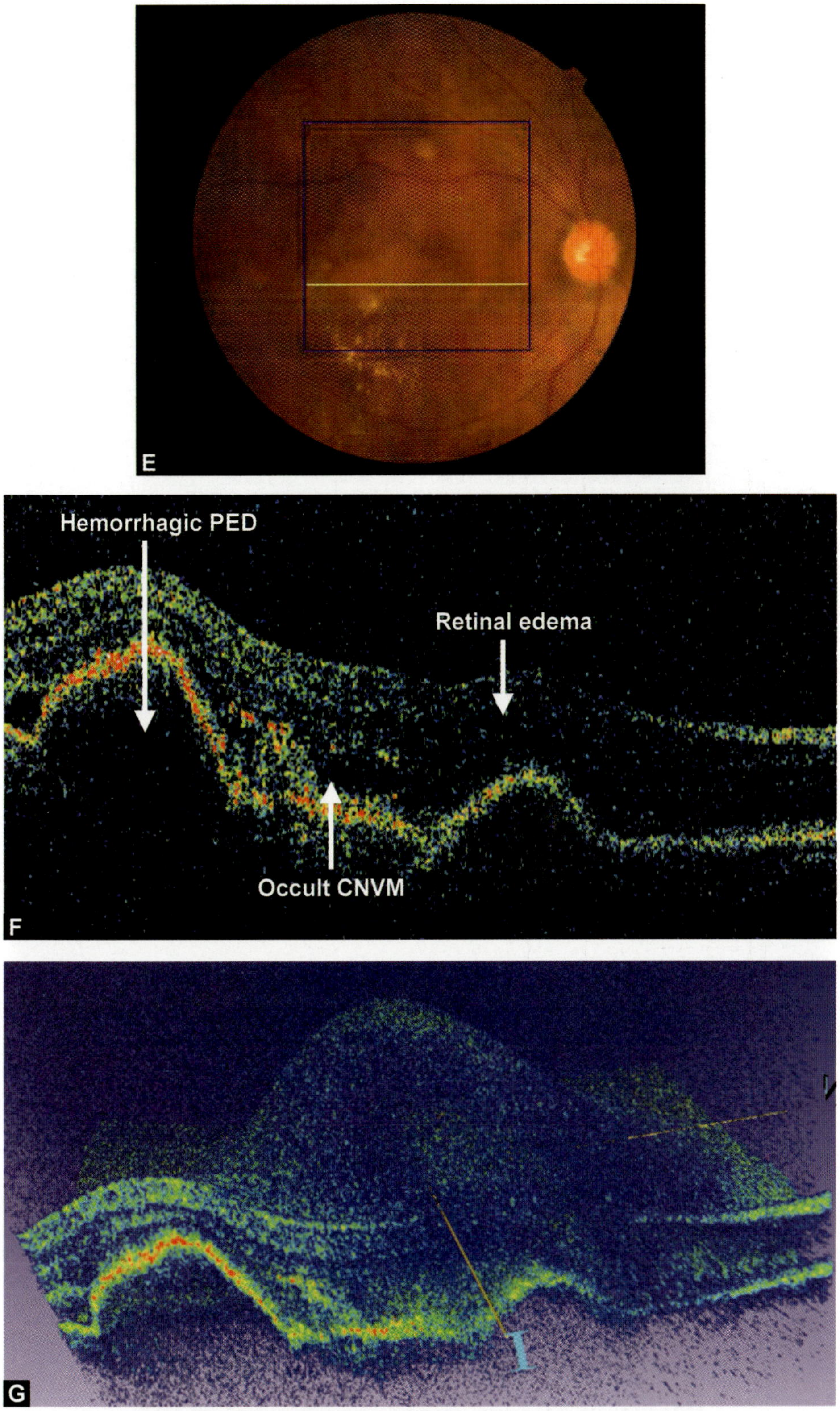

Figures 18.2.5E to G: (E) Color fundus photograph showing the horizontal line scan through the occult CNVM. (F) Horizontal line scan 2D image showing a hemorrhagic pigment epithelial detachment. On the right side of the detachment, the retinal pigment epithelium is disrupted due to the presence of a choroidal neovascular membrane. (G) Cropped 3D image showing a hemorrhagic pigment epithelial detachment. On the right side of the detachment, the retinal pigment epithelium is disrupted due to the presence of a choroidal neovascular membrane

CASE 18.3: NEOVASCULAR ARMD WITH RPE TEAR

Case Summary

A 65-year-old man presented with decreased vision in the left eye of 2 years duration. His best-corrected visual acuity in this eye was counting fingers. Fluorescein angiography showed a classic choroidal neovascular membrane (Figures 18.3.1 and 18.3.2).

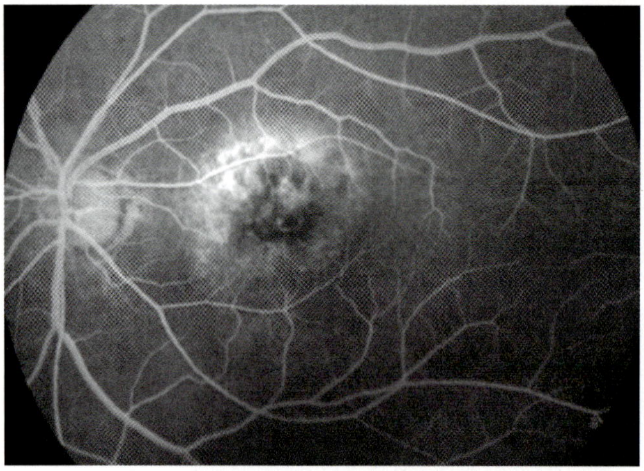

Figure 18.3.1: Early phase angiogram showing classic CNVM

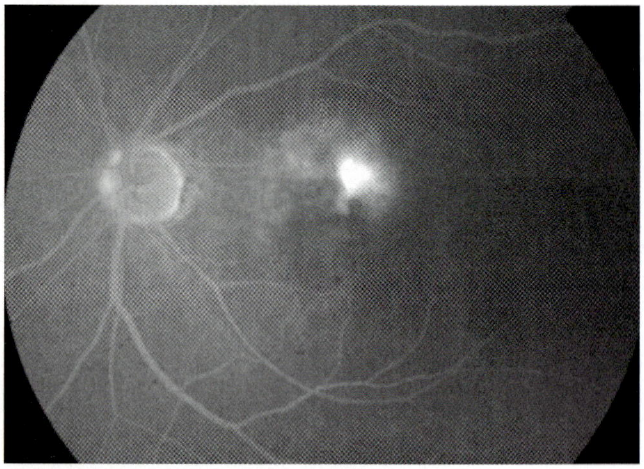

Figure 18.3.2: Late phase angiogram showing classic CNVM

Optical Coherence Tomography

Horizontal line scan showed an area of moderate reflectivity in front of the retinal pigment epithelium in the subfoveal region consistent with classic choroidal neovascularization. The cystic spaces with retinal thickening indicate that the CNV is active. A retinal pigment epithelial detachment with a tear was evident. The detachment contained blood cells that induced a dense shadow on the posterior layers. The detached posterior hyaloid was seen anterior to the retinal surface (Figures 18.3.3A to D).

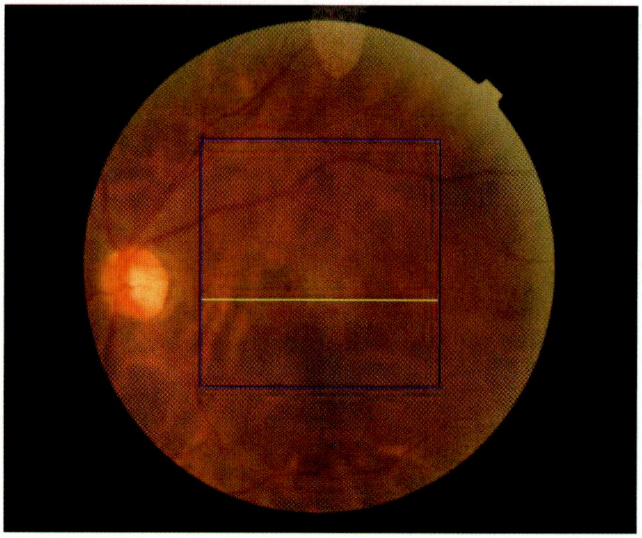

Figure 18.3.3A: Color fundus photograph showing the horizontal line scan through the fovea

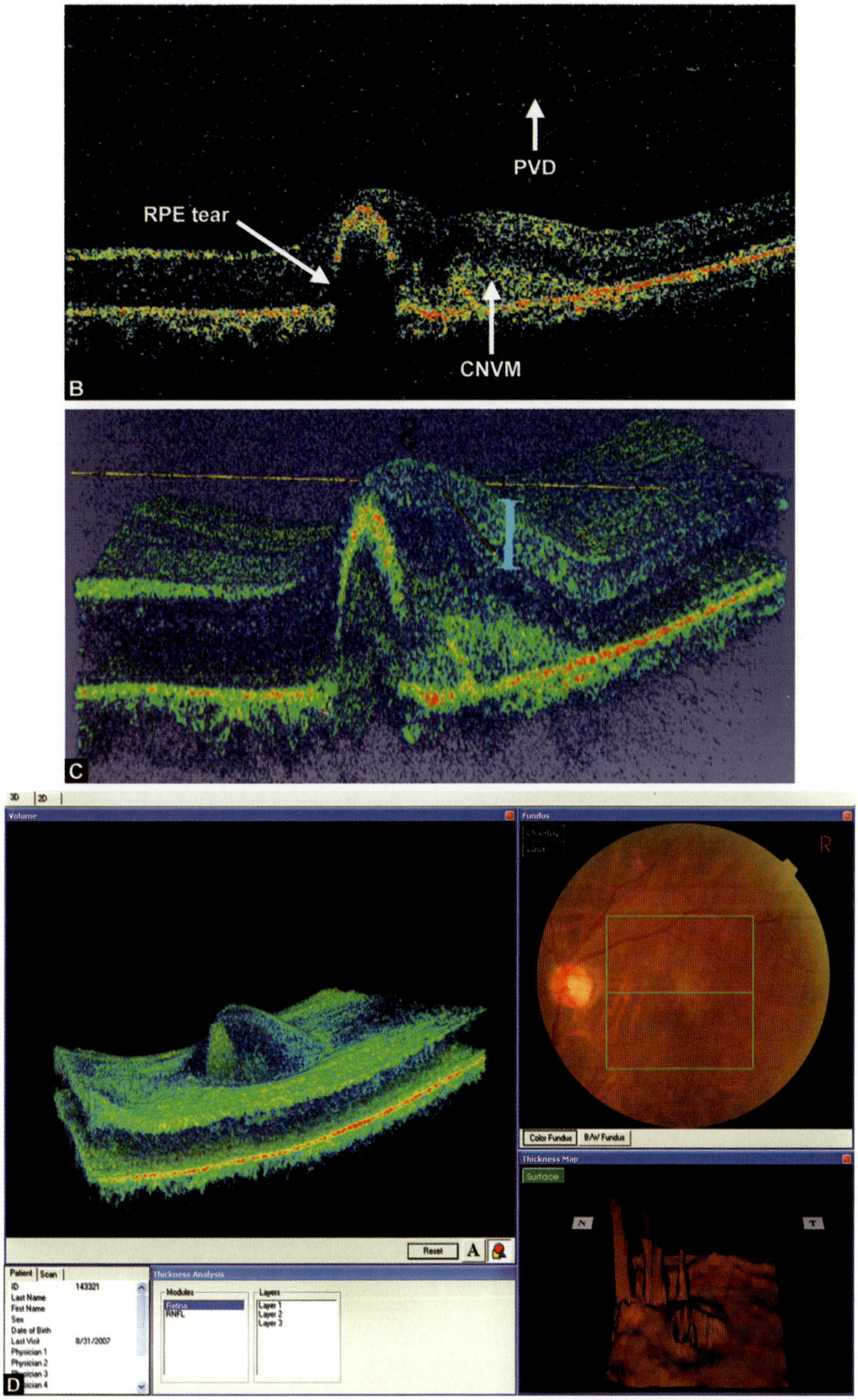

Figures 18.3.3B to D: (B) Horizontal line scan 2D image showing an area of moderate reflectivity, cystic spaces and a pigment epithelial detachment with a tear. The detachment contains blood cells that induce a dense shadow on the posterior layers. The detached posterior hyaloid is seen anterior to the retinal surface. (C) Cropped 3D image showing an area of moderate reflectivity, cystic spaces and a pigment epithelial detachment with a tear. The detachment contains blood cells that induce a dense shadow on the posterior layers. The detached posterior hyaloid is seen anterior to the retinal surface. (D) 3D image of Case 18.3

CASE 18.4: NEOVASCULAR ARMD TREATED WITH INDOCYANINE GREEN MEDIATED PHOTOTHROMBOSIS (i-MP)

Case Summary

A 68-year-old woman presented with decreased vision in the right eye. Her best-corrected visual acuity in this eye was 2/60. Fluorescein angiography showed an extensive area of increasing hyperfluorescence from RPE changes with dense areas within, suggestive of occult CNV (Figures 18.4.1 and 18.4.2).

Indocyanine green angiography confirmed the presence of CNV in the juxtafoveal area with an area of RPE change temporal to it with loss of choriocapillaris (Figures 18.4.3 and 18.4.4).

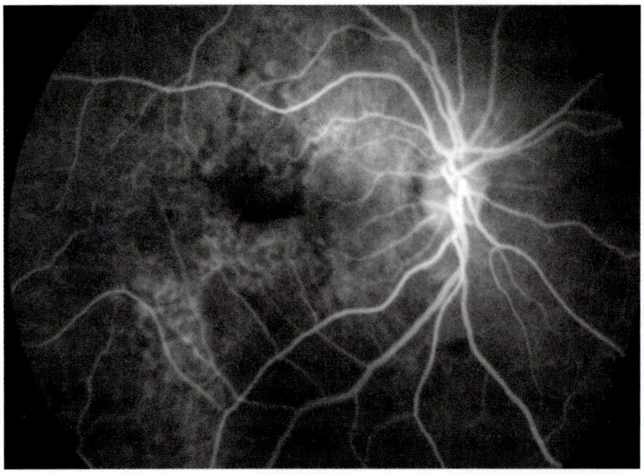

Figure 18.4.1: Early phase angiogram showing RPE mottling

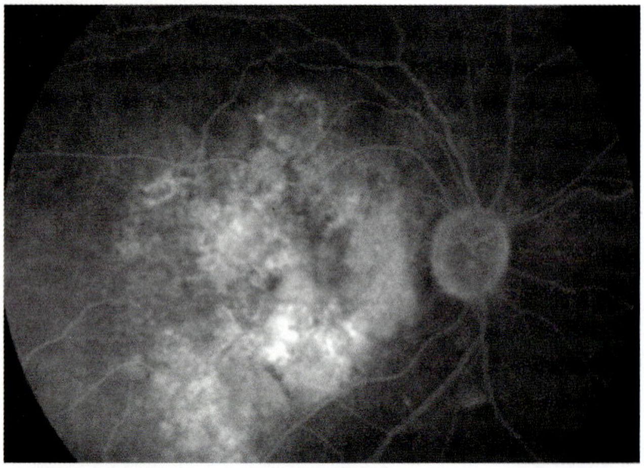

Figure 18.4.2: Late phase angiogram showing occult CNVM

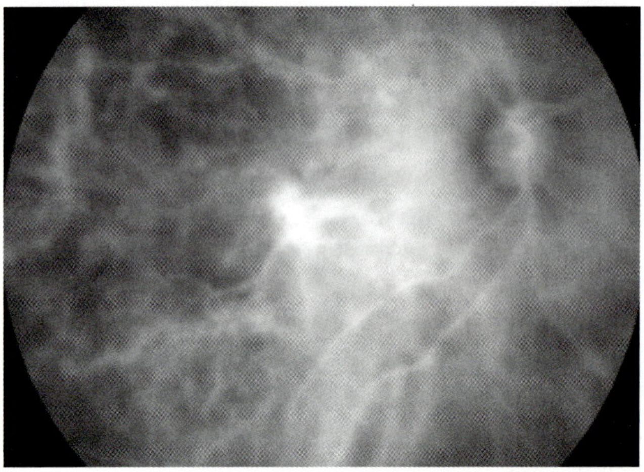

Figure 18.4.3: Early phase ICG showing CNVM

Figure 18.4.4: Late phase ICG showing CNVM

Optical Coherence Tomography

Horizontal line scan showed undulations in the RPE consistent with drusen.There were areas of severely disrupted and thickened RPE with poorly defined boundaries suggestive of an occult CNV with overlying retinal edema (Figures 18.4.5A to E). The patient was treated with Indocyanine green-mediated photothrombosis.

Follow-up

One month following i-MP, repeat OCT showed increase in retinal edema with reduction in the CNVM (Figures 18.4.6A to E).

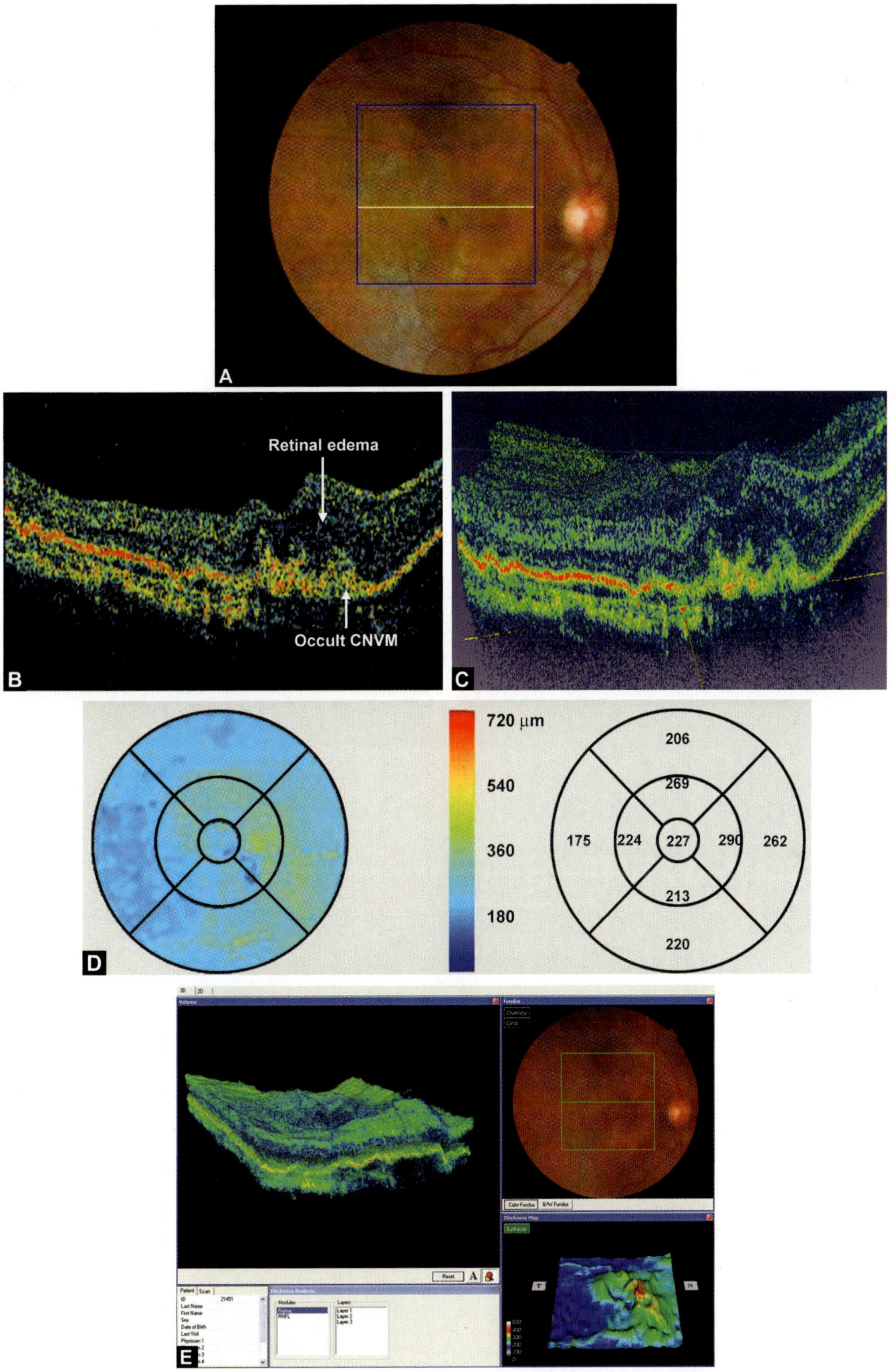

Figures 18.4.5A to E: (A) Color fundus photograph showing the horizontal line scan passing through the CNVM. (B) Horizontal line scan 2D image showing undulations in the RPE consistent with drusen. Areas of severely disrupted and thickened RPE with poorly defined boundaries suggestive of an occult CNV with overlying retinal edema is evident. (C) Cropped 3D image showing undulations in the RPE consistent with drusen. Areas of severely disrupted and thickened RPE with poorly defined boundaries suggestive of an occult CNV with overlying retinal edema is evident. (D) Macular thickness map showing foveal thickness measuring 227µm. (E) 3D image of Case 18.4

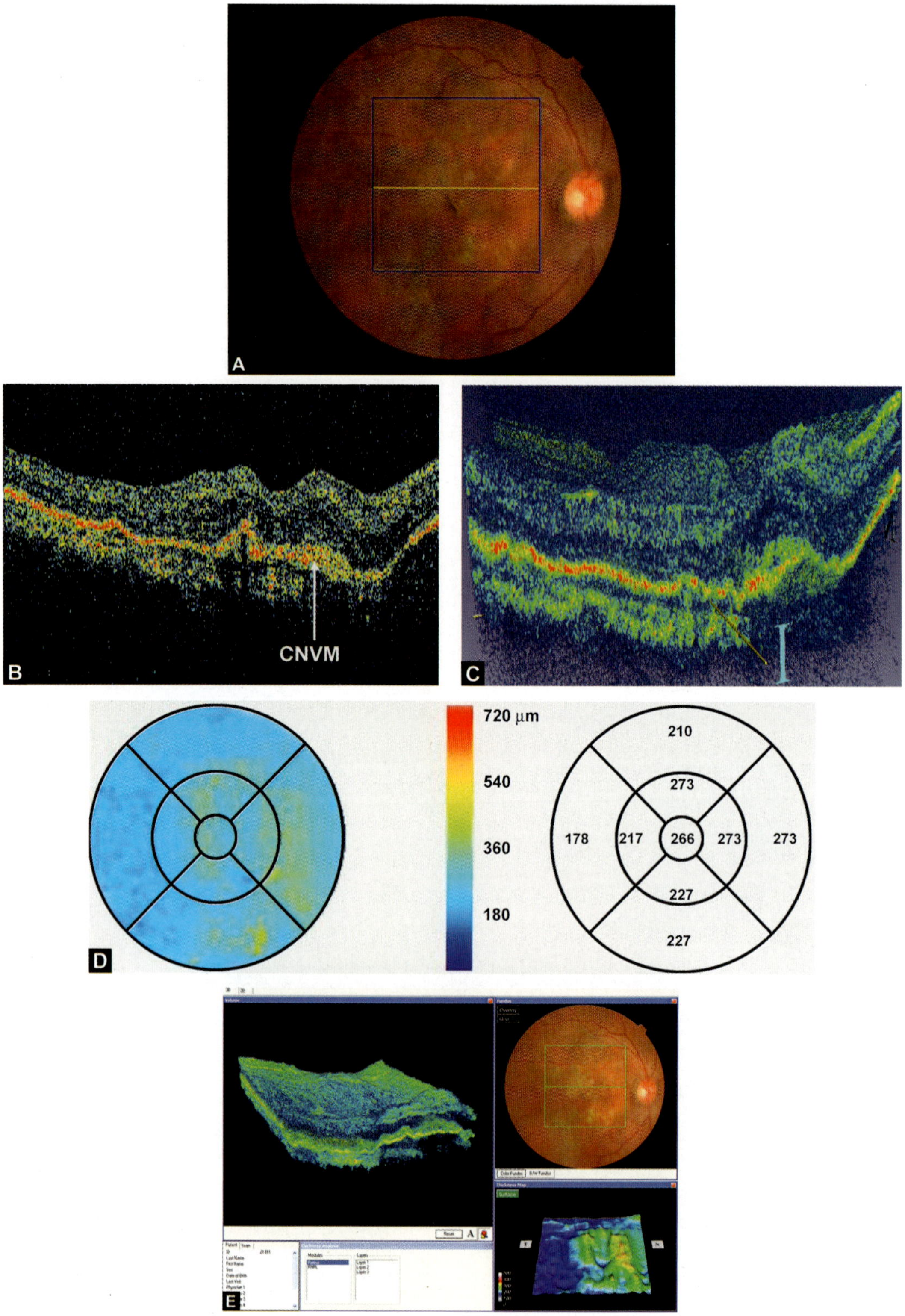

Figures 18.4.6A to E: (A) Color fundus photograph 1month following i-MP showing the horizontal line scan passing through the CNVM. (B) Horizontal line scan 2D image showing increase in retinal edema with reduction in the CNVM. (C) Cropped 3D image showing increase in retinal edema with reduction in the CNVM. (D) Macular thickness map showing increase in foveal thickness measuring 266 µm. (E) 3D image of Case 18.4, one month following i-MP

Repeat OCT done at 3 months follow-up showed reactionary edema with no evidence of CNV (Figure 18.4.7).

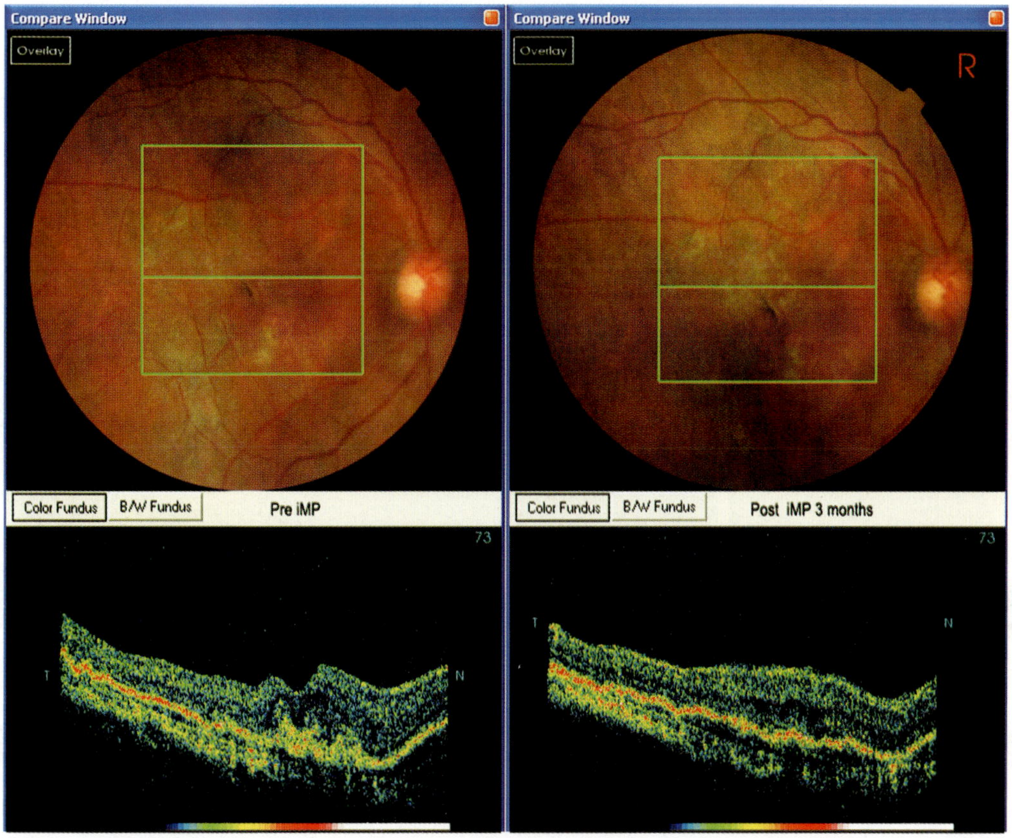

Figure 18.4.7: At 3 months post i-MP, reactionary edema with no evidence of CNV is seen

CASE 18.5: NEOVASCULAR ARMD (IMAGING WITH TOPCON 3D OCT-2000)

Case Summary

A 54-year-old man presented with decreased vision in the left eye of two months duration. His best-corrected visual acuity was 6/24 in this eye. Fluorescein angiography showed subretinal hemorrhage and a classic choroidal neovascular membrane (Figures 18.5.1 and 18.5.2)

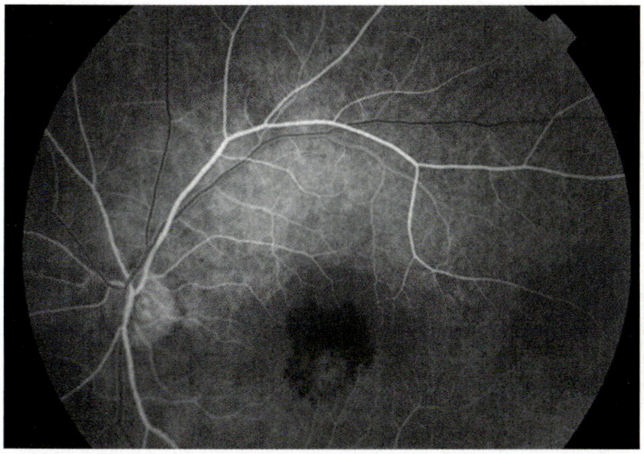

Figure 18.5.1: Early phase angiogram showing classic CNVM

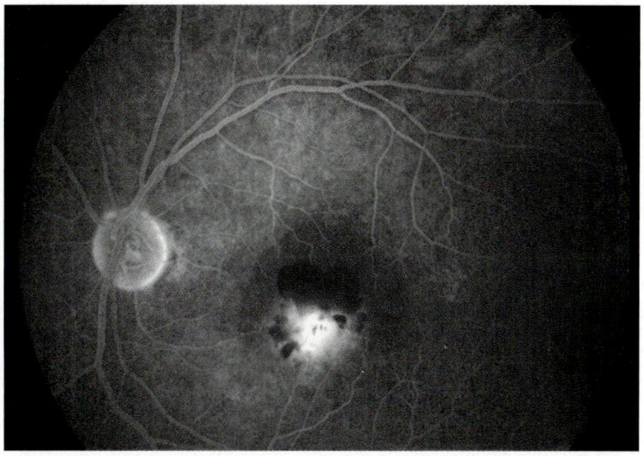

Figure 18.5.2: Late phase angiogram showing classic CNVM

Optical Coherence Tomography

Horizontal line scan showed the presence of a hyporeflective space consistent with serous retinal detachment (Figures 18.5.3A and B).

Horizontal line scan showed an area of moderate reflectivity underlying the external limiting membrane corresponding to the area of subretinal hemorrhage (Figures 18.5.3C and D).

Horizontal line scan showed disruption of the RPE with an overlying area of moderate reflectivity beneath an intact external limiting membrane consistent with choroidal neovascularization. In addition, serous fluid accumulation can be seen on either side of the lesion (Figures 18.5.3E and F).

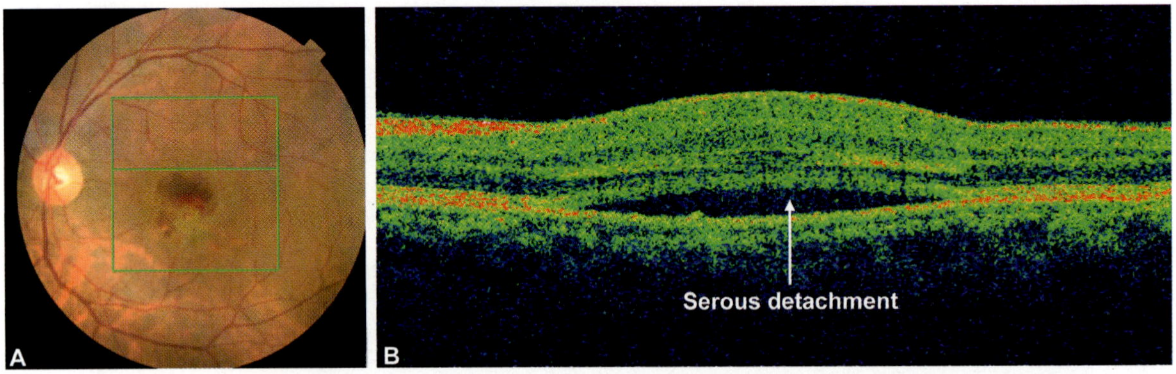

Figures 18.5.3A and B: (A) Color fundus photograph showing the horizontal line scan passing above the fovea. (B) Horizontal line scan 2D image showing the presence of a hyporeflective space consistent with serous retinal detachment

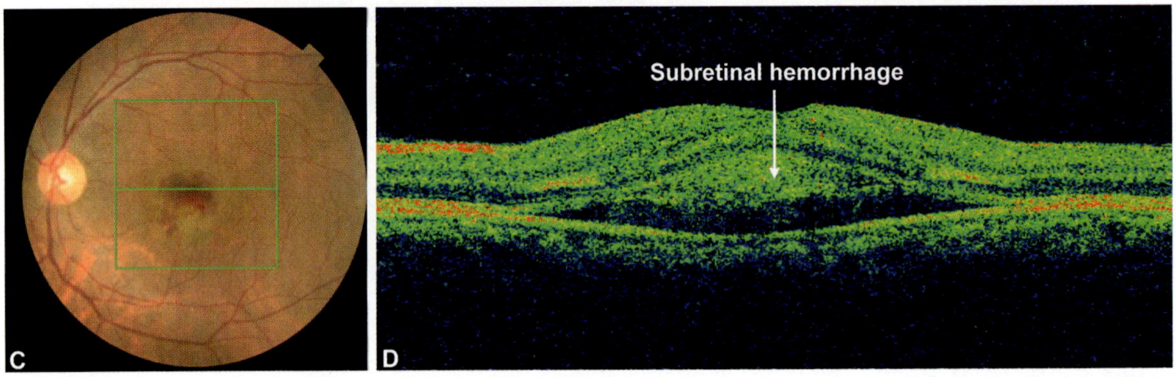

Figures 18.5.3C and D: (C) Color fundus photograph showing the horizontal line scan passing through the fovea. (D) Horizontal line scan 2D image showing an area of moderate reflectivity underlying the external limiting membrane corresponding to the area of subretinal hemorrhage.

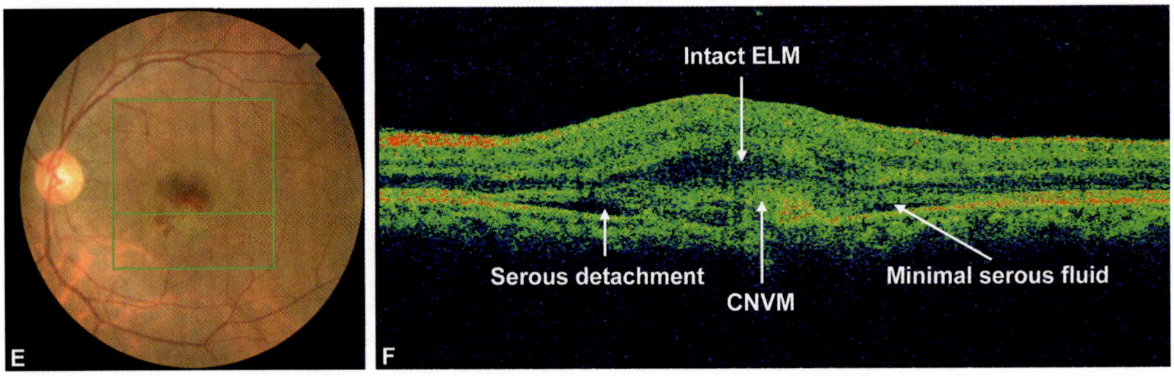

Figures 18.5.3E and F: (E) Color fundus photograph showing the horizontal line scan passing just below the fovea. (F) Horizontal line scan 2D image showing disruption of the RPE with an overlying area of moderate reflectivity beneath an intact external limiting membrane consistent with choroidal neovascularization. Serous fluid accumulation can be seen on either side of the lesion

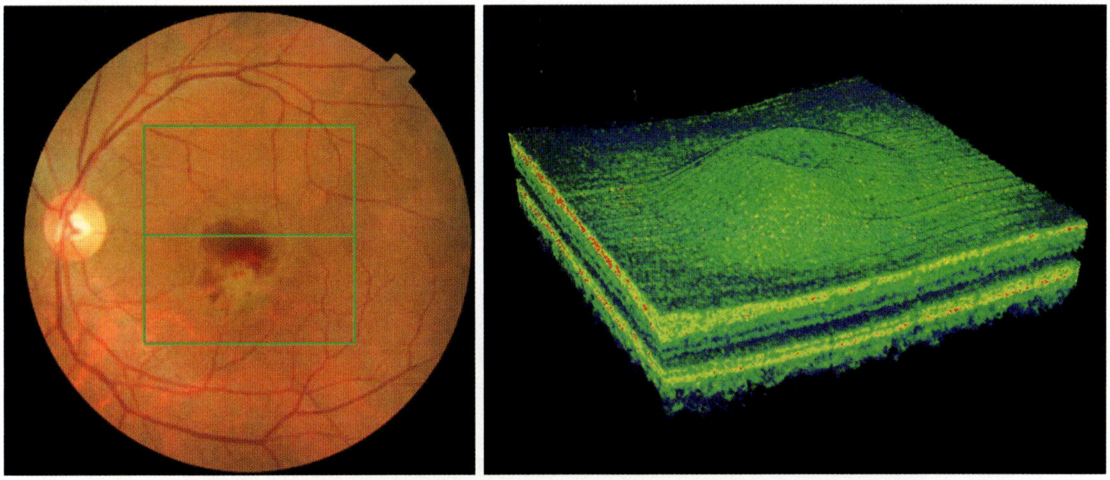

Figure 18.5.4: 3D image of the macula scan of Case 18.5

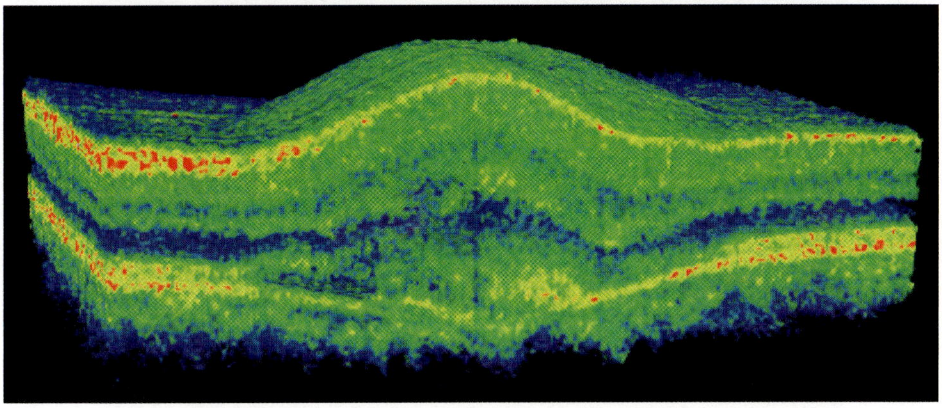

Figure 18.5.5: Cropped section of the 3D image of Case 18.5

CONCLUSIONS

1. OCT is, therefore, not only useful in the diagnosis of CNV but also in the follow-up of patients treated by various modes of therapy.
2. Imaging with 3D OCT-2000 gives better color contrast of the B scan images due to the new software algorithm that has been incorporated.

SUGGESTED READING

1. Costa RA, Farah ME, Cardillo JA, et al. Immediate indocyanine green angiography and optical coherence tomography evaluation after photodynamic therapy of subfoveal choroidal neovascularization. Retina 2003;23:159–65 [PubMed].
2. Farah ME, Cardillo JA, Luzardo AC, Calucci D, Williams GA, Costa RA. Indocyanine green-mediated photothrombosis for the management of predominantly classic choroidal neovascularization caused by age-related macular degeneration. Br J Ophthalmol 2004;88(8):1055-9 [PubMed].
3. TAP Study Group. Photodynamic therapy of subfoveal choroidal neovascularization in age-related macular degeneration with verteporfin. One-year results 2 randomized trials-Report 1. Arch Ophthalmol 1999;117:1329-45 [PubMed].
4. VIP Study Group. Verteporfin therapy of subfoveal choroidal neovascularization in age-related macular degeneration: two-year results of a randomized clinical trial including lesions with occult with no classic choroidal neovascularization-verteporfin in photodynamic therapy report 2. Am J Ophthalmol 2001;131:541-60 [PubMed].

19 Optic Nerve Disorders

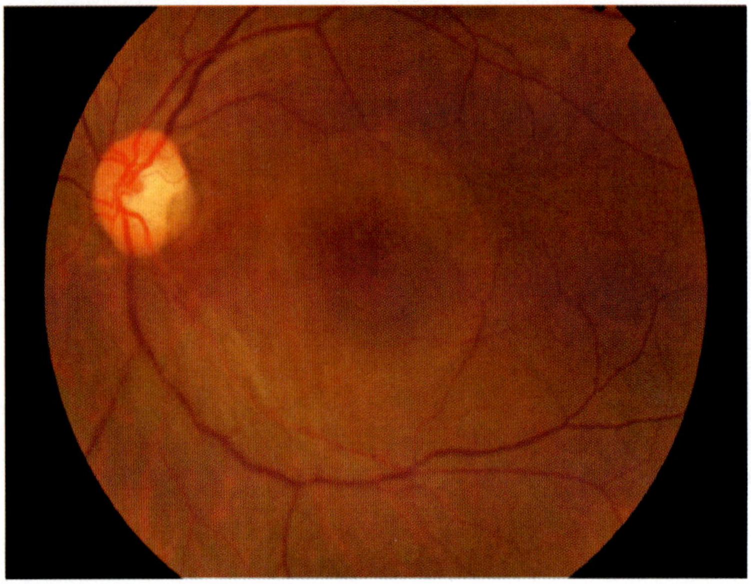

Optic Disc Pit

Optic disc pit is a rare congenital defect within the optic nerve head which is frequently associated with macular detachment in 25 to 75 percent cases. It is most frequently seen on the temporal aspect of the disc but can occur anywhere. It has been suspected that the subretinal fluid originates from the vitreous cavity via an inner retinoschisis-like separation within the papillomacular bundle between the optic disc pit and the central retinal detachment.

Fluorescein Angiography

The optic disc pit appears hypofluorescent in the early phase due to the absence of vessels in the pit and in the late phases it becomes hyperfluorescent due to staining of tissue at the pit.

Optical Coherence Tomography

The optic disc pit is seen as a defect in the optic nerve head. OCT of the associated maculopathy demonstrates a two layer structure. (1) a schisis-like separation of the inner layers of the retina (2) a detachment of the outer layers from the pigment epithelium.

CASE 19.1: OPTIC DISC PIT WITH SEROUS MACULAR DETACHMENT

Case Summary

A 55-year-old woman was referred for fluorescein angiography for complaints of defective vision in her left eye. Her best corrected visual acuity was counting fingers at one metre. Fluorescein angiography showed hypofluorescence of the optic pit in the early phase (arrow Figure 19.1.1) and hyperfluorescence in the late phase (Figure 19.1.2).

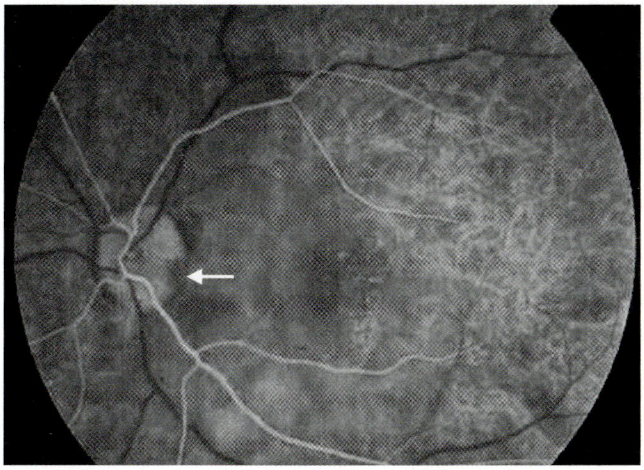

Figure 19.1.1: Early phase angiogram shows hypofluorescence of the optic pit

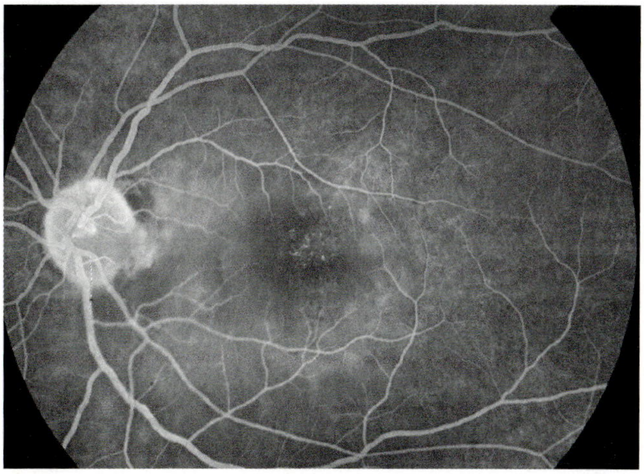

Figure 19.1.2: Late phase angiogram shows hyperfluorescence of the optic pit

Optical Coherence Tomography

Horizontal line scan passing through the optic pit showed a defect in the temporal aspect of the cup. The peripapillary temporal retina showed schisis in the inner retinal layers. The inner schisis communicates with the optic disc pit (Figures 19.1.3A and B).

Horizontal line scan passing through the macula showed inner schisis, schisis-like separation of the outer retinal layers, full thickness neurosensory retinal detachment and development of hole in the outer cavity (Figures 19.1.3C and D).

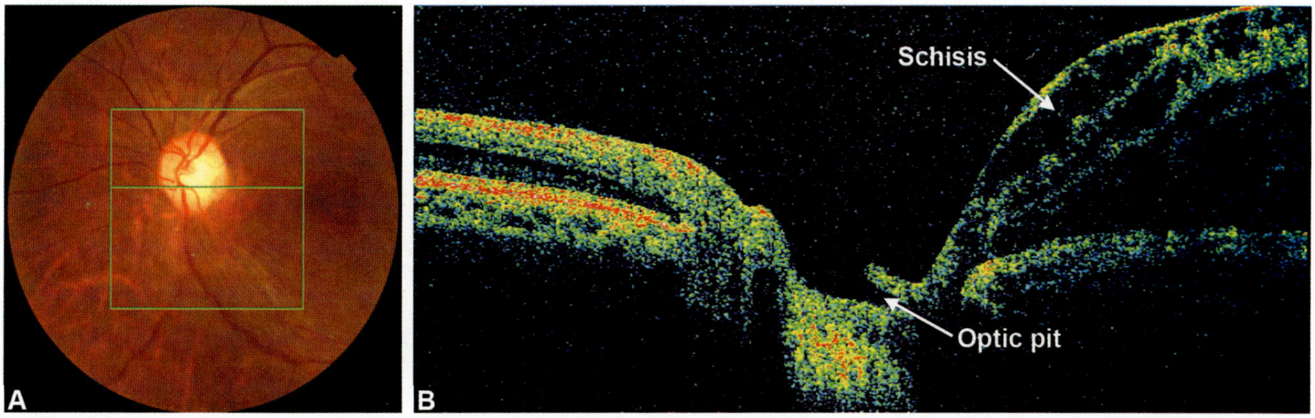

Figures 19.1.3A and B: (A) Color fundus photograph showing the horizontal line scan through the optic disc pit. (B) Horizontal line scan through the optic disc pit, 2D image showing a defect in the temporal aspect of the cup. The peripapillary temporal retina showed schisis in the inner retinal layers. The inner schisis communicates with the optic disc pit

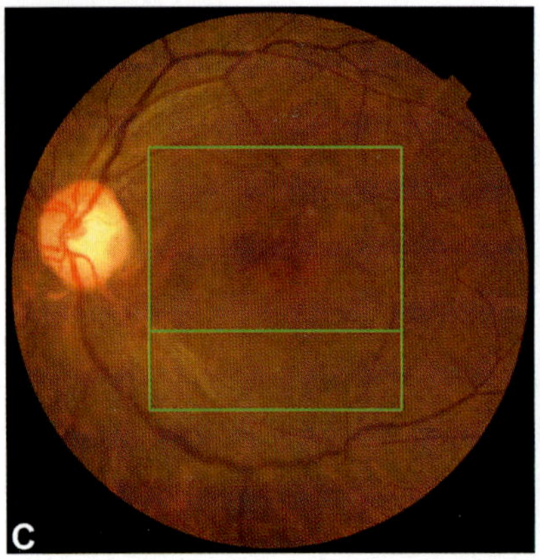

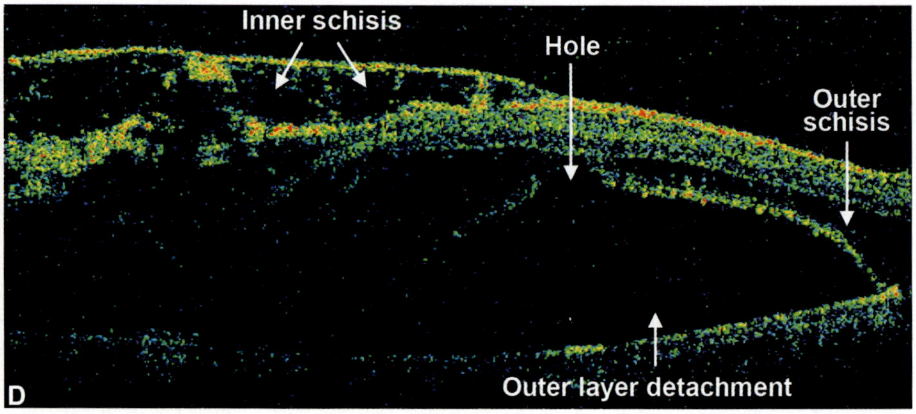

Figures 19.1.3C and D: (C) Color fundus photograph showing the horizontal line scan below the fovea. (D) Horizontal line scan through the macula showed inner schisis, schisis like separation of the outer retinal layers, full thickness neurosensory retinal detachment and development of hole in the outer cavity

CONCLUSIONS

1. OCT has shown that the inner layer separation provides a conduit for the continuous flow of fluid from the pit to the displaced retinal elevation.
2. It is also useful in monitoring the response of the maculopathy to various treatments.

SUGGESTED READING

1. Krivoy D, Gentile R, Liebmann JM, Stegman Z, Rosen R, Walsh JB, Ritch R. Imaging congenital optic disc pits and associated maculopathy using optical coherence tomography. Arch Ophthalmol 1996;114(2):165-70.
2. Linceff H, Kreissig I. Optical coherence tomography of pneumatic displacement of optic disc pit maculopathy. Br J Ophthalmol 1998;82(4):367-72.
3. Theodossiadis PG, Geigoropoulos VG, Emfietzoglon J, Theodossiadis GP. Vitreous finding in optic disc pit maculopathy based on optical coherence tomography. Graefes Arch Clin Exp Ophthalmol 2007;245(9):1311-8.

PAPILLEDEMA

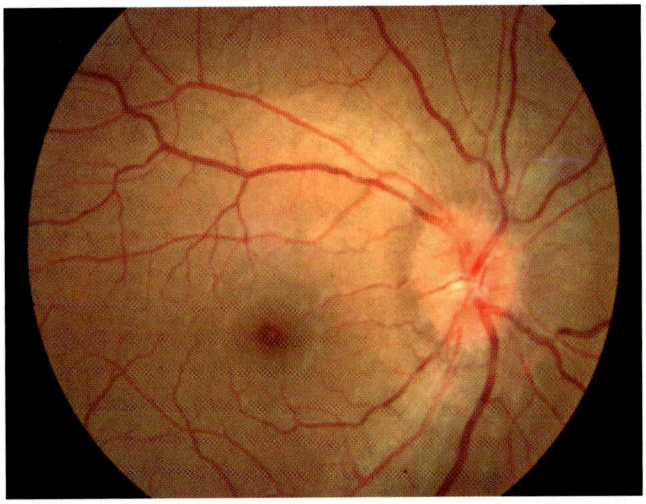

Papilledema is an optic disc swelling that is secondary to elevated intracranial pressure. In contrast to other causes of optic disc swelling, vision usually is well preserved with acute papilledema. It almost always presents as a bilateral phenomenon and may develop over hours to weeks.

CASE 19.2: PAPILLEDEMA

Case Summary

A 48-year-old lady diagnosed with viral encephalitis was referred with history of headache of one month duration. Her visual acuity in both eyes was 6/6. Fluorescein angiography showed splinter hemorrhage and dilated disc capillaries with late staining of the disc (Figures 19.2.1 and 19.2.2).

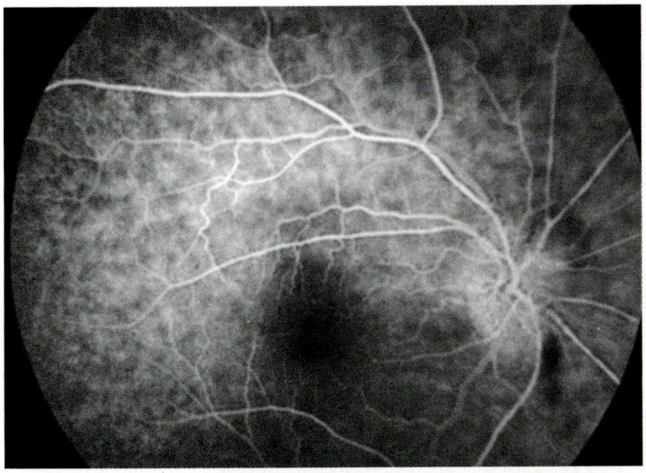

Figure 19.2.1: Early phase angiogram of the right eye shows splinter hemorrhage and dilated disc capillaries

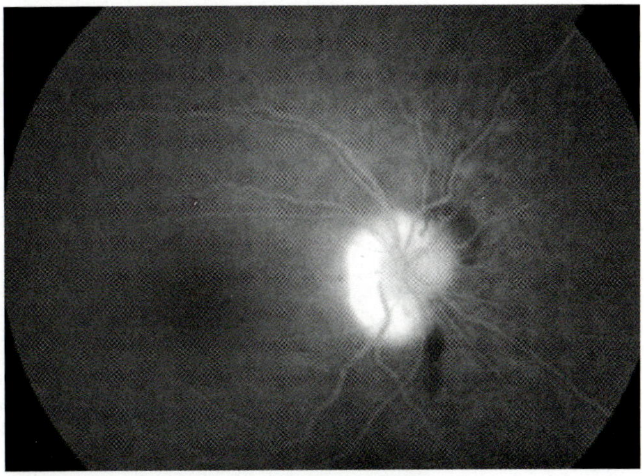

Figure 19.2.2: Late phase angiogram shows leakage from the disc capillaries

Optical Coherence Tomography

Horizontal line scan through the right optic disc showed substantial disc elevation with a clear optical space inside the disc because of the marked tissue thickening and fluid accumulation within it (Figures 19.2.3A to D).

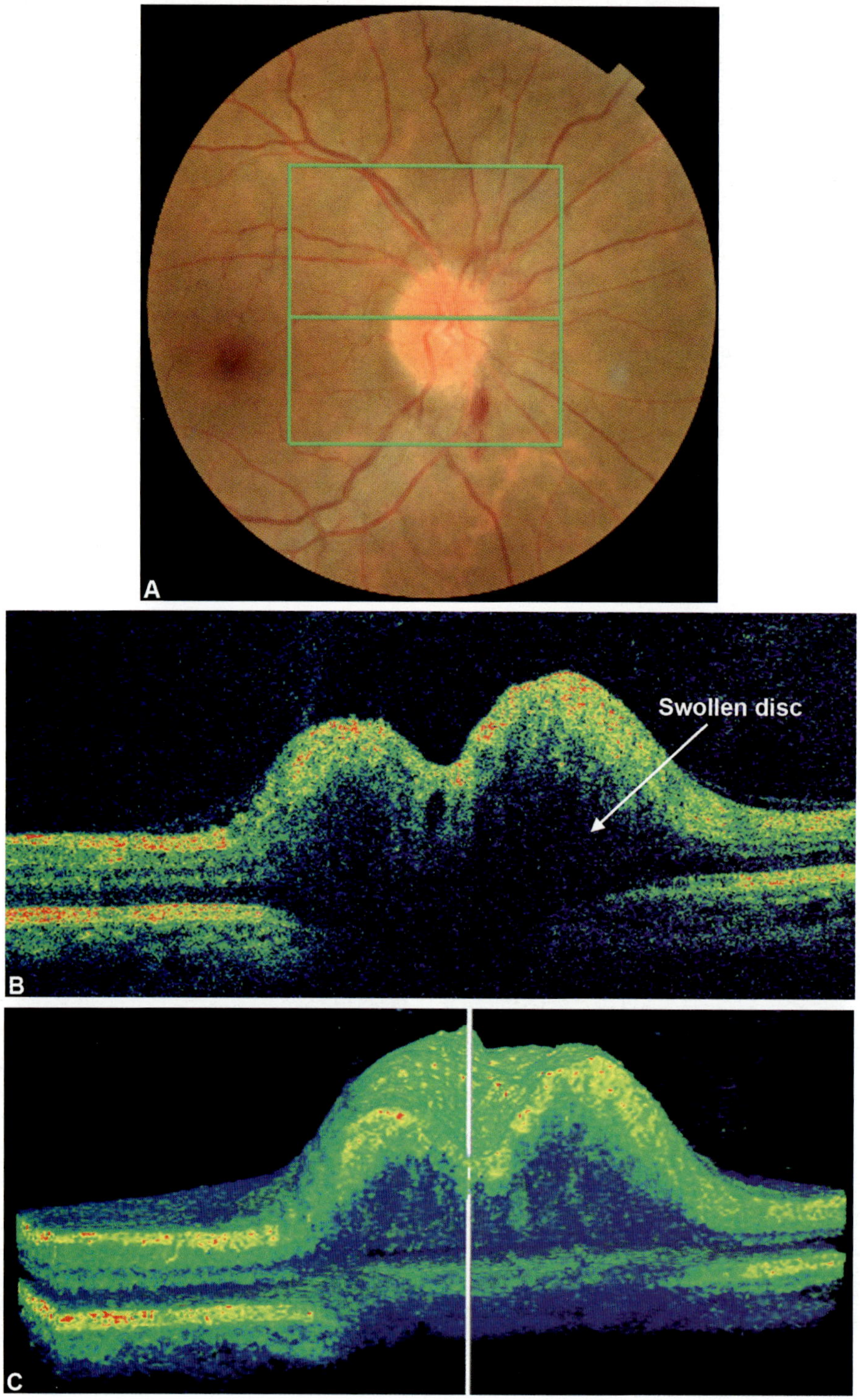

Figures 19.2.3A to C: (A) Color fundus photograph of the right eye showing the horizontal line scan through the optic disc. (B) Horizontal line scan, 2D image showing substantial disc elevation with a clear optical space inside the disc because of the marked tissue thickening and fluid accumulation within it. (C) Cropped 3D image showing substantial disc elevation with a clear optical space inside the disc because of the marked tissue thickening and fluid accumulation within it.

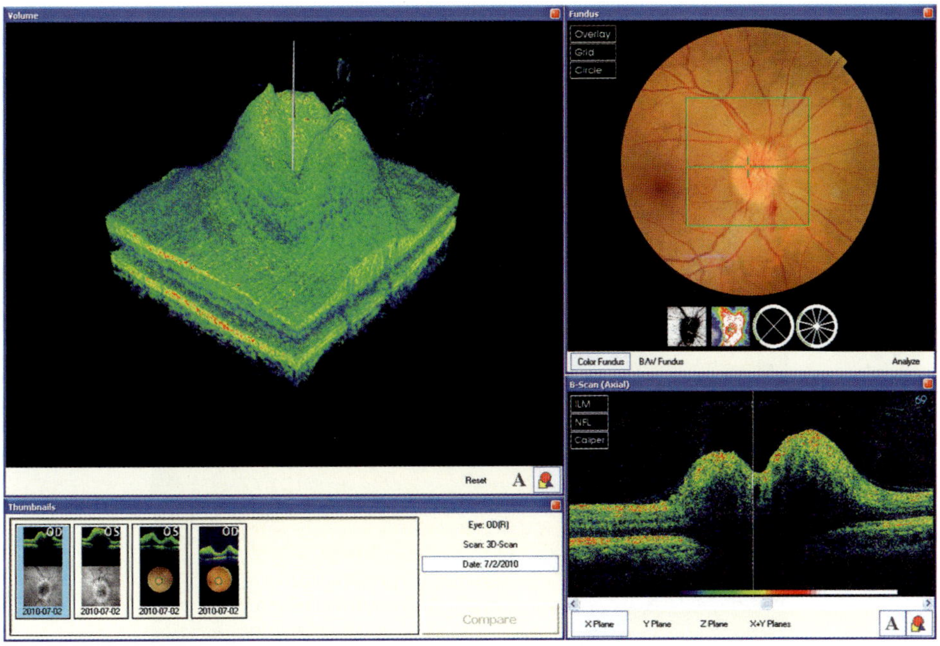

Figure 19.2.3D: 3D image of the right eye of Case 19.2 **(Images with Topcon 3D OCT-2000)**

Fluorescein angiography of the left eye also showed dilated disc capillaries with late staining of the disc (Figures 19.2.4 and 19.2.5).

Optical Coherence Tomography

Horizontal line scan through the left optic disc showed substantial disc elevation with a clear optical space within due to marked tissue thickening and fluid accumulation (Figures 19.2.6A to D). RNFL analysis showed increased thickness of the RNFL in both eyes (Figure 19.2.6E).

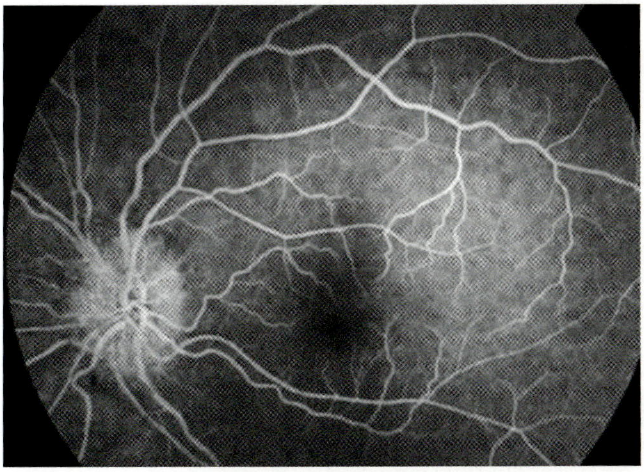

Figure 19.2.4: Early phase angiogram of the left eye shows splinter hemorrhage and dilated disc capillaries

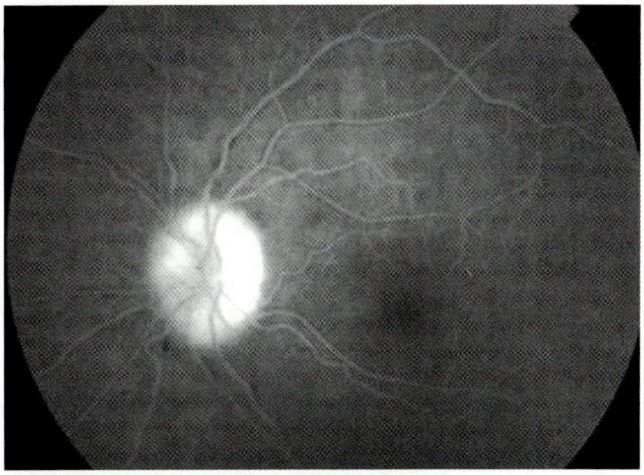

Figure 19.2.5: Late phase angiogram shows leakage from the disc capillaries

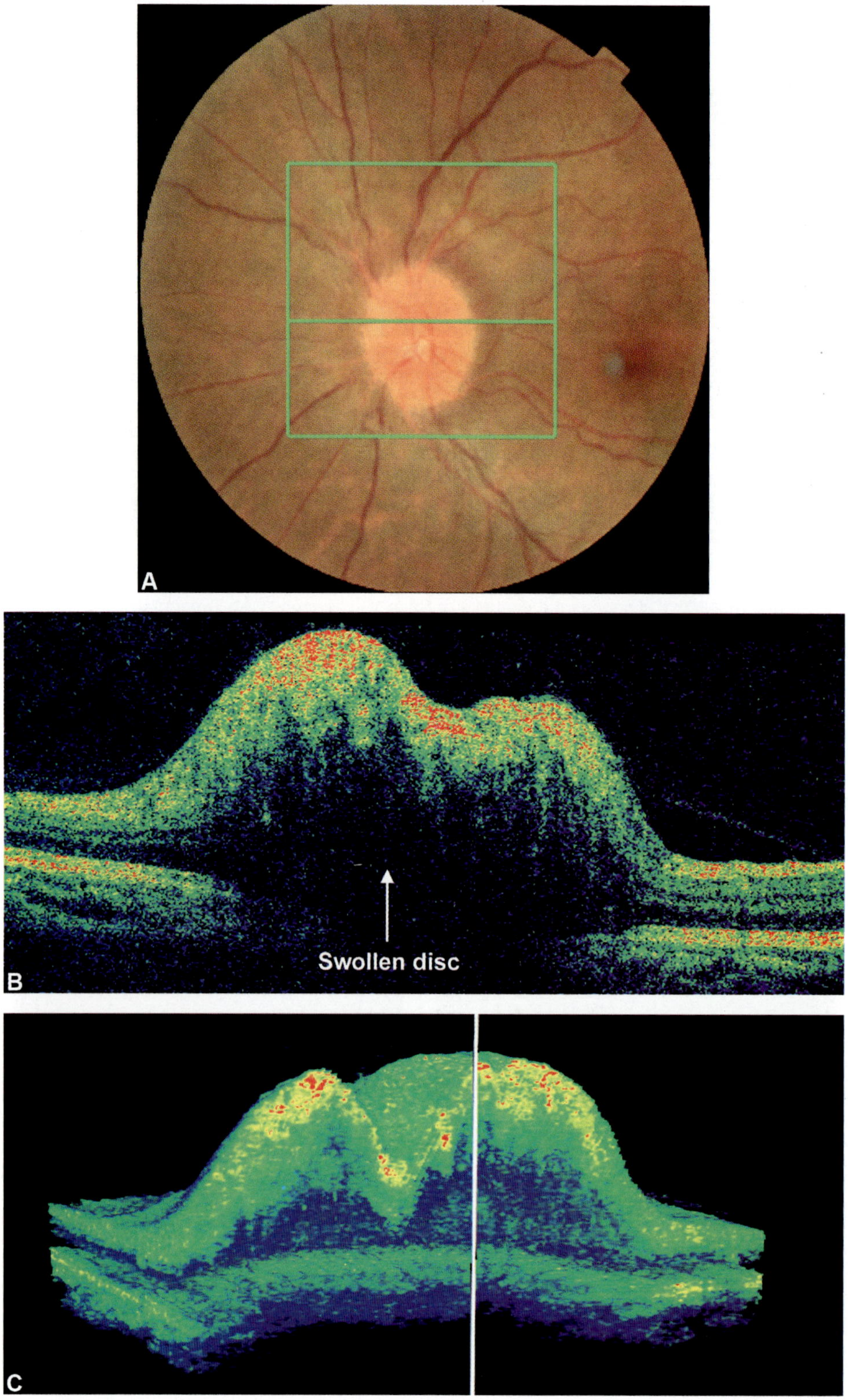

Figures 19.2.6A to C: (A) Color fundus photograph of the left eye showing the horizontal line scan through the optic disc. (B) Horizontal line scan, 2D image showing substantial disc elevation with a clear optical space inside the disc because of the marked tissue thickening and fluid accumulation within it. (C) Cropped 3D image showing substantial disc elevation with a clear optical space inside the disc because of the marked tissue thickening and fluid accumulation within it **(Images with Topcon 3D OCT-2000)**

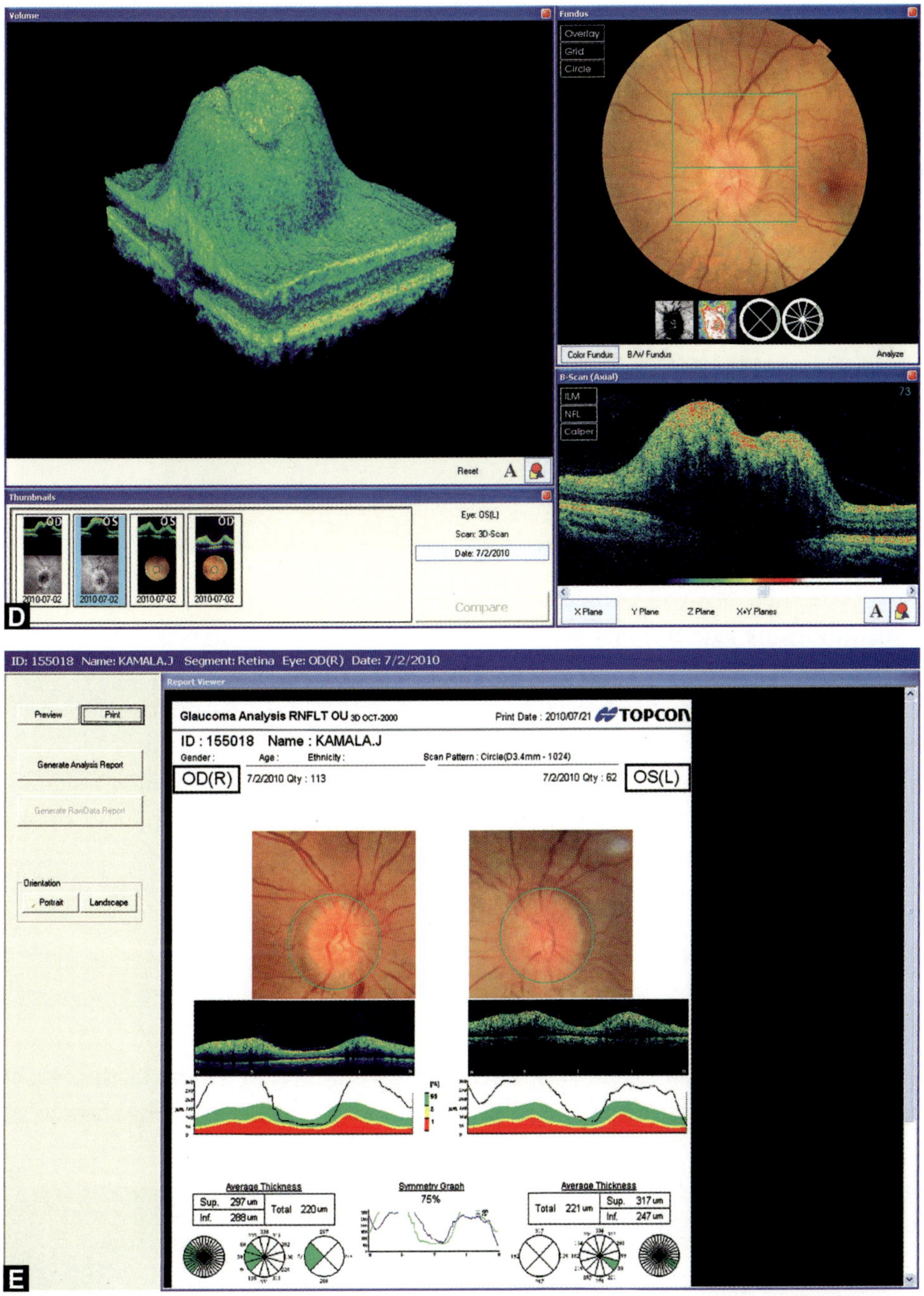

Figures 19.2.6D and E: (D) 3D image of the left eye of Case 19.2 (E) RNFL analysis showing increased RNFL thickness in both eyes **(Images with Topcon 3D OCT-2000)**

CONCLUSION

OCT is useful in cases of papilledema to document and follow the course of the disease.

OPTIC DISC DRUSEN

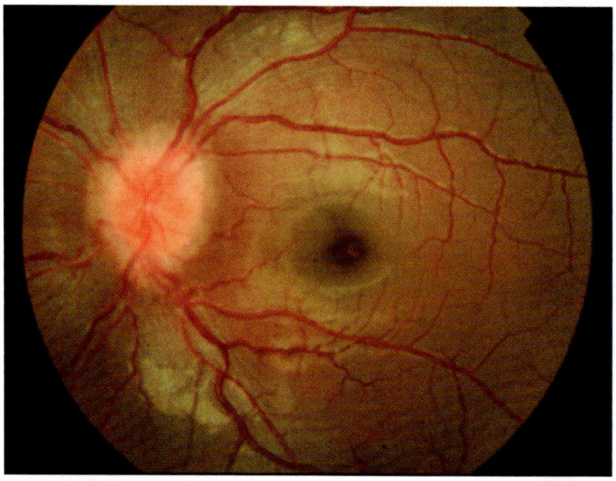

Optic disc drusen is composed of small conglomerates of mucopolysaccharides and proteinaceous material that become calcified with advancing age. It is bilateral in 70 percent of cases and can occur at any age in both sex. They may be inherited as an autosomal trait with irregular penetrance.

Majority of patients are asymptomatic, however, some may experience transient visual obscurations. Gradual loss of the peripheral visual field may occur. Patients may eventually lose central acuity.

Drusen may either be superficial when they appear as small, white-to-yellow, granular bulgings of the substance of the disc or they can be deeply buried in the substance of the nerve. Superficial drusen may exhibit autofluorescence whereas buried disc drusen do not autofluoresce.

Disc drusen may be associated with retinitis pigmentosa and pseudoxanthoma elasticum.

CASE 19.3: OPTIC DISC DRUSEN

Case Summary

A 17-year-old girl presented with complaints of transient obscurations of vision in the left eye of two weeks duration. Her best-corrected visual acuity in this eye was 6/6. Fluorescein angiography showed staining of the disc (Figures 19.3.1 and 19.3.2).

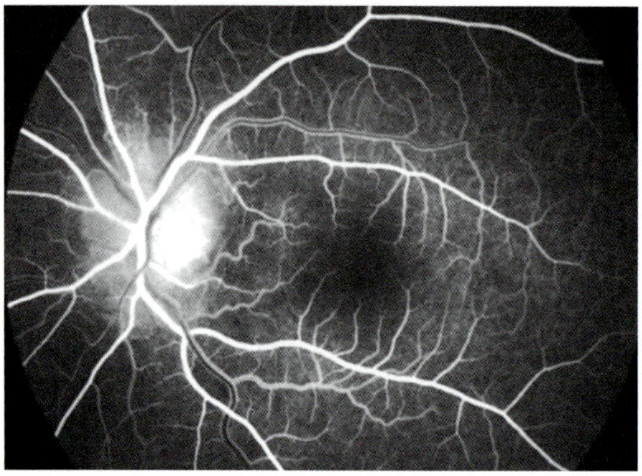

Figure 19.3.1: Early phase angiogram shows optic disc drusen

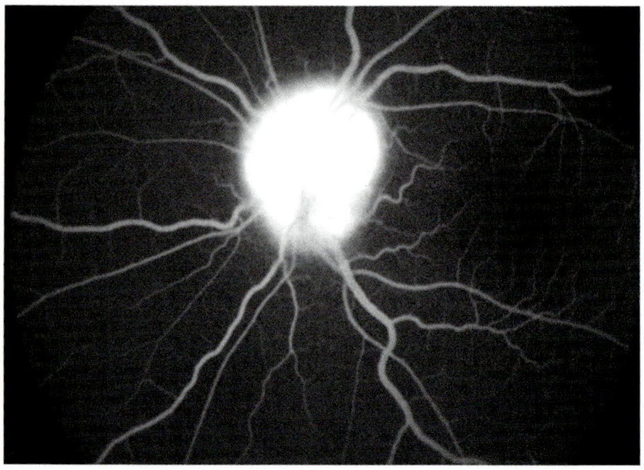

Figure 19.3.2: Late phase angiogram shows staining of the disc

Optical Coherence Tomography

Horizontal line scan showed elevation of the disc with dense finger like shadowing underneath the disc (Figures 19.3.3A to D). Marked thinning of the RNFL was evident (Figure 19.3.3E).

Ultrasonography showed an area of moderate reflectivity at the optic nerve head thus confirming the diagnosis of optic disc drusen (Figure 19.3.3F).

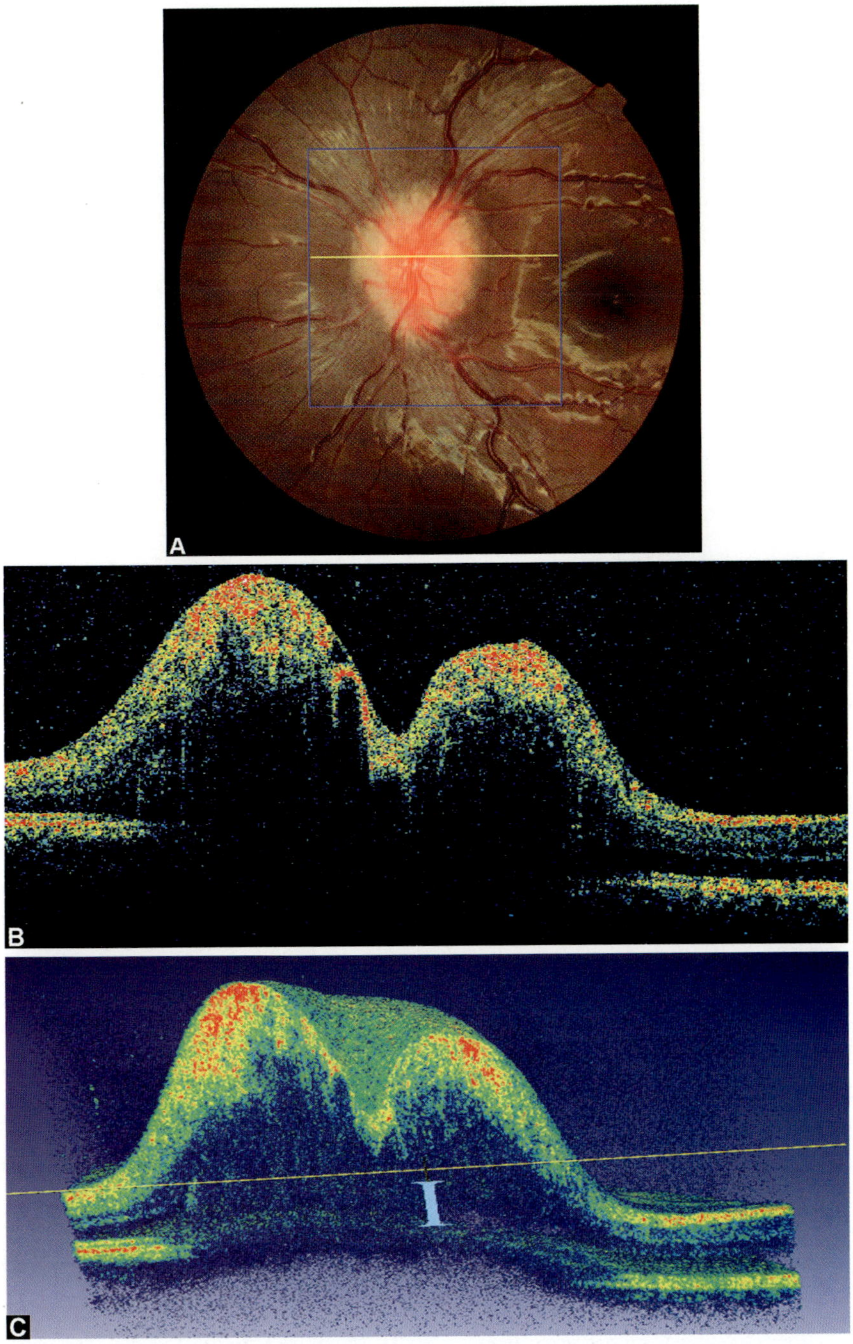

Figures 19.3.3A to C: (A) Color fundus photograph of the left eye showing the horizontal line scan through the optic disc. (B) Horizontal line scan, 2D image showing elevation of the disc with dense finger like shadowing underneath the disc. (C) Cropped 3D image showing elevation of the disc with dense finger like shadowing underneath the disc

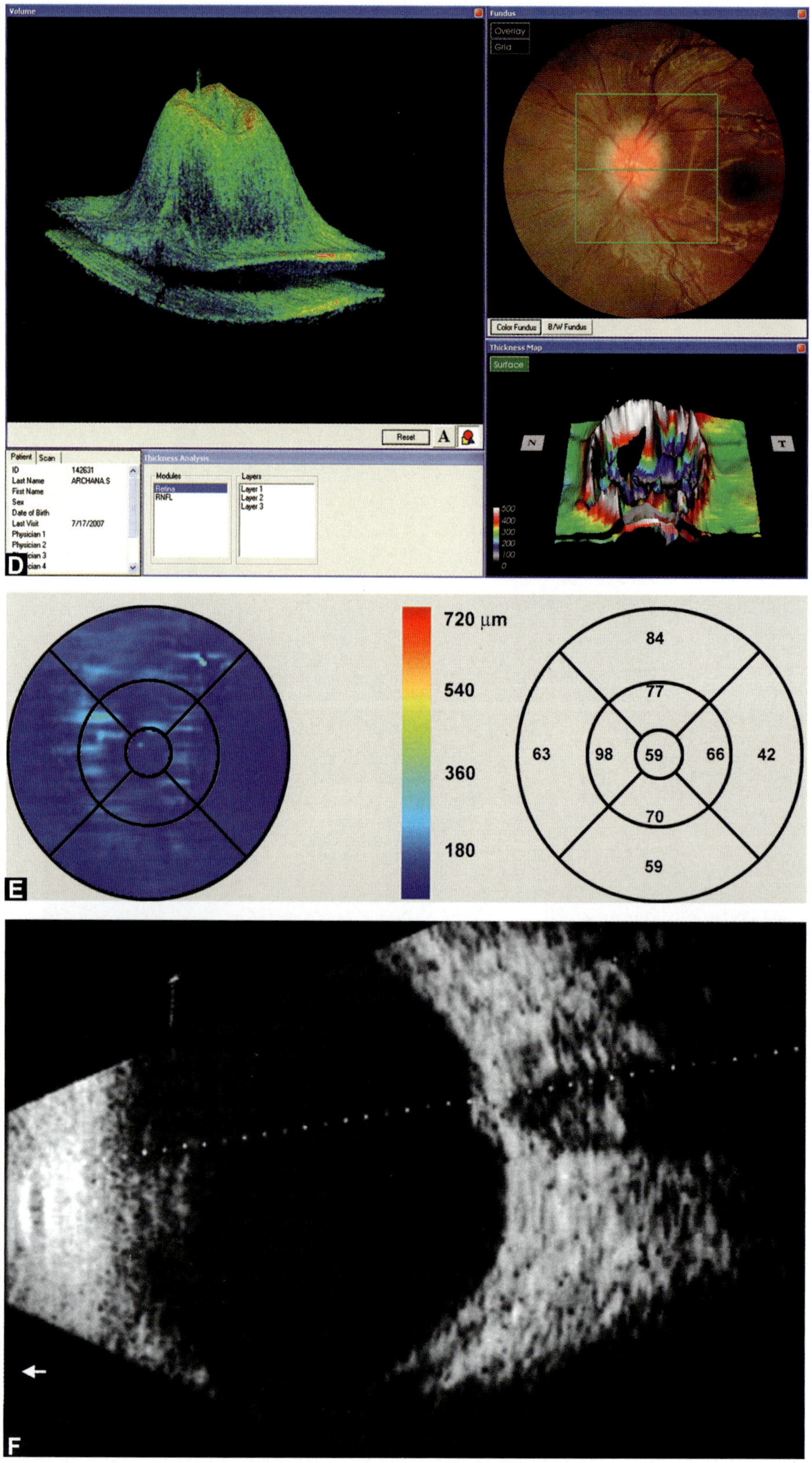

Figures 19.3.3D to F: (D) 3D image of Case 19.3. (E) RNFL thickness map showing marked thinning of the RNFL. (F) Ultrasound B scan shows an area of moderate reflectivity at the optic nerve head thus confirming the diagnosis of optic disc drusen

CONCLUSION

OCT findings may be specially beneficial in cases where the clinical optic nerve head assessment does not detect drusen.

SUGGESTED READING

1. Katz BJ, Pomeranz HD. Visual field defects and retinal nerve fiber layer defects in eyes with buried optic nerve drusen. Am J Ophthalmol 2006;141(2):248-53.
2. Roh S, Noecker RJ, Schuman JS, Hedges TR 3rd, Weiter JJ, Mattox C. Effect of optic nerve head drusen on nerve fiber layer thickness. Ophthalmology 1998;105(5):878-85.

OPTIC DISC MELANOCYTOMA

Optic disc melanocytoma is a benign brown-to-black tumor that involves the substance of the optic disc and the adjacent retina. It can enlarge slowly and produce visual loss due to compression of the optic disc.

Fluorescein Angiography

The melanocytoma shows hypofluorescence through all phases of the angiogram.

CASE 19.4: OPTIC DISC MELANOCYTOMA

Case Summary

A 58-year-old male presented with history of seeing a black patch in his right eye of three days duration. His best-corrected visual acuity was 6/6 in the right eye.

Optical Coherence Tomography

Horizontal line scan through the optic disc showed an area of hyper-reflectivity with underlying shadowing corresponding to the optic disc melanocytoma. In addition, there was evidence of fibrin within the neurosensory detachment temporal to the disc (Figures 19.4.1A and B).

Horizontal line scan passing inferior to the optic disc showed exudation and a hypo-reflective space within the neurosensory detachment. In addition, a small pigment epithelial detachment was evident (Figures 19.4.1C and D).

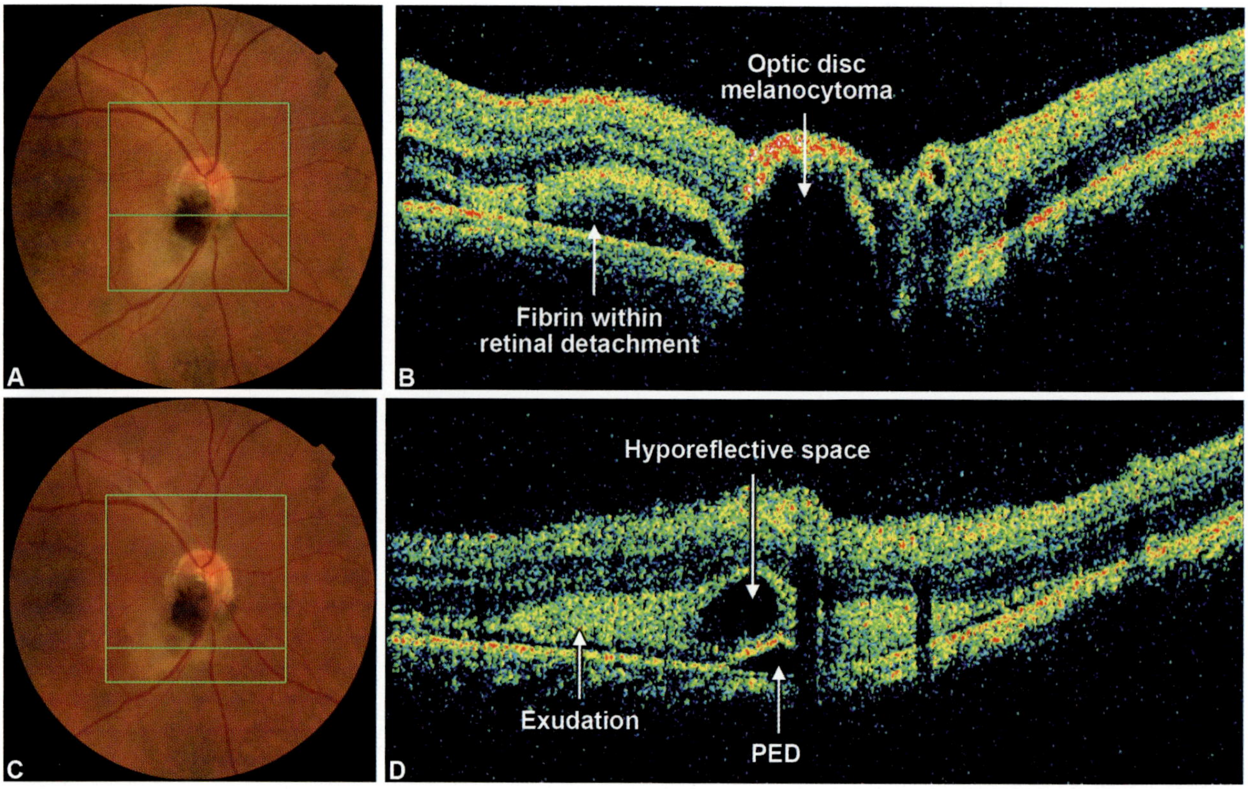

Figures 19.4.1A to D: (A) Color fundus photograph showing the horizontal line scan through the optic disc melanocytoma. (B) Horizontal line scan, 2D image showing an area of hyper-reflectivity with underlying shadowing corresponding to the optic disc melanocytoma. There was evidence of fibrin within the neurosensory detachment temporal to the disc. (C) Color fundus photograph showing the horizontal line scan inferior to the disc. (D) Horizontal line scan, 2D image showing exudation and a hypo-reflective space within the neurosensory detachment. A small pigment epithelial detachment was evident

Horizontal line scan through the fovea showed a hyporeflective space consistent with serous retinal detachment (Figures 19.4.1E and F).

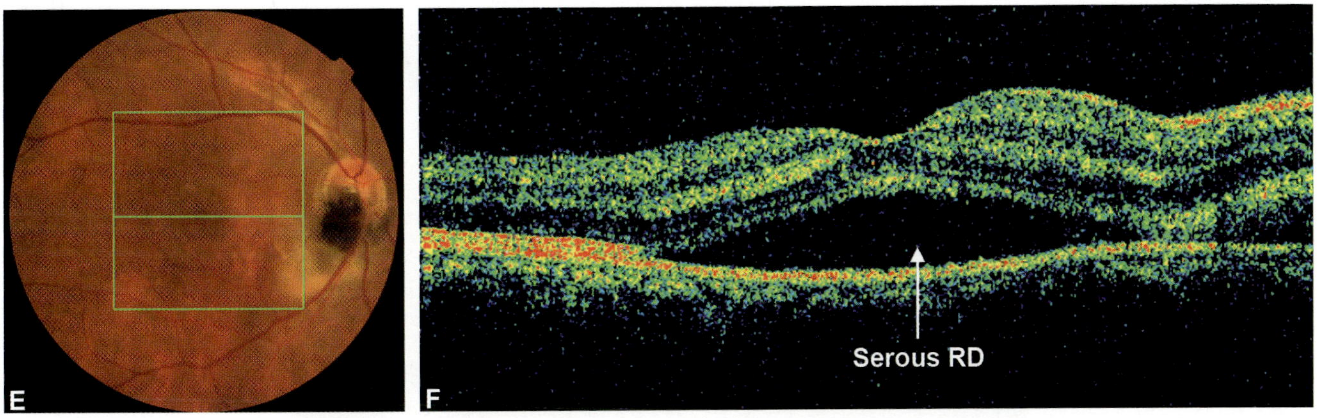

Figures 19.4.1E and F: (E) Color fundus photograph showing the horizontal line scan through the fovea. (F) Horizontal line scan, 2D image showing a hyporeflective space consistent with serous retinal detachment

SUGGESTED READING

1. Antcliff RJ, Ffytche TJ, Shilling JS, Marshall J. Optical coherence tomography of melanocytoma. Am J Ophthalmol 2000;130: 845-7
2. Chaudhary R, Arora R, Mehta DK, et al. Optical coherence tomography study of optic disc melanocytoma. Ophthalmic Surg Lasers Imaging 2006;37:58-61.
3. Shields CL, Perez B, Benavides, Materin MA, Shields JA. Optical coherence tomography of optic disc melanocytoma in 15 cases. Retina 2008;28:441-6.

20 Polypoidal Choroidal Vasculopathy

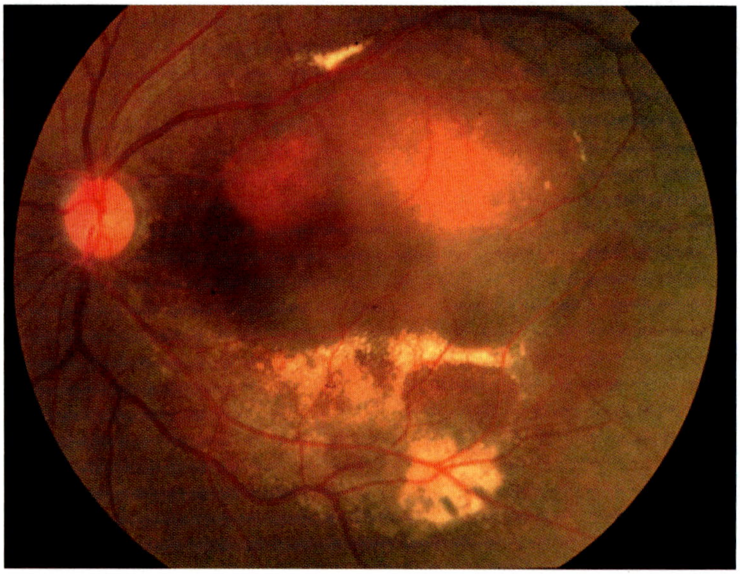

Polypoidal choroidal vasculopathy is a peculiar form of choroidal vascular abnormality associated with multiple recurrent hemorrhagic, serous or serosanguineous pigment epithelial detachments and serous retinal detachments. It is characterized by the presence of branching vascular networks that terminate in polypoidal lesions located under the retinal pigment epithelium.

Indocyanine green angiography confirms the diagnosis by demonstrating the polyps as hyperfluorescent areas at the end of branching choroidal vascular networks.

Optical Coherence Tomography

1. Spectral Domain OCT shows that the polypoidal lesions correspond to areas of moderate reflectivity located between the undulating RPE and thin straight reflective Bruch's membrane line.
2. Double reflective layers consisting of retinal pigment epithelium (RPE) and another highly reflective layer beneath the RPE (double-layer sign) is seen frequently in the area of the vascular network.
3. It helps in differentiating the various types of pigment epithelial detachments.
4. It demonstrates the presence of serous retinal detachments.

CASE 20.1: POLYPOIDAL CHOROIDAL VASCULOPATHY

Case Summary

A 58-year-old male presented with diminished vision in the left eye of one month duration. His best-corrected vision in this eye was 6/18;N18.

Early-phase ICG showed the branching vascular pattern with polypoidal structures at the border of the vascular network. The late phase ICG showed staining in the region of the vascular network, leakage of dye from the polyps and hemorrhagic PED (Figures 20.1.1 and 20.1.2).

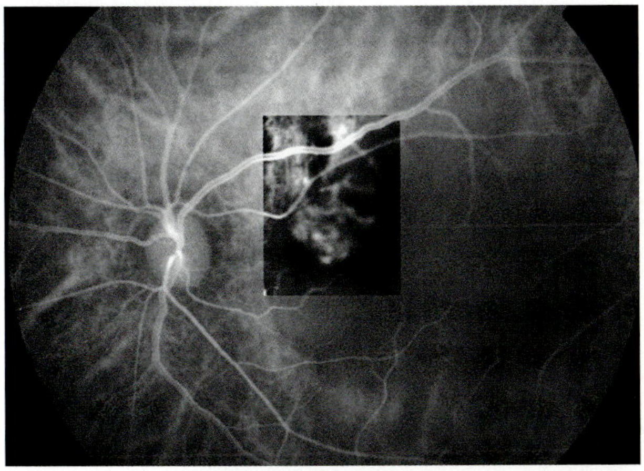

Figure 20.1.1: Early phase ICG shows the branching vascular pattern with polypoidal structures at the border of the vascular network

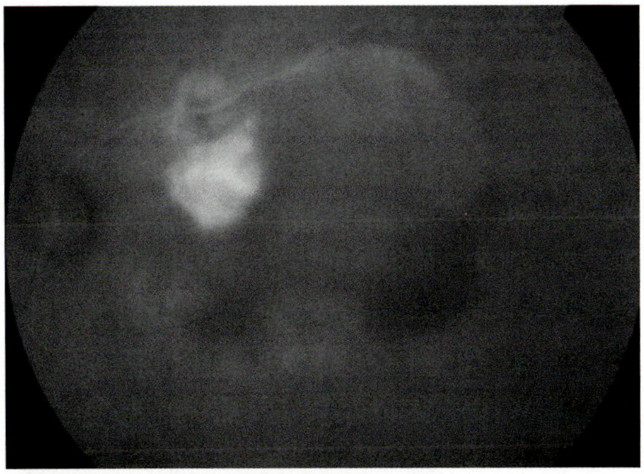

Figure 20.1.2: Late phase ICG shows staining in the region of the vascular network, leakage of dye from the polyps and hemorrhagic PED

Optical Coherence Tomography

Horizontal line scan showed the polypoidal lesions as areas of moderate reflectivity (denoted by red asterisks) located between the undulating RPE and thin straight reflective Bruch's membrane line (BM). Serous retinal detachment was also evident (Figures 20.1.3A and B).

Horizontal line scan passing through the orange colored lesion showed a large elevation of the RPE consistent with RPE detachment. The detachment contained blood cells which induced a shadow effect that prevented the choriocapillaris from being seen. In addition, undulations of the RPE were evident (Figures 20.1.4A to D).

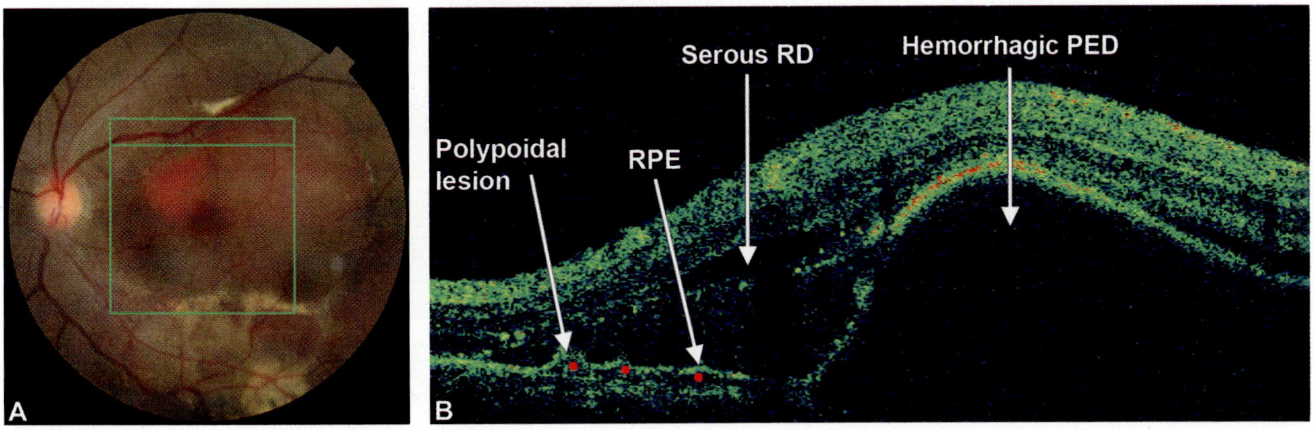

Figures 20.1.3A and B: (A) Color fundus photograph showing the horizontal line scan above the fovea. (B) Horizontal line scan above the fovea 2D image showing the polypoidal lesions as areas of moderate reflectivity (denoted by red asterisks) located between the undulating RPE and thin straight reflective Bruch's membrane line(BM). Serous retinal detachment is also evident

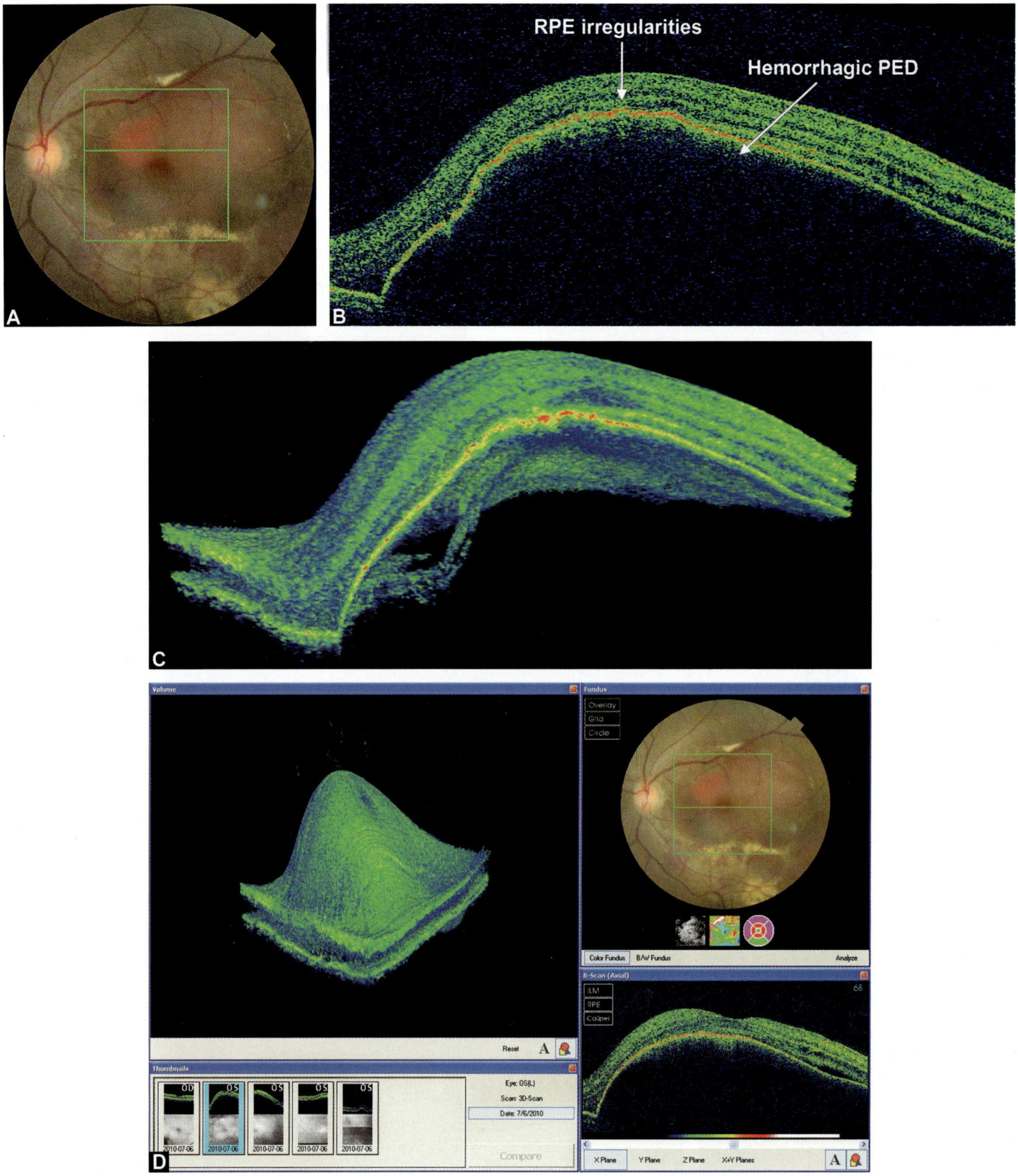

Figures 20.1.4A to D: (A) **C**olor fundus photograph showing the horizontal line scan through the orange colored lesion. (B) Horizontal line scan passing through the orange colored lesion, 2D image showing a large elevation of the RPE consistent with RPE detachment. The detachment contains blood cells which induces a shadow effect that prevents the choriocapillaris from being seen. Undulations of the RPE are evident. (C) Cropped 3D image showing a large elevation of the RPE consistent with RPE detachment. The detachment contains blood cells which induces a shadow effect that prevents the choriocapillaris from being seen. Undulations of the RPE are evident. (D) 3D image of Case 20.1 **(Images with Topcon 3D OCT 2000)**

CASE 20.2: POLYPOIDAL CHOROIDAL VASCULOPATHY

Case Summary

A 62-year-old male presented with complaints of seeing a black patch of five days duration. His best-corrected vision in this eye was counting fingers 1 meter.

Fluorescein angiography showed subretinal hemorrhage and areas of leakage within it (Figures 20.2.1 and 20.2.2).

Indocyanine green angiography showed a single polyp with branching vascular network. The late-phase ICG showed hypofluorescence in the center of the polyp with staining of the wall of the polyp. In addition, there was leakage of dye into the PED (Figures 20.2.3 and 20.2.4).

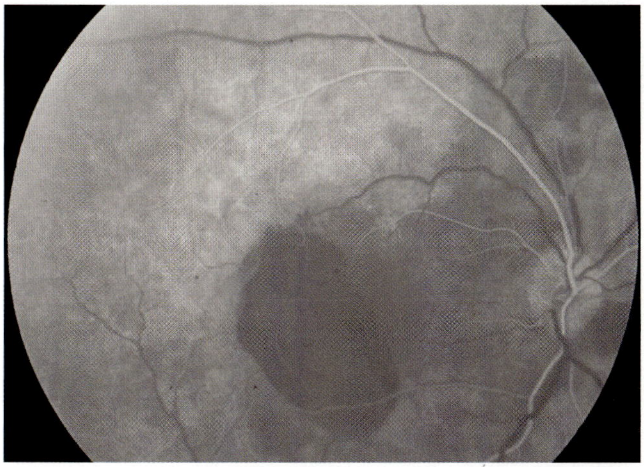

Figure 20.2.1: Early phase angiogram shows a large patch of blocked fluorescence due to subretinal hemorrhage

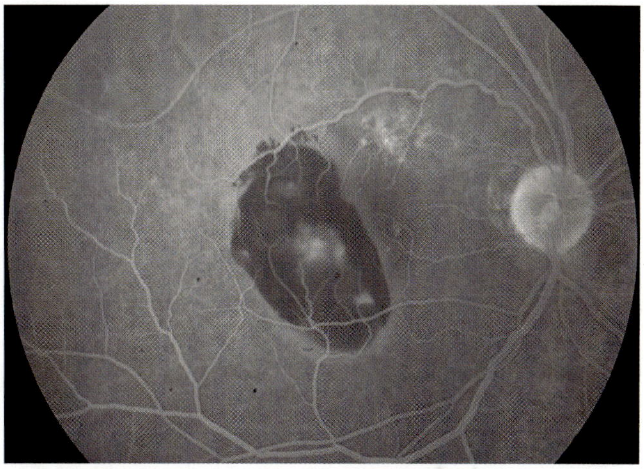

Figure 20.2.2: Late phase angiogram shows areas of leakage

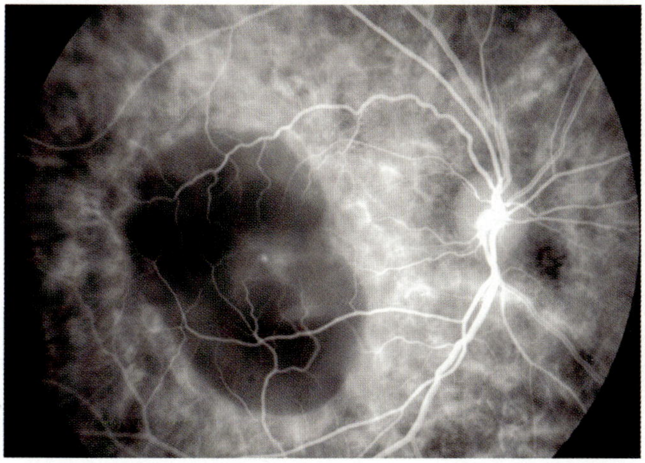

Figure 20.2.3: Early phase ICG shows a single polyp with branching vascular network

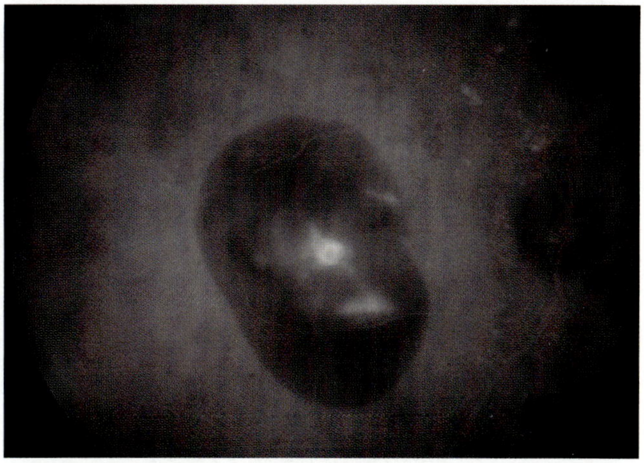

Figure 20.2.4: Late phase ICG shows hypofluorescence in the center of the polyp with staining of the wall of the polyp. Leakage of dye into the PED is also seen

Optical Coherence Tomography

Horizontal line scan showed accumulation of blood beneath the photoreceptor layer (Figures 20.2.5A and B).

Horizontal line scan showed a large elevation of the RPE consistent with RPE detachment. The detachment contained blood cells which induced a shadow effect that prevented the choriocapillaris from being seen (Figures 20.2.5C and D).

Horizontal line scan showed another hemorrhagic pigment epithelial detachment (Figure 20.2.5E and F).

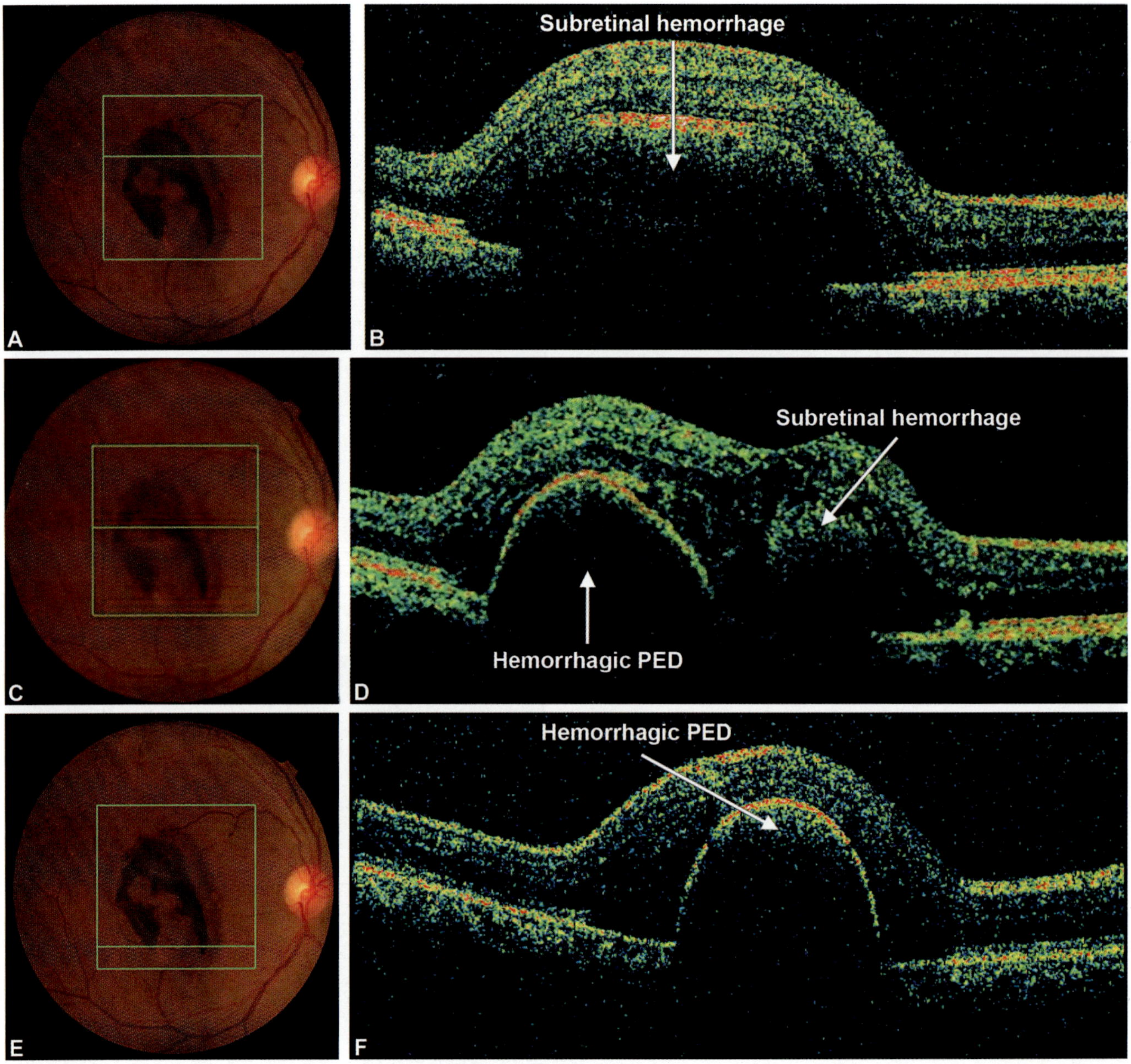

Figures 20.2.5A to F: (A) Color fundus photograph showing the horizontal line scan above the fovea. (B) Horizontal line scan above the fovea 2D image showing accumulation of blood beneath the photoreceptor layer. (C) Color fundus photograph showing the horizontal line scan through the fovea. (D) Horizontal line scan through the fovea 2D image showing a large elevation of the RPE consistent with RPE detachment. The detachment contains blood cells which induces a shadow effect that prevents the choriocapillaris from being seen. (E) Color fundus photograph showing the horizontal line scan below the fovea. (F) Horizontal line scan below the fovea 2D image showing hemorrhagic pigment epithelial detachment

CASE 20.3: POLYPOIDAL CHOROIDAL VASCULOPATHY

Case Summary

A 50-year-old male presented with diminished vision in the left eye of one month duration. His best-corrected vision in this eye was 6/12. Fluorescein angiography showed two pigment epithelial detachments, one of which showed leakage of dye from the underlying polyps. In addition, serous retinal elevation was also evident (Figures 20.3.1 and 20.3.2).

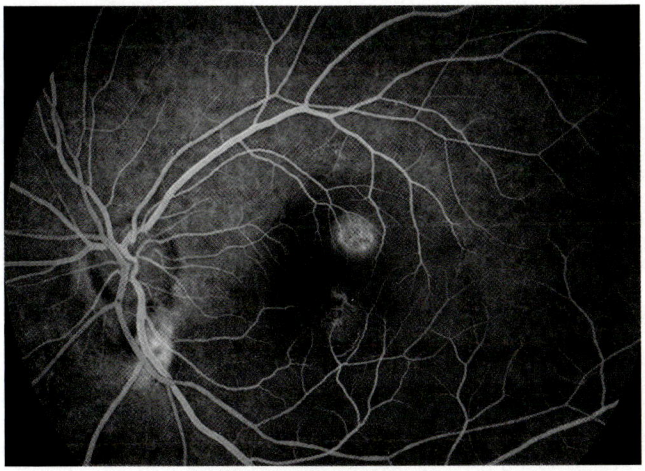

Figure 20.3.1: Early phase angiogram shows two pigment epithelial detachments

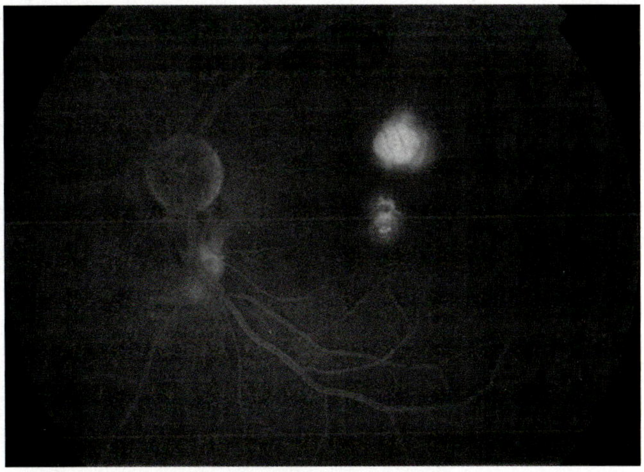

Figure 20.3.2: Late phase angiogram shows leakage of dye from the underlying polyps and serous retinal elevation

Optical Coherence Tomography

Horizontal line scan revealed double reflective layers that consisted of retinal pigment epithelium (RPE) and another highly reflective layer beneath the RPE (double-layer sign). Serous retinal detachment was also evident (Figures 20.3.3A and B).

Horizontal line scan passing below the fovea showed a large serous pigment epithelial detachment within the serous retinal detachment (Figures 20.3.3C and D).

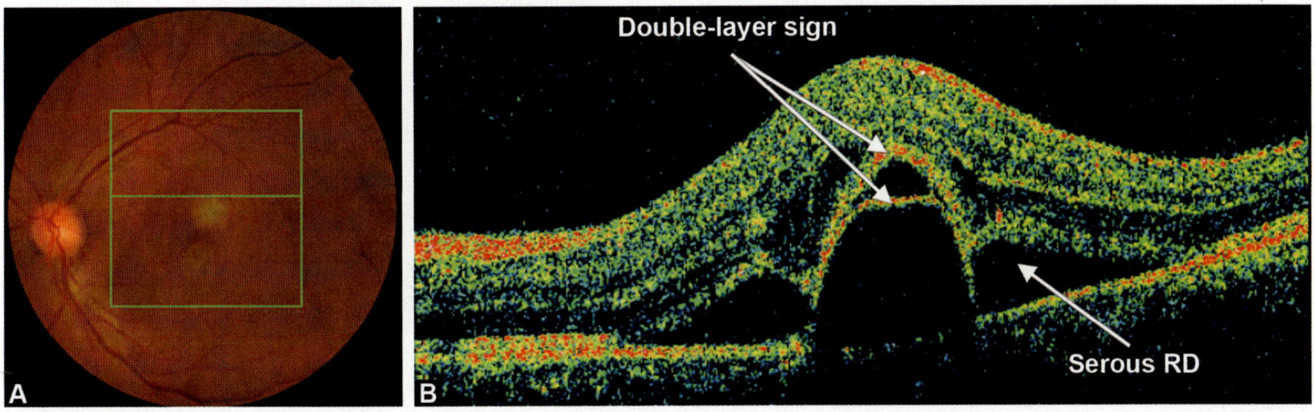

Figures 20.3.3A and B: (A) Color fundus photograph showing the horizontal line scan above the fovea. (B) Horizontal line scan above the fovea 2D image showing double reflective layers consisting of retinal pigment epithelium (RPE) and another highly reflective layer beneath the RPE ("double-layer sign"). Serous retinal detachment is also evident.

Figure 20.3.3E shows the cropped 3D image of Figure 20.3.3B.

The inner retinal layers have been peeled away to demonstrate the two pigment epithelial detachments (Figure 20.3.3F).

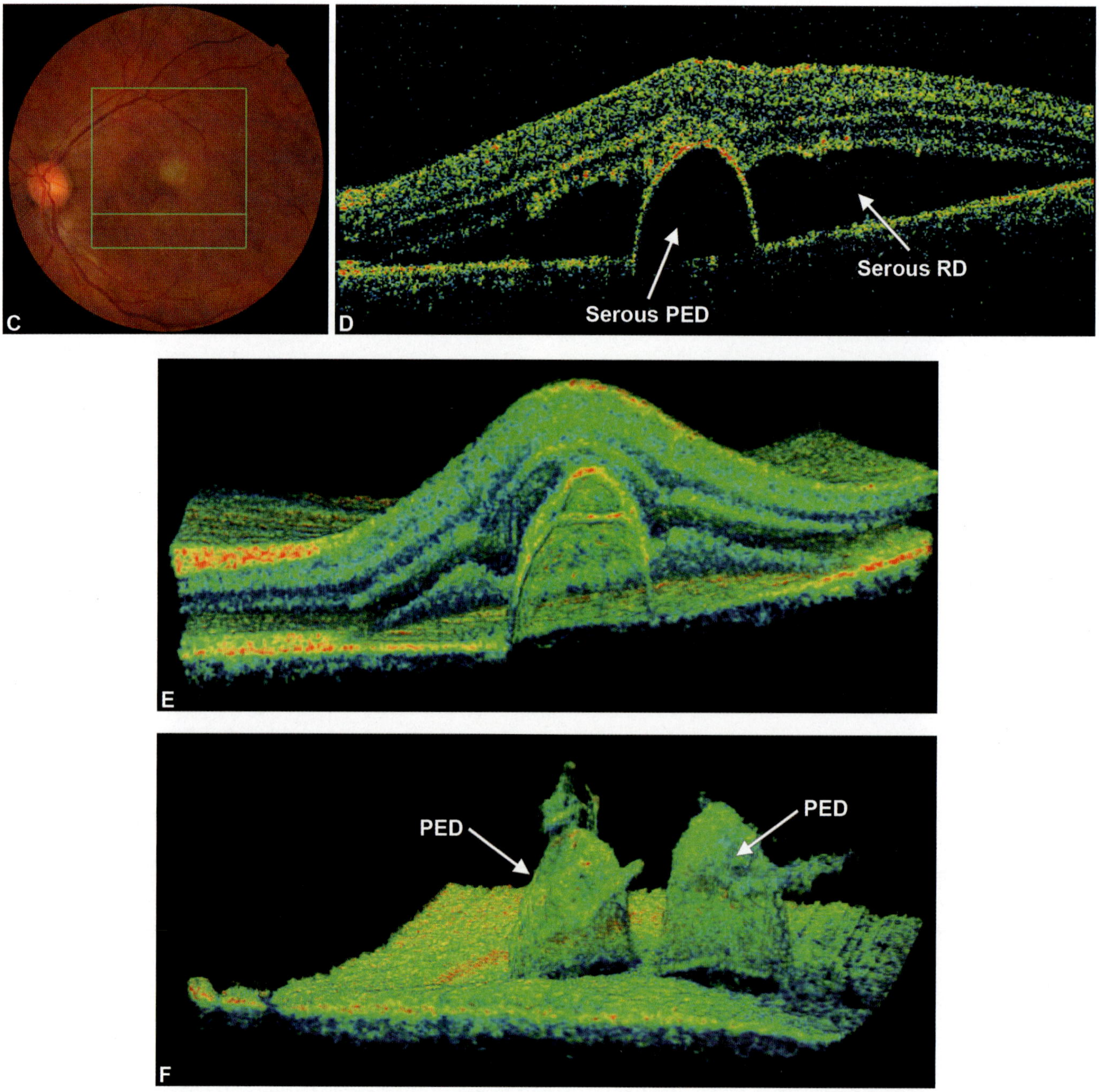

Figures 20.3.3C to F: (C) Color fundus photograph showing the horizontal line scan below the fovea. (D) Horizontal line scan below the fovea 2D image showing a large serous pigment epithelial detachment within the serous retinal detachment. (E) Cropped 3D image showing double reflective layers consisting of retinal pigment epithelium(RPE) and another highly reflective layer beneath the RPE ("double-layer sign"). Serous retinal detachment is also evident. (F) The inner retinal layers have been peeled away to demonstrate the two pigment epithelial detachments

CONCLUSION

Spectral Domain OCT is a valuable tool for establishing the diagnosis of polypoidal choroidal vasculopathy.

SUGGESTED READING

1. Yumiko Ojima, Masanori Hangai, Atsushi Sakamoto, et al. Improved visualization of Polypoidal Choroidal Vasculopathy lesions using Spectral Domain Optical Coherence Tomography. Retina 2009;29(1):52-9.
2. Sato T, Kishi S, Watanabe G, Matsumoto H, Mukai R. Tomographic features of branching vascular networks in polypoidal choroidal vasculopathy. Retina 2007;27(5):589-94.

21 Retinal Arterial Occlusion

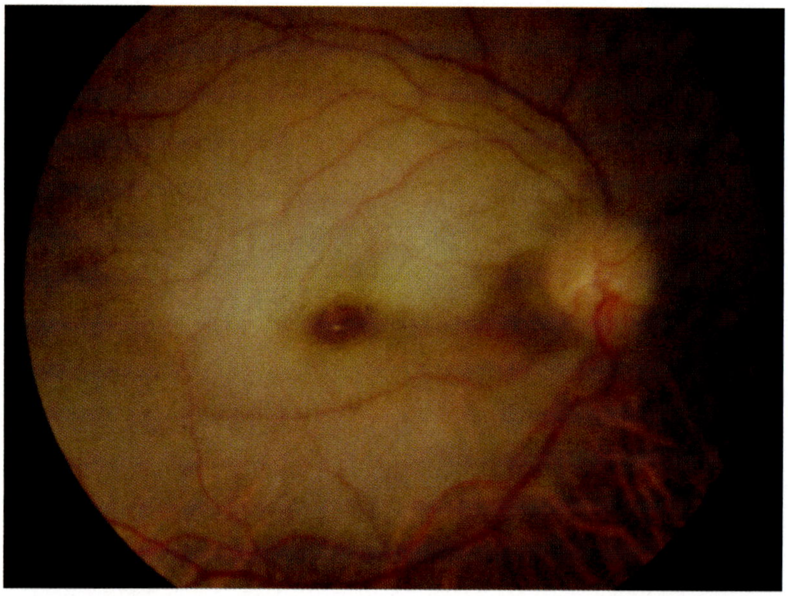

OCT is helpful in retinal arterial occlusions to document either macular edema or atrophy. The ischemic retina shows increased reflectivity in the inner retinal layers with decreased reflectivity of the photoreceptor layer and retinal pigment epithelium in the perifoveolar region secondary to the shadowing effect. The ischemic retina, however, regains its reflectivity over a period of time.

CASE 21.1: BRANCH ARTERY OCCLUSION WITH STAGE 4 MACULAR HOLE

Case Summary

A 72-year-old woman presented with sudden loss of vision in the right eye of one week duration. Her best-corrected visual acuity was perception of light in this eye. Fluorescein angiography showed delayed arterial filling with hyperfluorescence at the fovea which faded in the late phase (Figures 21.1.1 and 21.1.2).

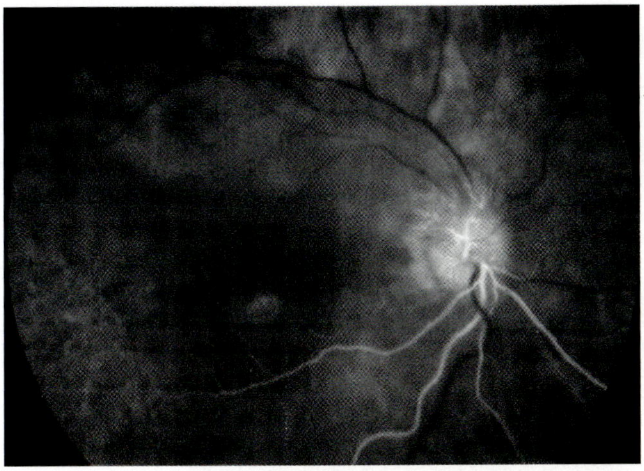

Figure 21.1.1: Early phase angiogram shows delayed arterial filling with hyperfluorescence at the fovea

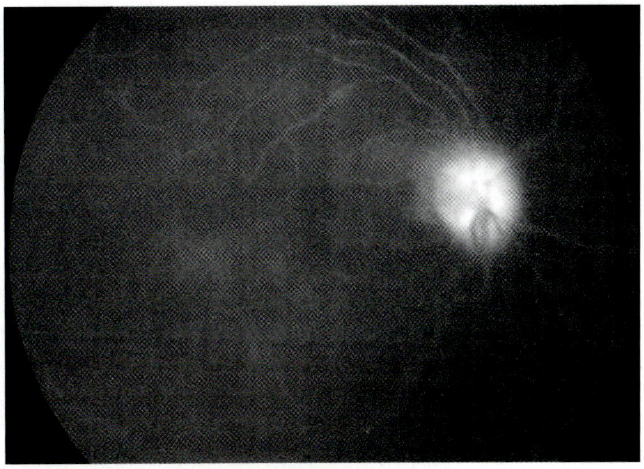

Figure 21.1.2: Late phase angiogram shows fading away of the hyperfluorescence

Optical Coherence Tomography–1

Horizontal line scan showed hyper-reflectivity in the inner retinal layers corresponding to the opaque retina clinically. There was a hyper-reflective membrane intimately adherent to the underlying retina. The posterior hyaloid membrane was seen anterior to the retina (Figures 21.1.3A to C).

Optical Coherence Tomography–2

Horizontal line scan through the fovea showed the presence of full thickness retinal dehiscence and epiretinal membrane. The posterior hyaloid membrane was seen anterior to the retina (Figures 21.1.3D to F).

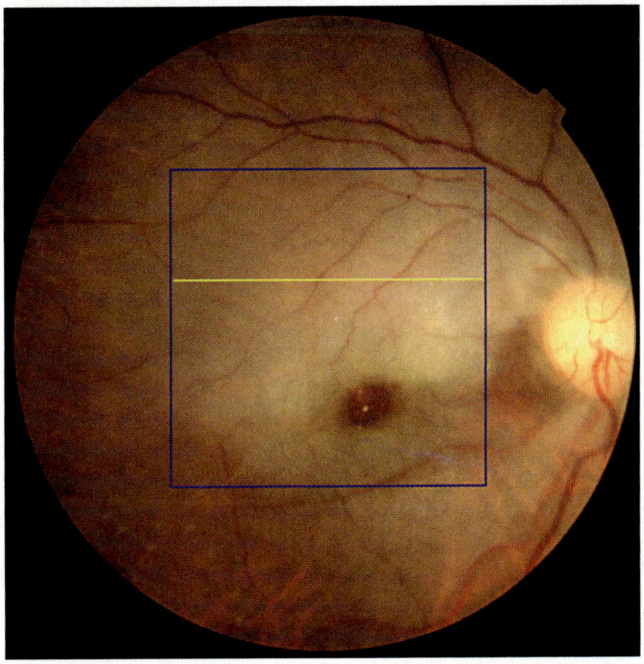

Figure 21.1.3A: Color fundus photograph showing the horizontal line scan through the opaque retina

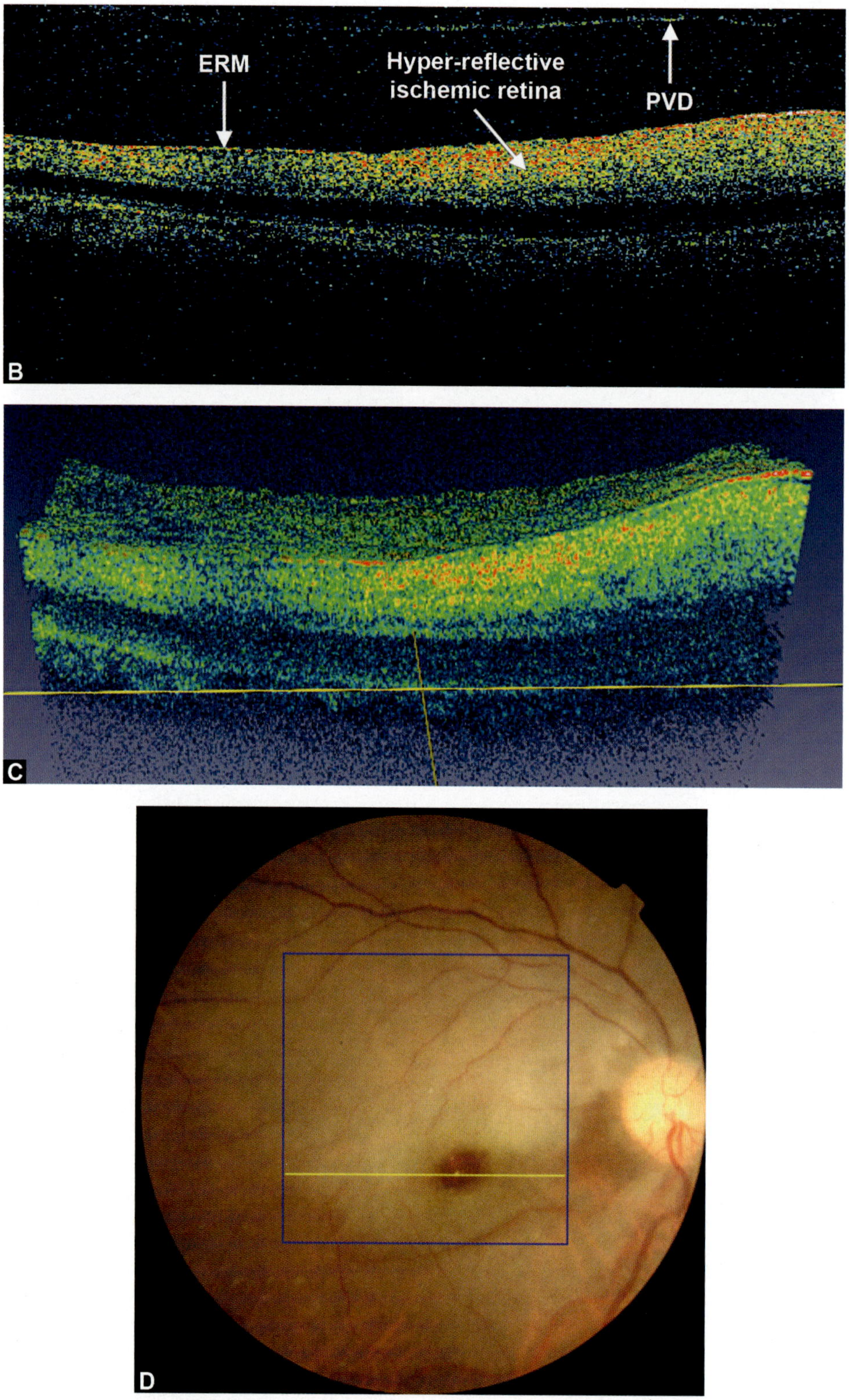

Figures 21.1.3B to D: (B) Horizontal line scan 2D image showing hyper-reflectivity in the inner retinal layers corresponding to the opaque retina clinically. Epiretinal membrane and posterior vitreous detachment are also evident. (C) Cropped 3D image showing hyper-reflectivity in the inner retinal layers corresponding to the opaque retina clinically. Epiretinal membrane and posterior vitreous detachment are also evident. (D) Color fundus photograph showing the horizontal line scan through the fovea

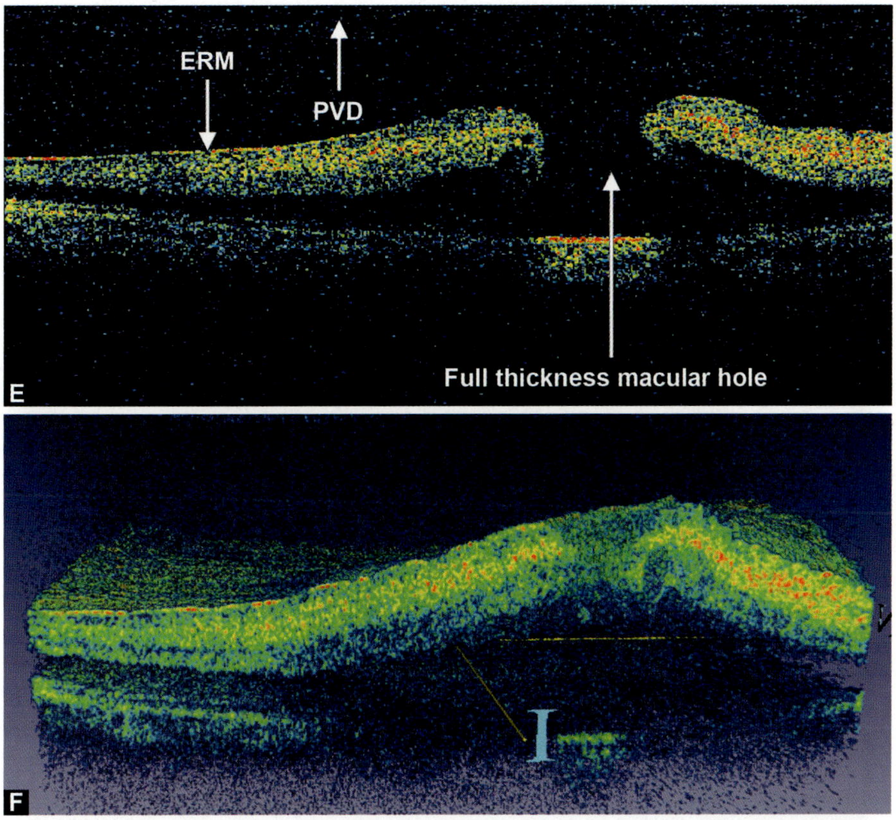

Figures 21.1.3E and F: (E) Horizontal line scan 2D image showing the presence of full thickness retinal dehiscence, epiretinal membrane and posterior hyaloid membrane. (F) Cropped 3D image showing the presence of full thickness retinal dehiscence, epiretinal membrane and posterior hyaloid membrane

CASE 21.2: CENTRAL RETINAL ARTERY OCCLUSION WITH CILIORETINAL ARTERY SPARING

Case Summary

A 60-year-old male presented with sudden loss of vision in the left eye of two days duration. His best-corrected visual acuity was hand movements in this eye. Fluorescein angiography showed arm to retina time of 25.8 secs, patchy choroidal filling, cilioretinal artery filling and delayed arterial filling in the early phase angiogram (Figure 21.2.1). The late phase angiogram showed complete filling of the retinal vessels (Figure 21.2.2).

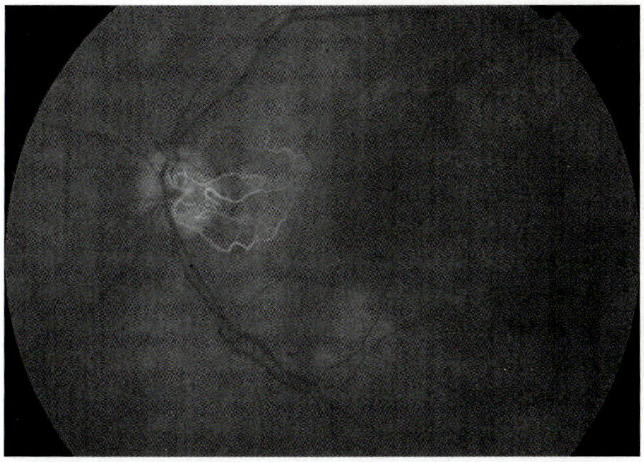

Figure 21.2.1: Early phase angiogram shows patchy choroidal filling, cilioretinal artery filling and delayed arterial filling

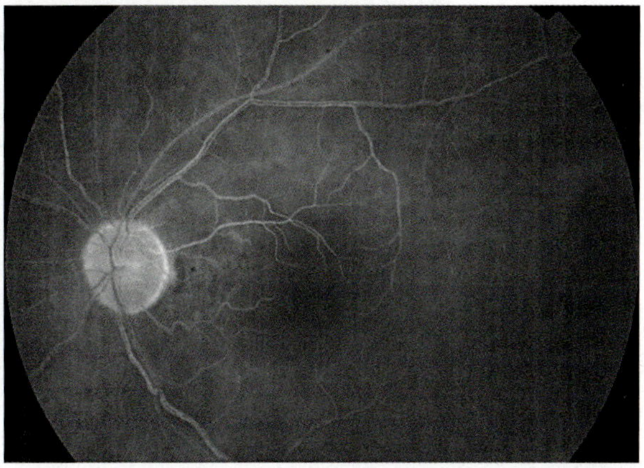

Figure 21.2.2: Late phase angiogram shows complete filling of the retinal vessels

Optical Coherence Tomography

Horizontal line scan showed hyper-reflectivity in the inner retinal layers corresponding to the opaque retina clinically with decreased reflectivity of the photoreceptor layer and retinal pigment epithelium in the perifoveolar region secondary to the shadowing effect (Figures 21.2.3A to D).

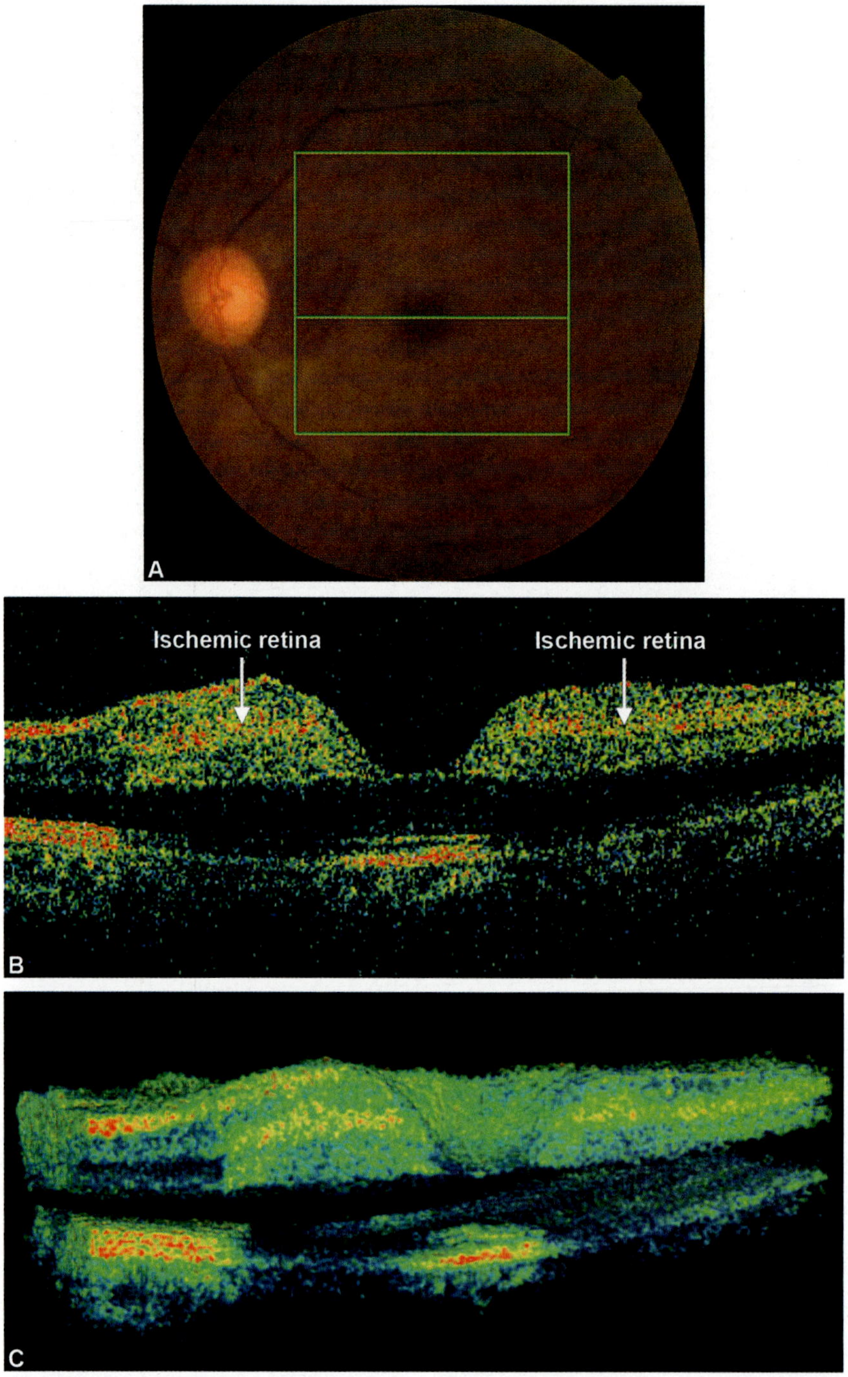

Figures 21.2.3A to C: (A) Color fundus photograph showing the horizontal line scan through the fovea. (B) Horizontal line scan 2D image showing hyper-reflectivity in the inner retinal layers corresponding to the opaque retina clinically with decreased reflectivity of the photoreceptor layer and retinal pigment epithelium in the perifoveolar region. (C) Cropped 3D image showing hyper-reflectivity in the inner retinal layers corresponding to the opaque retina clinically with decreased reflectivity of the photoreceptor layer and retinal pigment epithelium in the perifoveolar region.

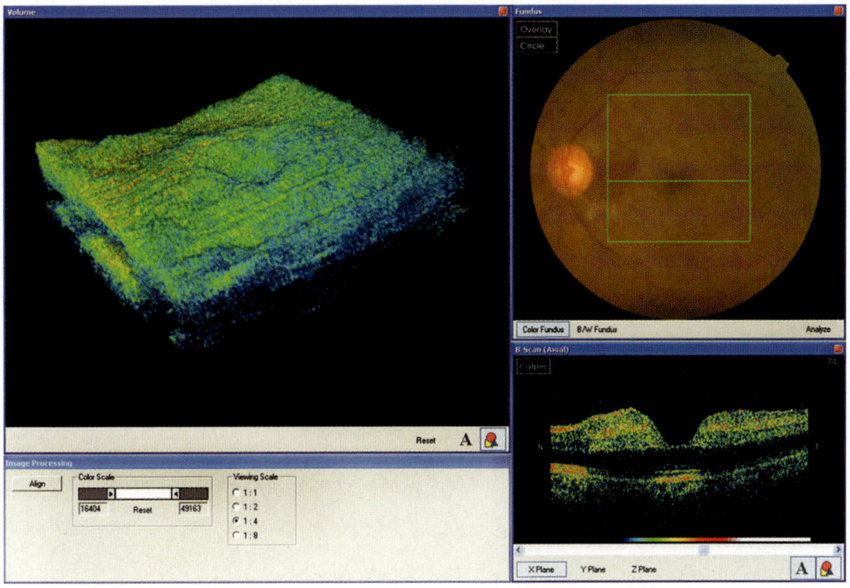

Figure 21.2.3D: 3D image of Case 21.2

SUGGESTED READING

1. Ozdemir H, Karacorlu S, Karacorlu M. Optical coherence tomography findings in central retinal artery occlusion. Retina 2006;26:110-2.
2. Spaide RF, Lee JK, Klancnik JM, Gross NE. Optical coherence tomography of branch retinal vein occlusion. Retina 2003;23: 343-7.

22 Retinal Detachment

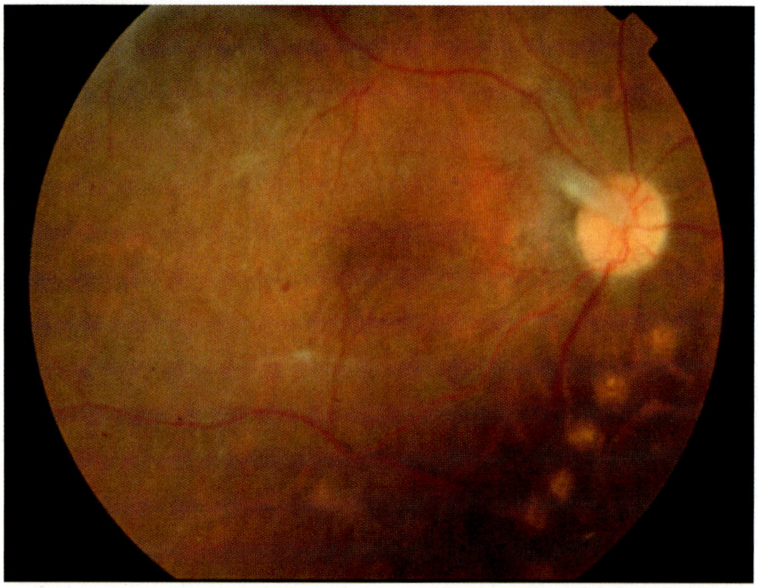

Retinal detachments at the posterior pole, in particular traction detachments can be readily detected by OCT. Preretinal and epiretinal membranes and the vitreoretinal traction that subtend them can easily be delineated.

CASE 22.1: TRACTIONAL RETINAL DETACHMENT

Case Summary

A 68-year-old man with proliferative diabetic retinopathy presented with diminished vision in the right eye. He gave a past history of laser photocoagulation. His best-corrected visual acuity in this eye was 2/60.

Optical Coherence Tomography

Horizontal line scan revealed a shallow cleavage at the level of the RPE-choriocapillaris complex with an optically clear cavity of subretinal fluid (Figures 22.1.1A to C).

OCT line scan through the fovea showed normal foveal contour without evidence of retinal detachment. There were cyst like spaces in the neurosensory retina suggestive of retinal edema (Figures 22.1.2A to D).

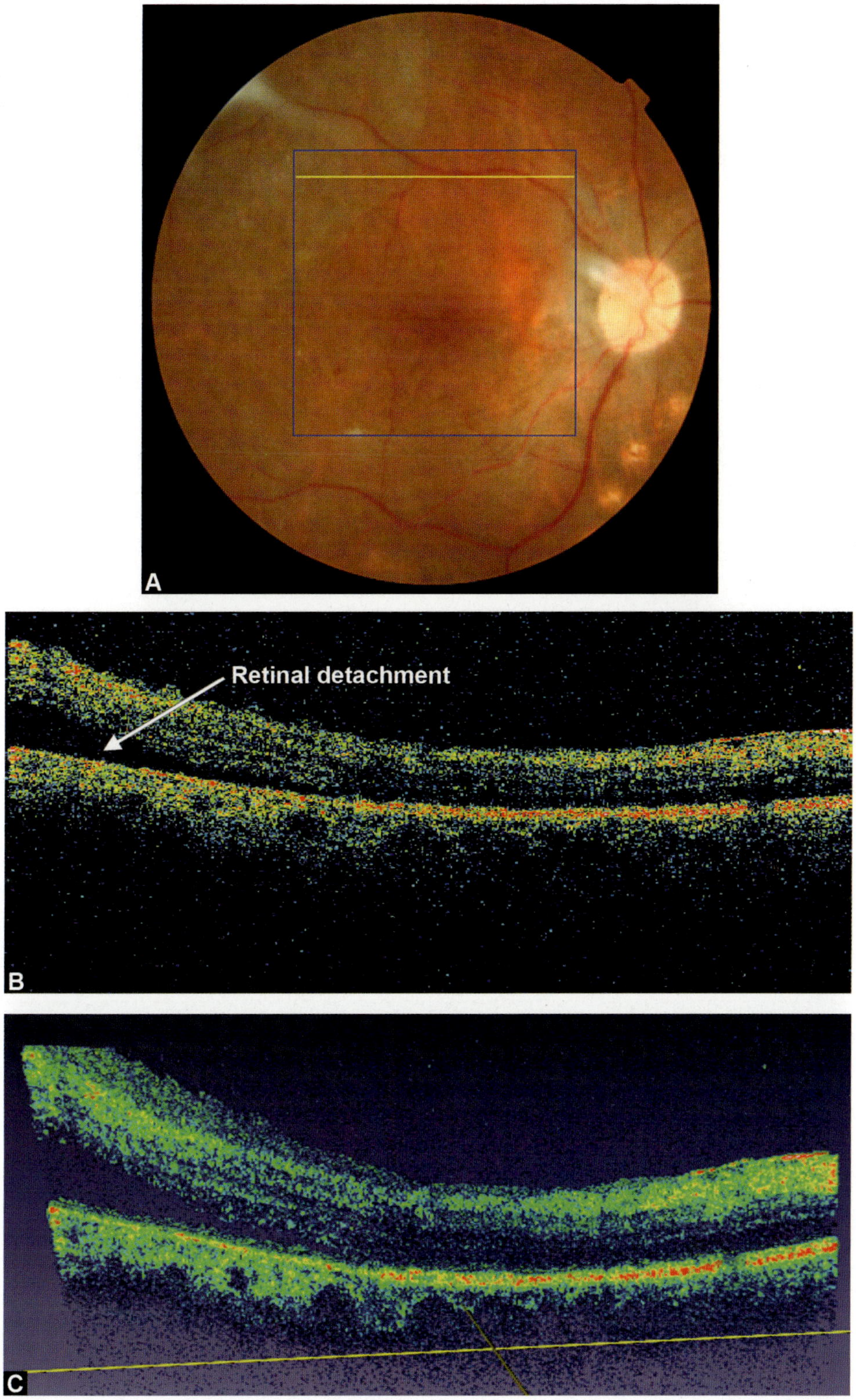

Figures 22.1.1A to C: (A) Color fundus photograph showing the horizontal line scan above the fovea. (B) Horizontal line scan 2D image showing shallow cleavage at the level of the RPE-choriocapillaris complex with an optically clear cavity of subretinal fluid. (C) Cropped 3D image showing shallow cleavage at the level of the RPE-choriocapillaris complex with an optically clear cavity of subretinal fluid

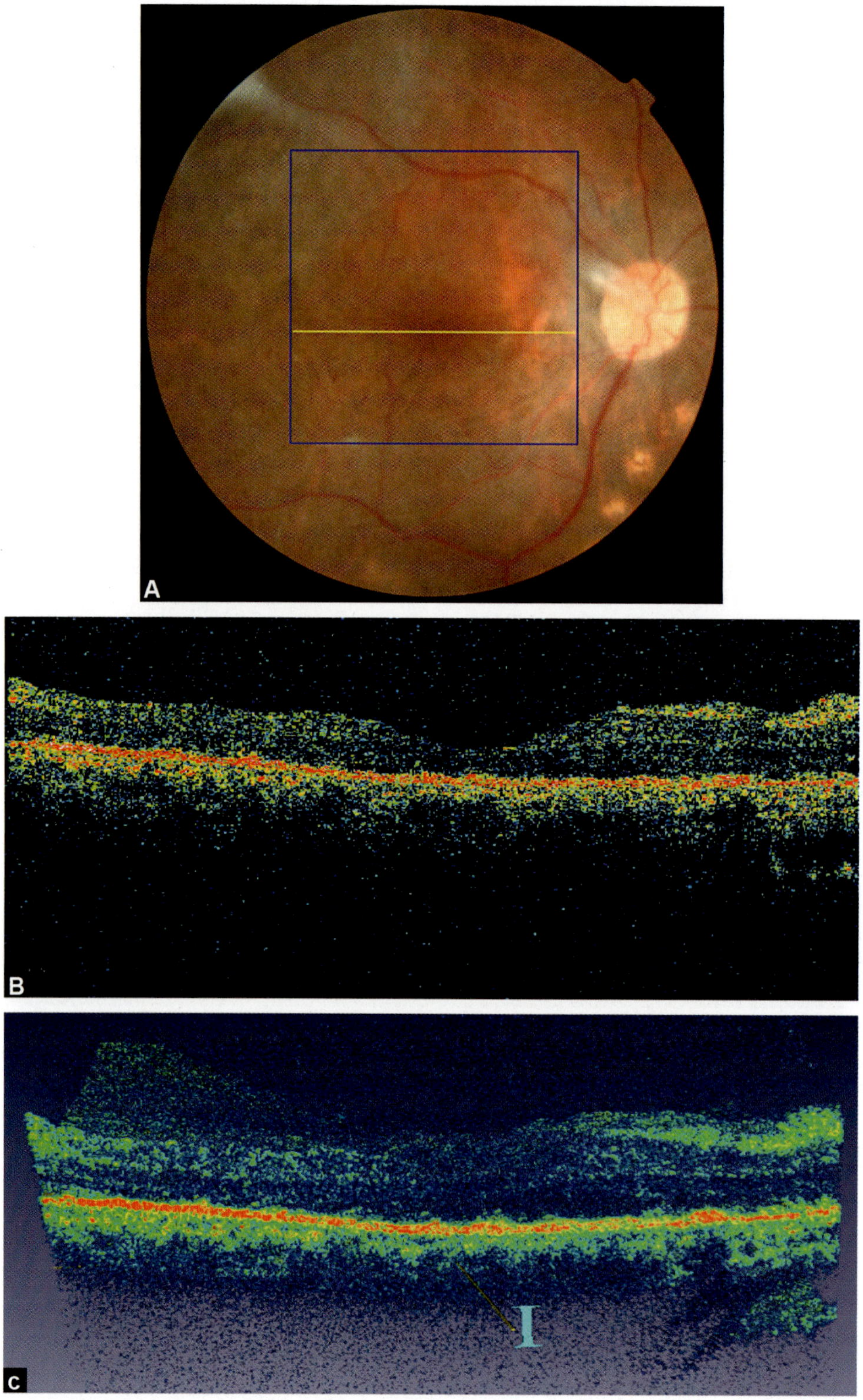

Figures 22.1.2A to C: (A) Color fundus photograph showing the horizontal line scan through the fovea. (B) Horizontal line scan, 2D image showing normal foveal contour without evidence of retinal detachment. Cyst like spaces in the neurosensory retina are suggestive of retinal edema. (C) Cropped 3D image showing normal foveal contour and cyst like spaces in the neurosensory retina suggestive of retinal edema

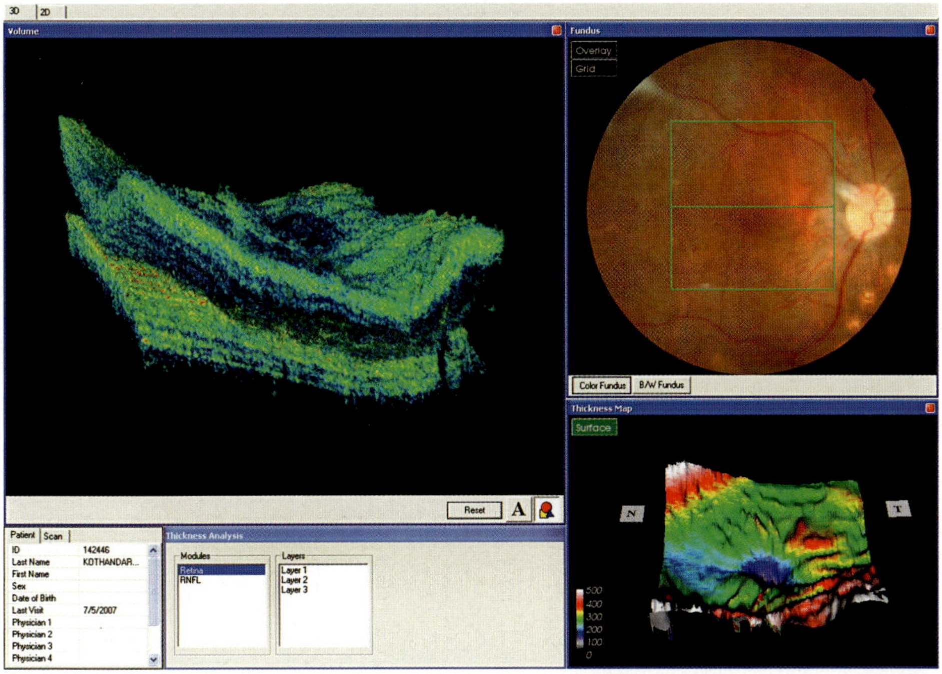

Figure 22.1.2D: 3D image of Case 22.1

Horizontal line scan below the fovea showed evidence of retinal detachment. The undulations on the retinal surface indicate traction (Figures 22.1.3A to C). Thus, the 3D OCT with its ability to scan at different levels, helped in confirming the extent of the retinal detachment at the posterior pole, which was thereby useful in predicting the surgical outcome in this case.

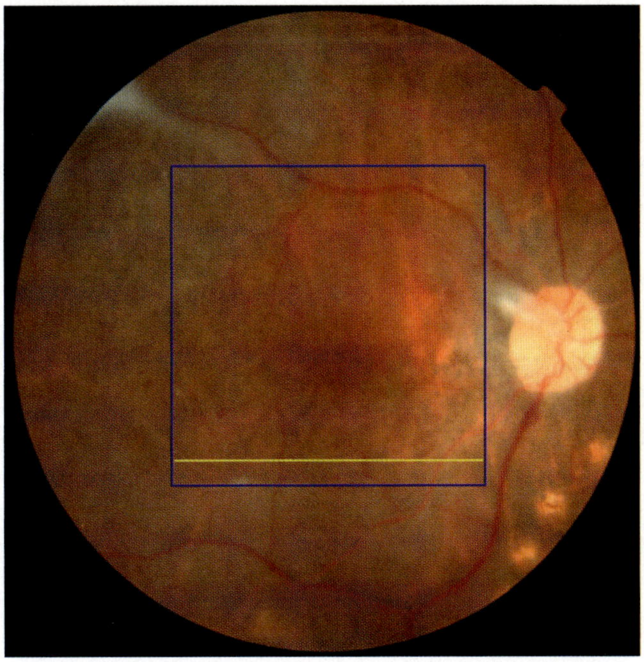

Figure 22.1.3A: Color fundus photograph showing the horizontal line scan below the fovea

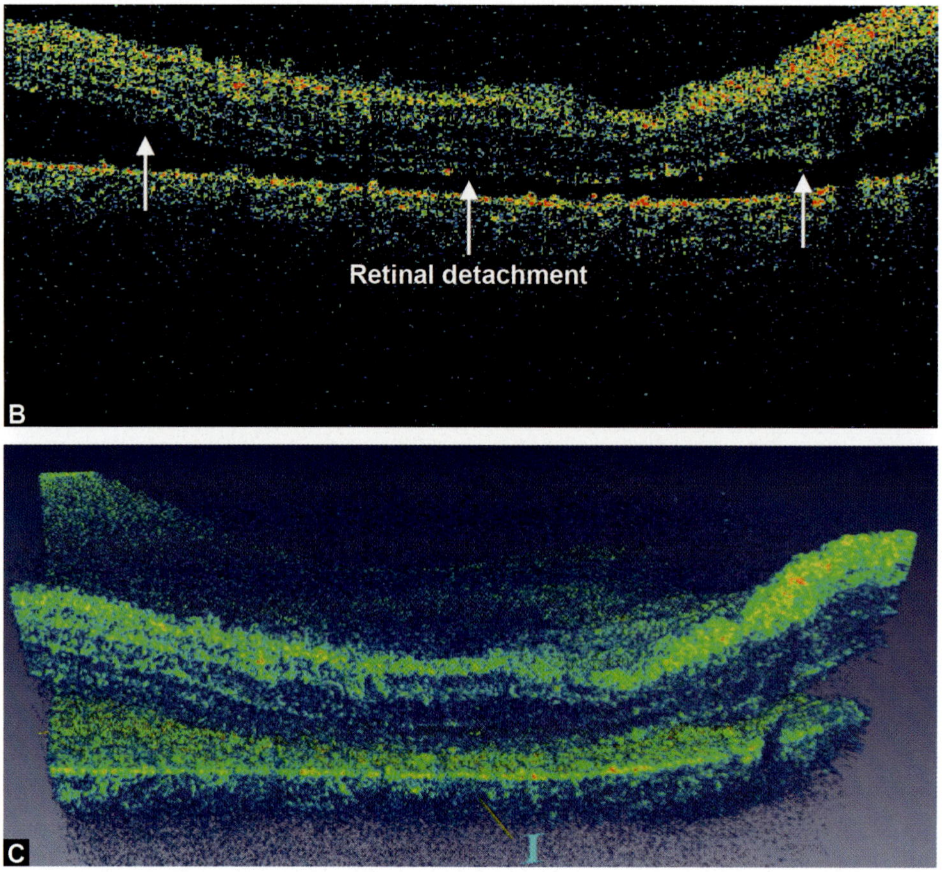

Figures 22.1.3B and C: (B) Horizontal line scan 2D image showing evidence of retinal detachment. (C) Cropped 3D image showing evidence of retinal detachment

CASE 22.2: RETINAL DETACHMENT

Case Summary

A 53-year-old man presented with diminished vision in the right eye of 4 days duration. His best-corrected visual acuity in this eye was 6/18.

Optical Coherence Tomography

Horizontal line scan revealed a shallow cleavage at the level of the RPE-choriocapillaris complex with an optically clear cavity of subretinal fluid (Figures 22.2.1A to D).

Horizontal line scan through the fovea showed increased retinal thickening with evidence of retinal detachment and schisis. (Figures 22.2.2A to C)

Horizontal line scan below the fovea showed increased retinal thickness and evidence of retinal detachment. The undulations on the retinal surface indicate traction. The poor reflectivity of the RPE is due to the height of the detachment (Figures 22.2.3A to C).

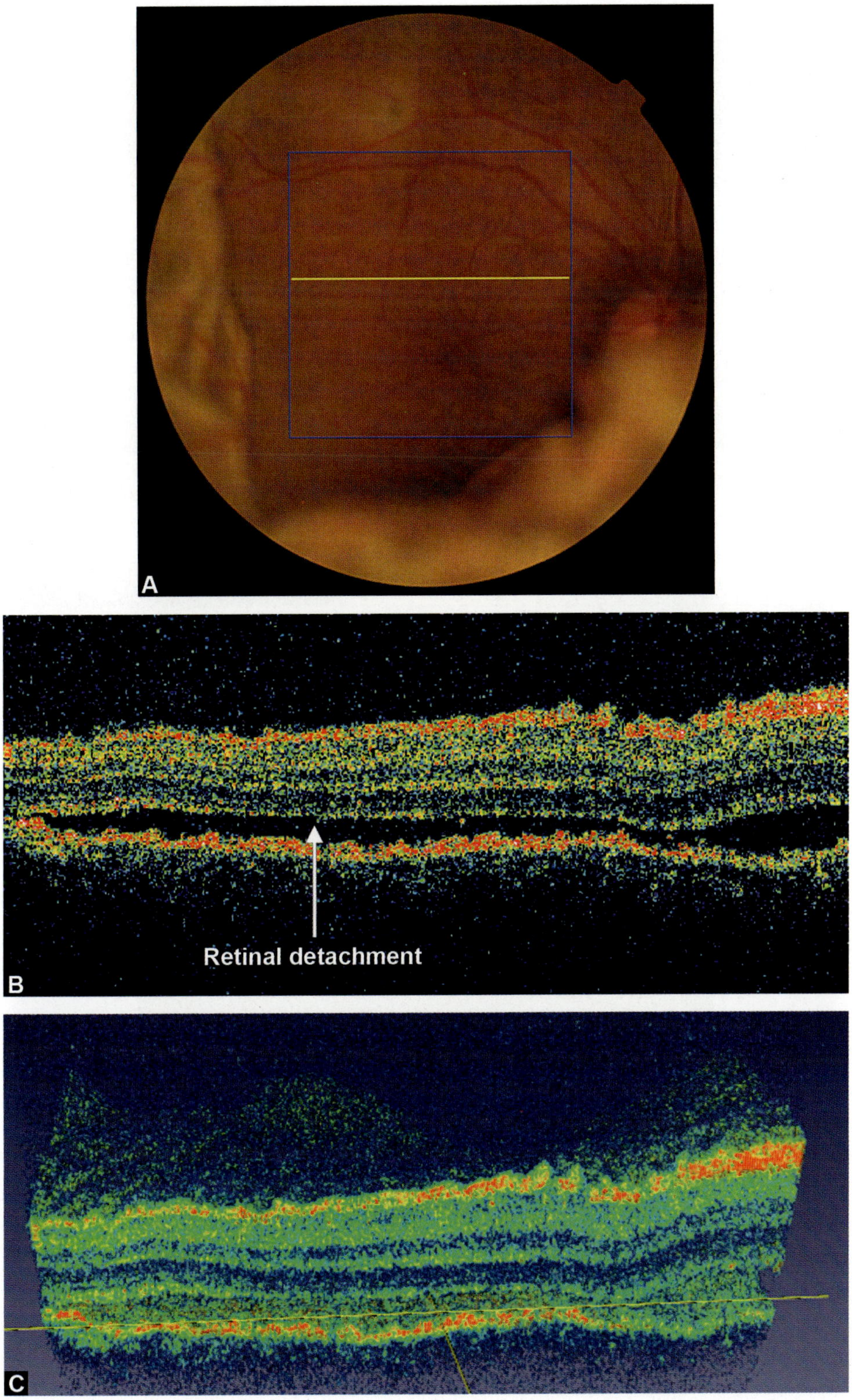

Figures 22.2.1A to C: (A) Color fundus photograph showing the horizontal line scan above the fovea. (B) Horizontal line scan, 2D image showing a shallow cleavage at the level of the RPE-choriocapillaris complex with an optically clear cavity of subretinal fluid. (C) Cropped 3D image showing a shallow cleavage at the level of the RPE-choriocapillaris complex with an optically clear cavity of subretinal fluid

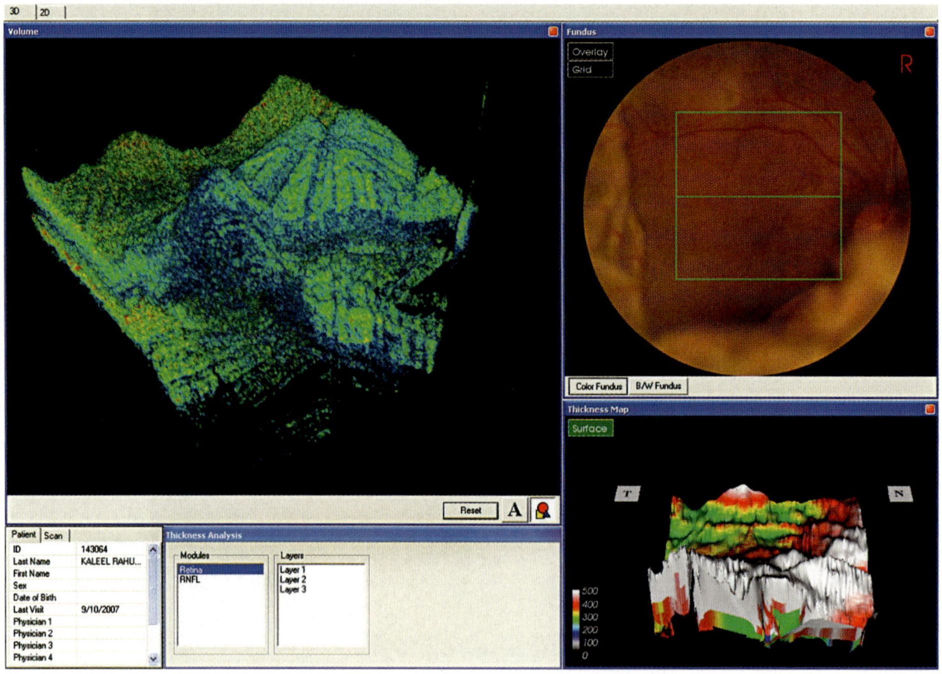

Figure 22.2.1D: 3D image of Case 22.2

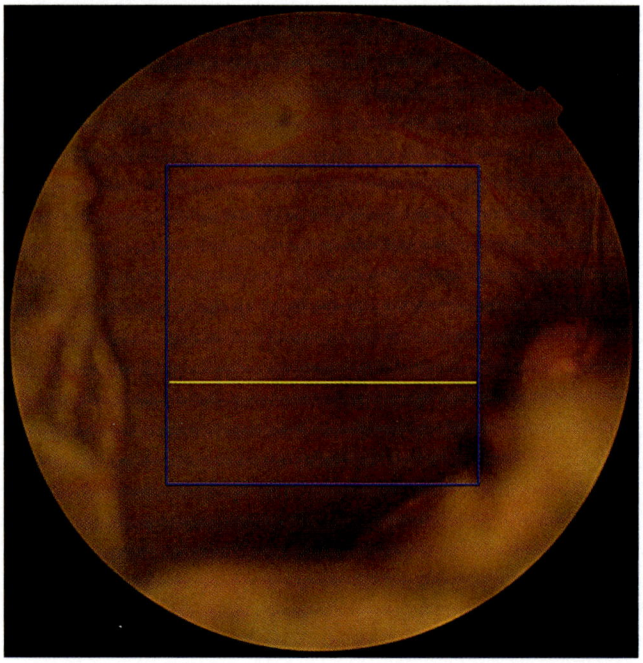

Figure 22.2.2A: Color fundus photograph showing the horizontal line scan through the fovea

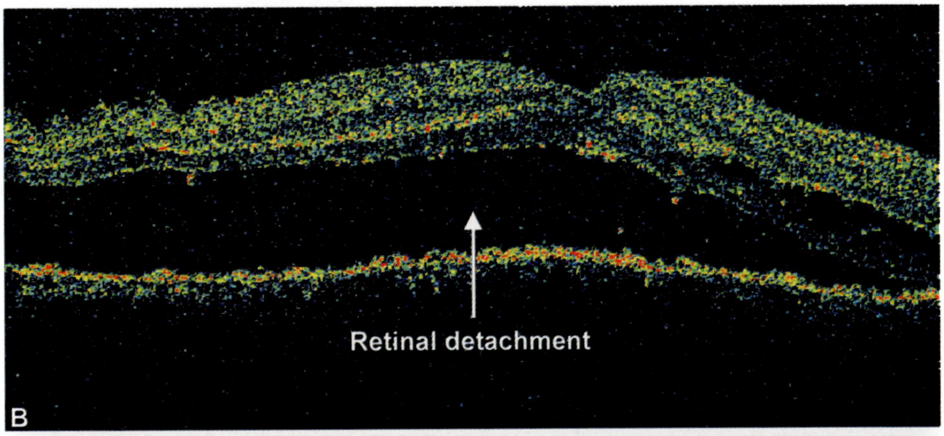

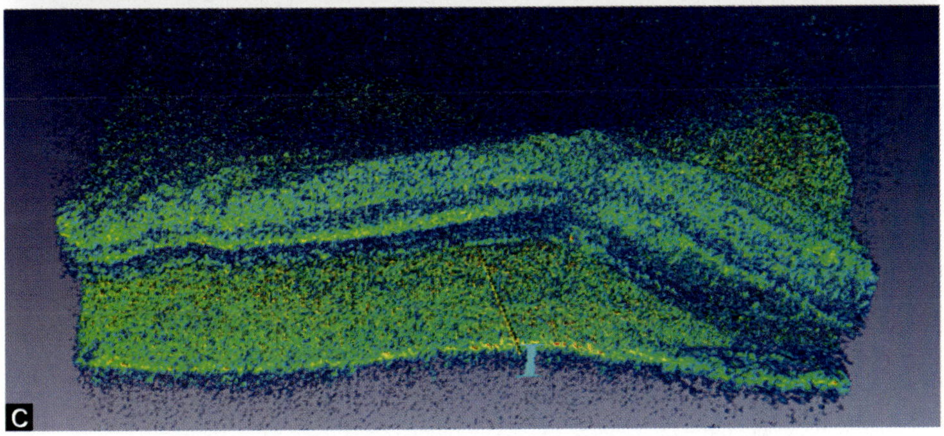

Figures 22.2.2B and C: (B) Horizontal line scan 2D image showing increased retinal thickening with evidence of retinal detachment and schisis. (C) Cropped 3D image showing increased retinal thickening with evidence of retinal detachment and schisis

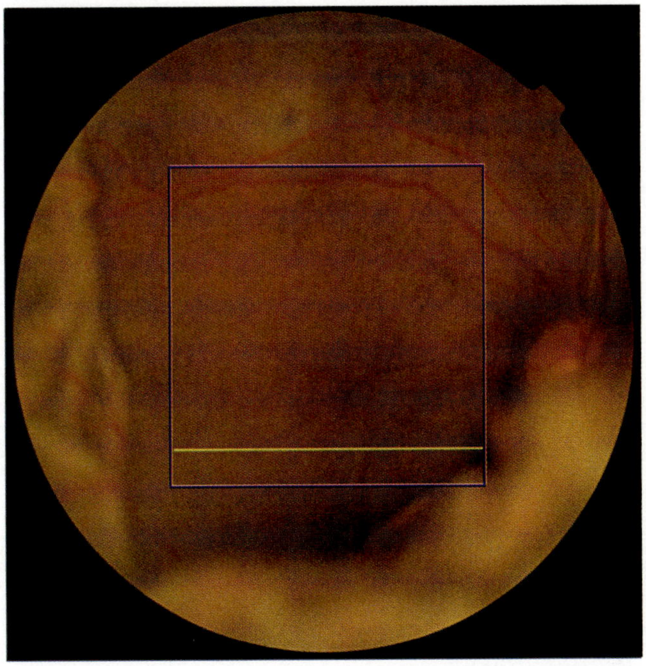

Figure 22.2.3A: Color fundus photograph showing the horizontal line scan below the fovea

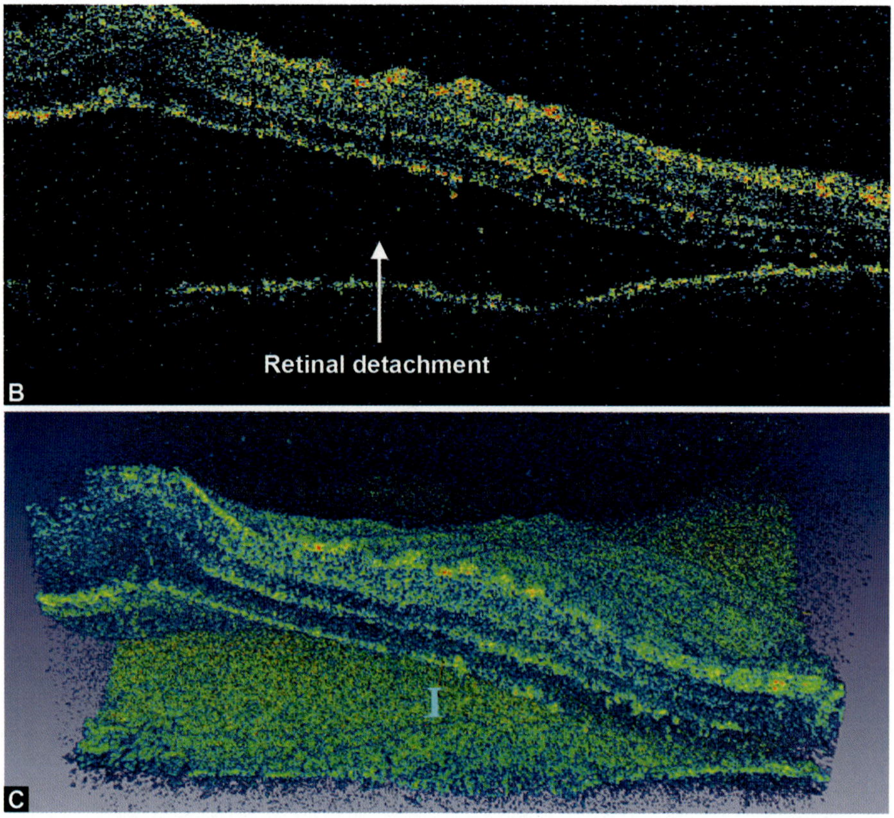

Figures 22.2.3B and C: Horizontal line scan 2D image showing increased retinal thickness, evidence of retinal detachment and undulations on the retinal surface. The poor reflectivity of the RPE is due to the height of the detachment. (C) Cropped 3D image showing increased retinal thickness, evidence of retinal detachment and undulations on the retinal surface

CASE 22.3: RETINOSCHISIS

Case Summary

A 17-year-old male with high myopia presented with diminished vision in the left eye of three months duration. His best-corrected visual acuity in this eye was 6/24. Fluorescein angiography showed peripapillary atrophy with progressive hyperfluorescence at the posterior pole (Figures 22.3.1 and 22.3.2).

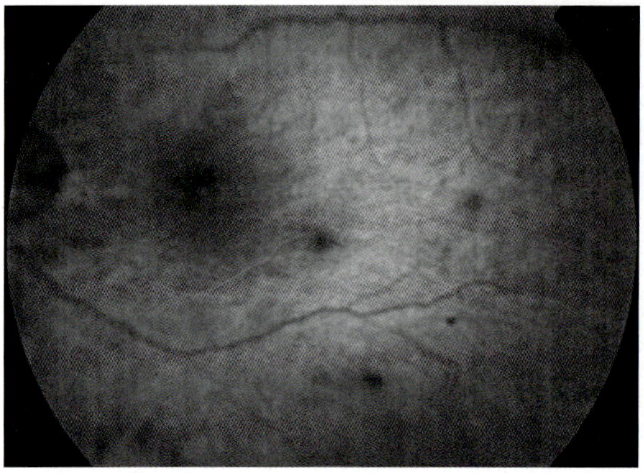

Figure 22.3.1: Early phase angiogram shows progressive hyperfluorescence

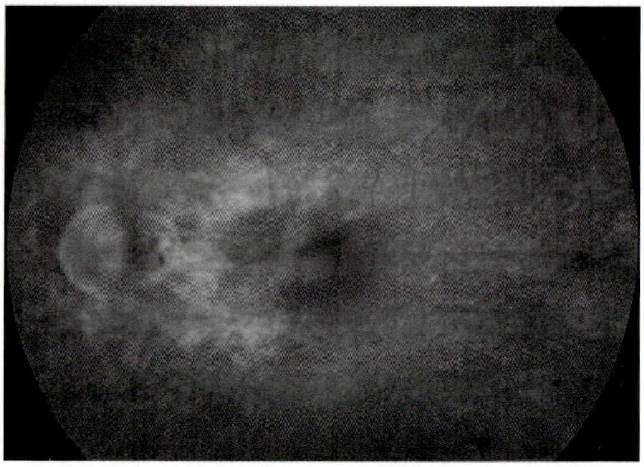

Figure 22.3.2: Late phase angiogram shows increasing hyperfluorescence

Optical Coherence Tomography

Horizontal line scan below the fovea showed splitting of the neurosensory retina indicating the presence of retinoschisis. Thus, the 3D OCT with its ability to continuously scan the area within the blue square was able to detect the retinoschisis, inferior to the fovea (Figures 22.3.3A to C).

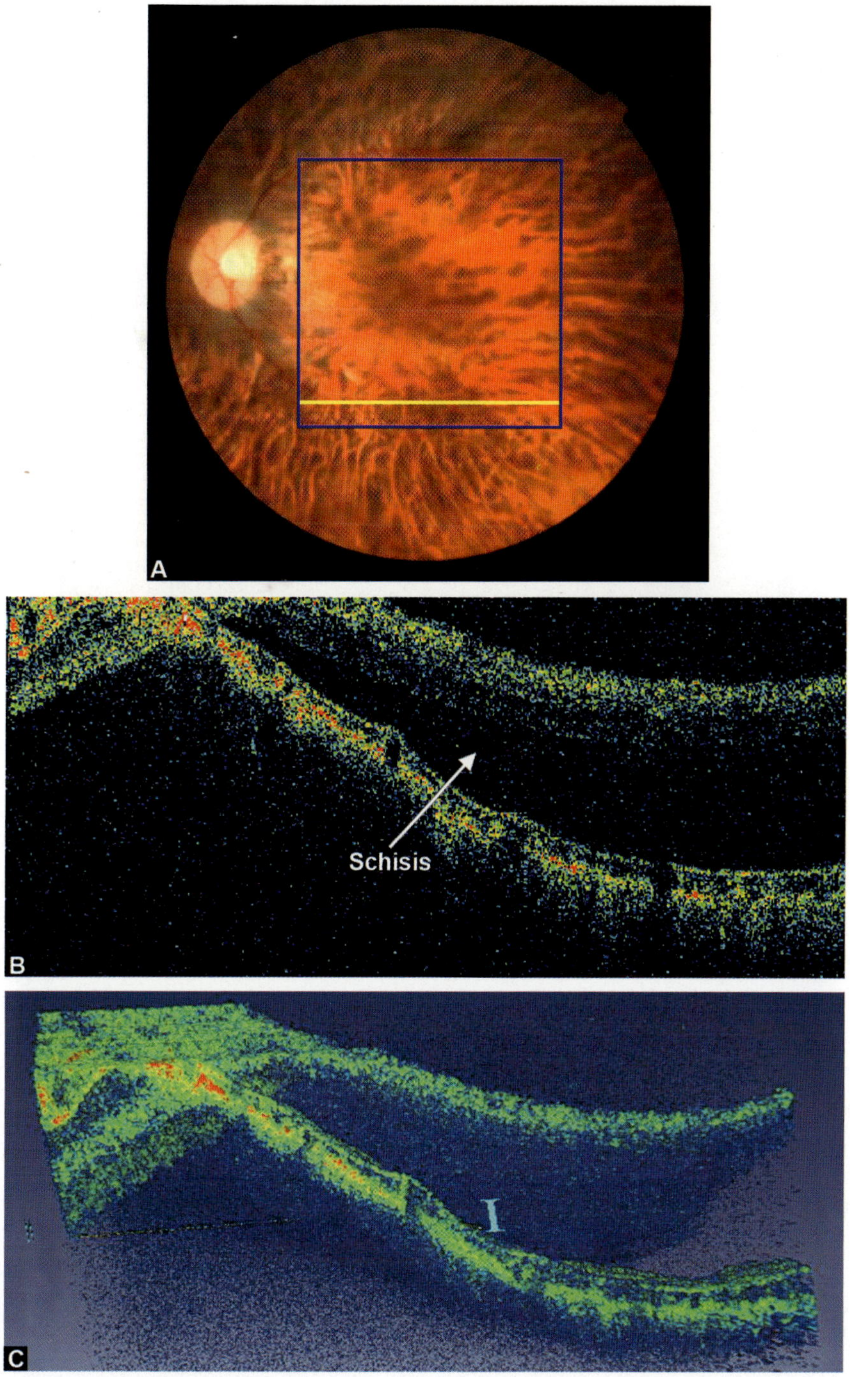

Figures 22.3.3A to C: (A) Color fundus photograph showing the horizontal line scan below the fovea. (B) Horizontal line scan 2D image showing splitting of the neurosensory retina indicating the presence of retinoschisis. (C) Cropped 3D image showing splitting of the neurosensory retina indicating the presence of retinoschisis

23 Retinal Vein Occlusion

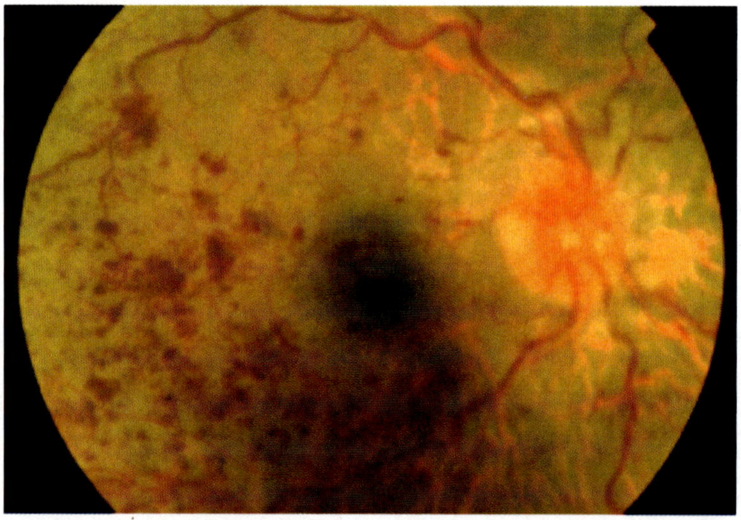

Retinal vein occlusion (branch and central) is the second most common retinal vascular diseases after diabetic retinopathy. Patients affected are usually in their fifth to sixth decade of life. The 10-year risk of developing cardiovascular complications is higher in patients with BRVO (Branch retinal vein occlusion) than CRVO (Central retinal vein occlusion).

Fluorescein angiography helps to determine the cause of visual loss - macular edema and/or macular ischemia.

Optical coherence tomography enables detection of subtle macular edema even in the presence of significant hemorrhage. It shows the presence of cystoid spaces, serous retinal detachment, epiretinal membranes and macular hole. It plays an important role in monitoring the response to the various treatment modalities employed, thereby reducing the need for repeated angiograms.

CASE 23.1: CENTRAL RETINAL VEIN OCCLUSION

Case Summary

A 62-year-old woman was seen with decreased vision in the right eye of one month duration. Her best-corrected visual acuity in this eye was 6/60. Fluorescein angiography showed non-ischemic central retinal vein occlusion with leakage of dye at the fovea and disc (Figures 23.1.1 and 23.1.2).

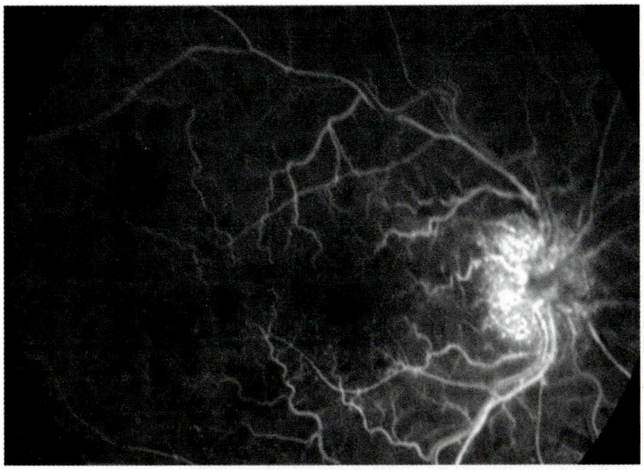

Figure 23.1.1: Early phase angiogram shows non-ischemic central retinal vein occlusion

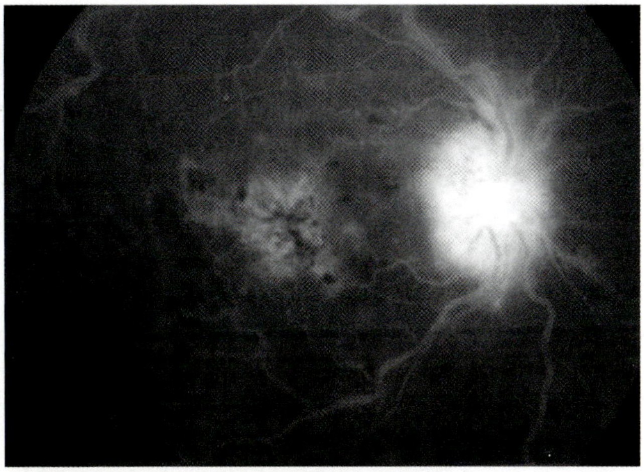

Figure 23.1.2: Late phase shows leakage at the disc and macula

Optical Coherence Tomography

Horizontal line scan showed loss of foveal contour, central retinal thickening and hyporeflective areas with intervening hyper-reflective septae suggestive of cystoid macular spaces. In addition, there was an area of hyporeflectivity in the subfoveal region consistent with subfoveal serous retinal detachment (Figures 23.1.3A to D).

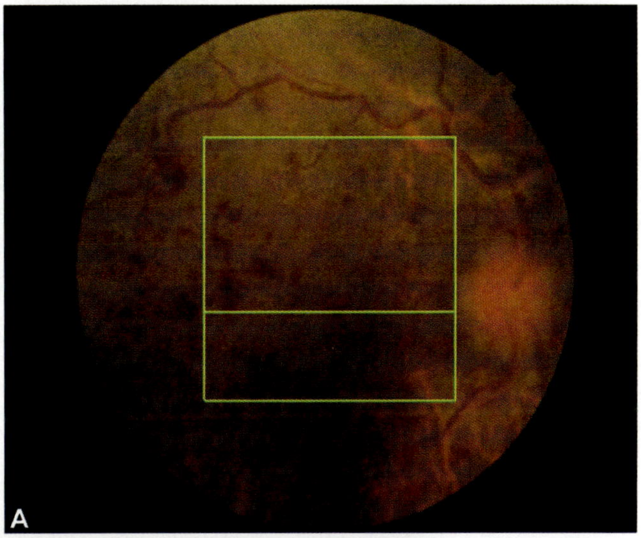

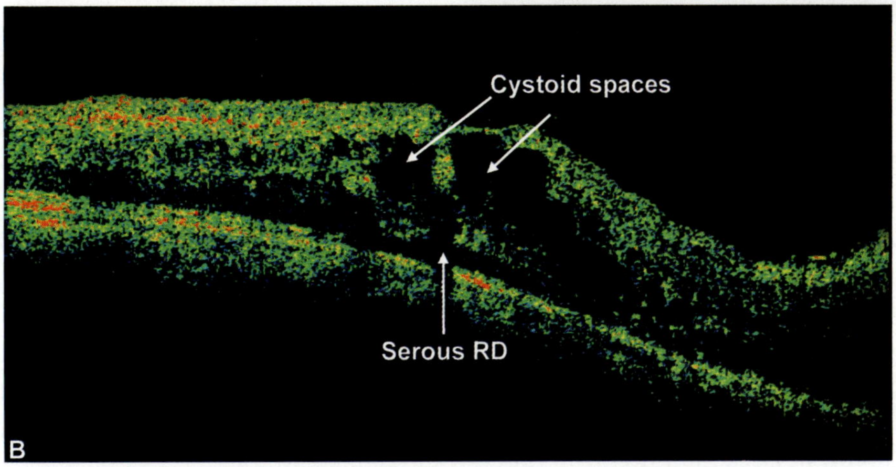

Figures 23.1.3A and B: (A) Color fundus photograph showing the horizontal line scan through the fovea. (B) Horizontal line scan, 2D image showing loss of foveal contour, central retinal thickening and hyporeflective areas with intervening hyper-reflective septae suggestive of cystoid macular spaces. An area of hyporeflectivity in the subfoveal region consistent with subfoveal serous retinal detachment is evident

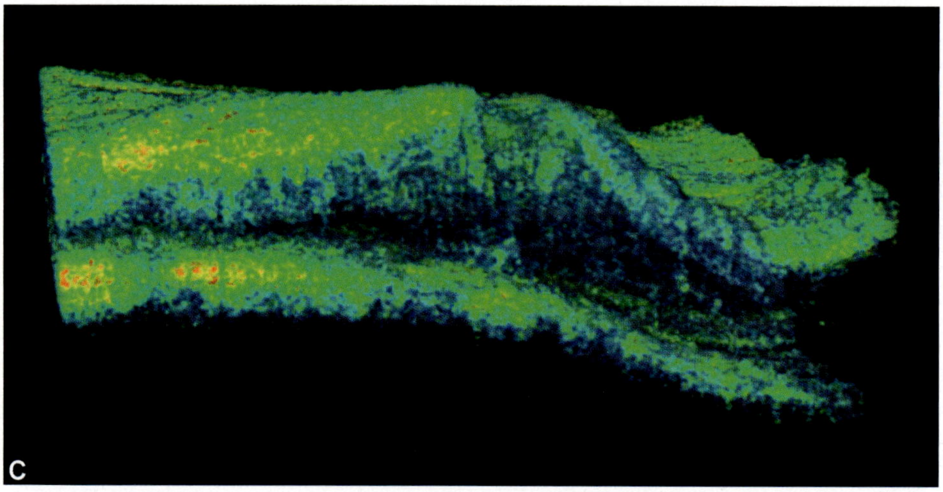

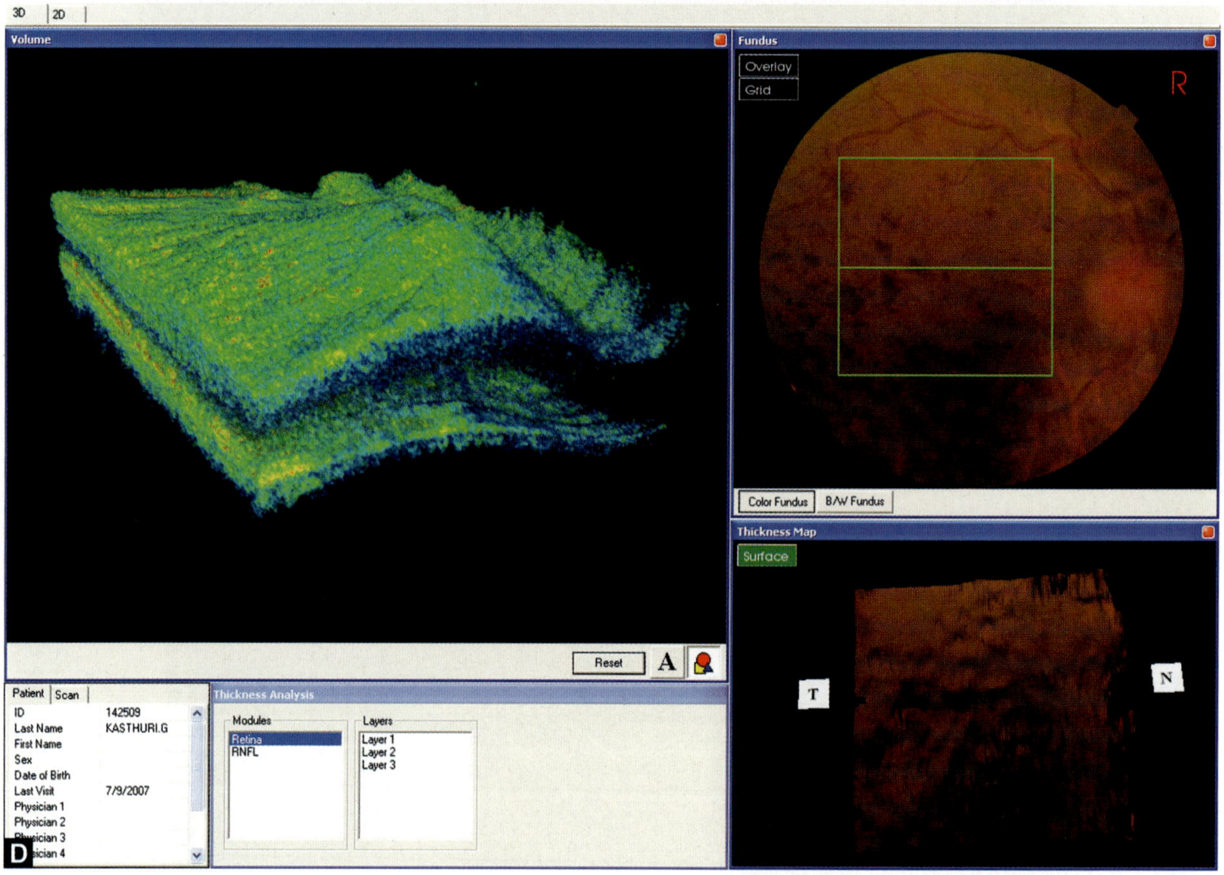

Figures 23.1.3C and D: (C) Cropped 3D image showing loss of foveal contour, central retinal thickening and hyporeflective areas with intervening hyper-reflective septae suggestive of cystoid macular spaces. An area of hyporeflectivity in the subfoveal region consistent with subfoveal serous retinal detachment is evident. (D) 3D image of Case 23.1

Optical Coherence Tomography

Horizontal line scan through the right optic disc showed substantial disc elevation with a clear optical space inside the disc because of the marked tissue thickening and fluid accumulation within it (Figures 23.1.4 and 23.1.5).

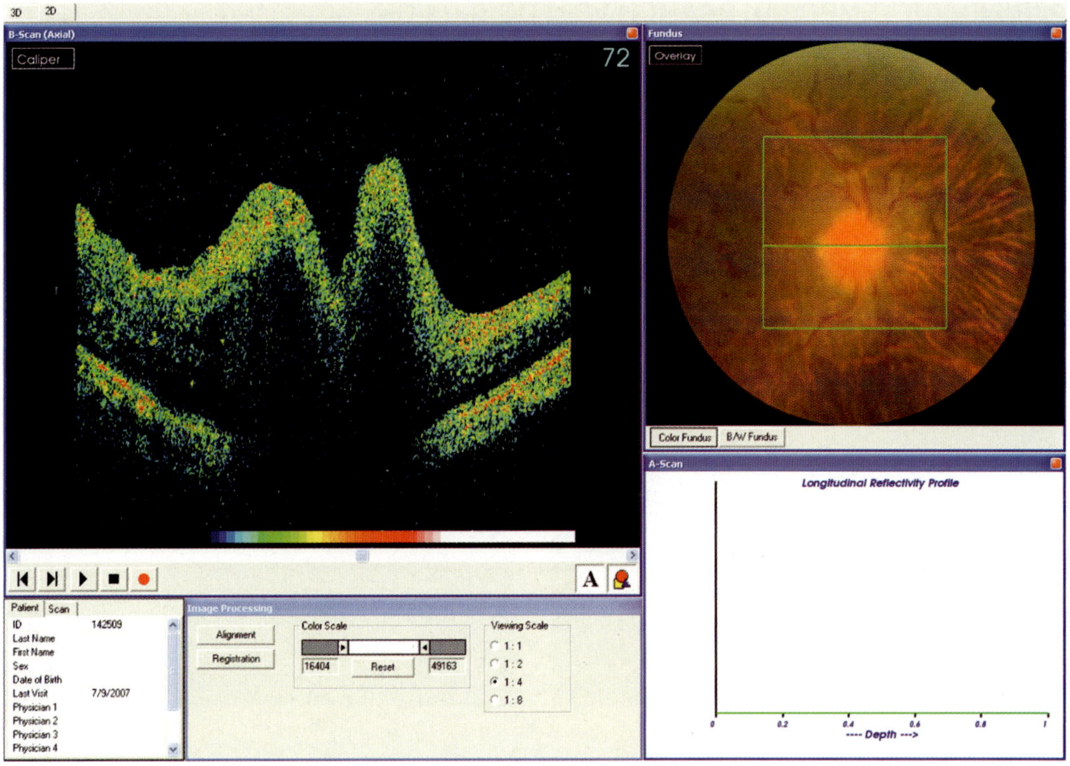

Figure 23.1.4: Color fundus photograph showing the horizontal line scan through the optic disc. Horizontal line scan 2D image showing substantial disc elevation with a clear optical space inside the disc because of the marked tissue thickening and fluid accumulation within it

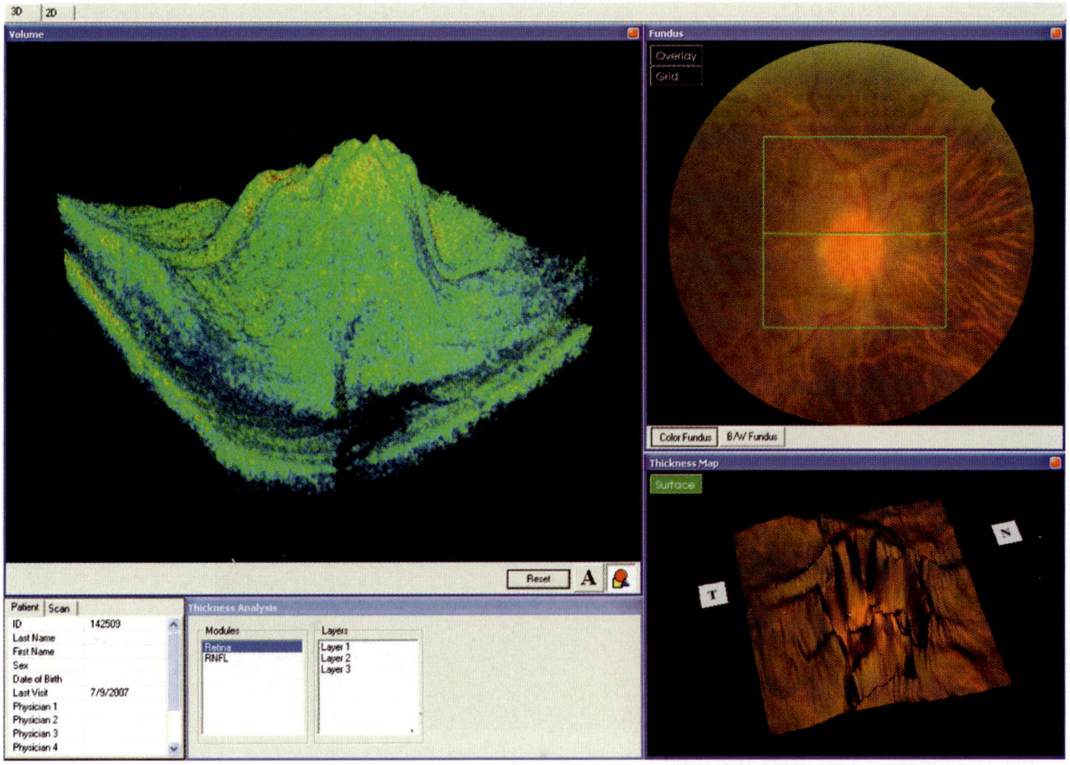

Figure 23.1.5: 3D image of the optic disc of Case 23.1

CASE 23.2: INFERIOR TEMPORAL BRANCH VEIN OCCLUSION

Case Summary

A 55-year-old woman was seen with decreased vision in the left eye of 15 days duration. Her best-corrected visual acuity in the left eye was 6/36. Fluorescein angiography showed inferior temporal branch retinal vein occlusion with leakage of dye (Figures 23.2.1 and 23.2.2).

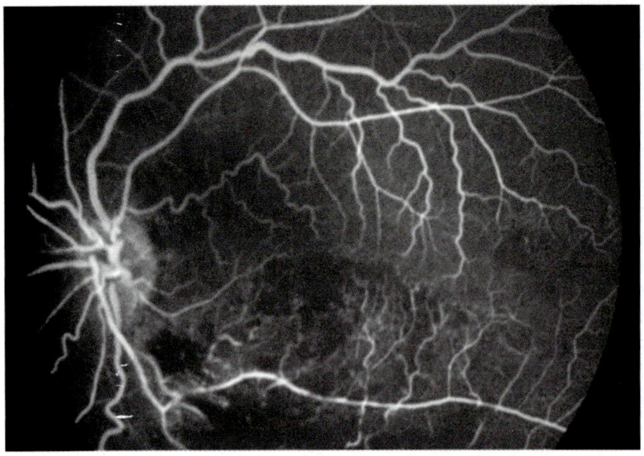

Figure 23.2.1: Early phase angiogram shows inferior temporal branch retinal vein occlusion

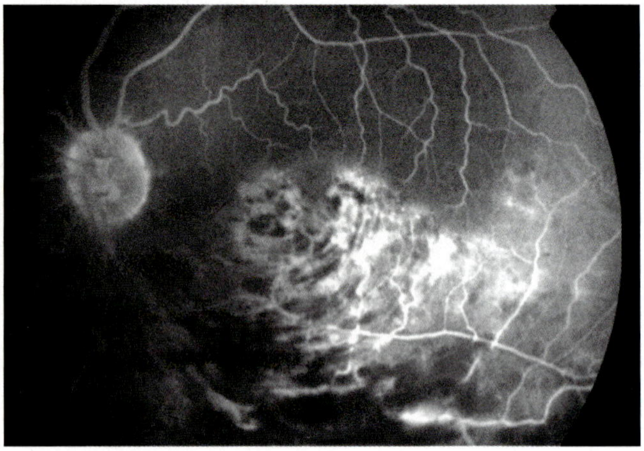

Figure 23.2.2: Late phase shows dilated leaking capillaries

Optical Coherence Tomography

Horizontal line scan showed loss of foveal contour, central retinal thickening and multiple hyporeflective areas with intervening hyper-reflective septae consistent with cystoid macular edema. Another hyporeflective area under the fovea was suggestive of serous retinal detachment (Figures 23.2.3A to D).

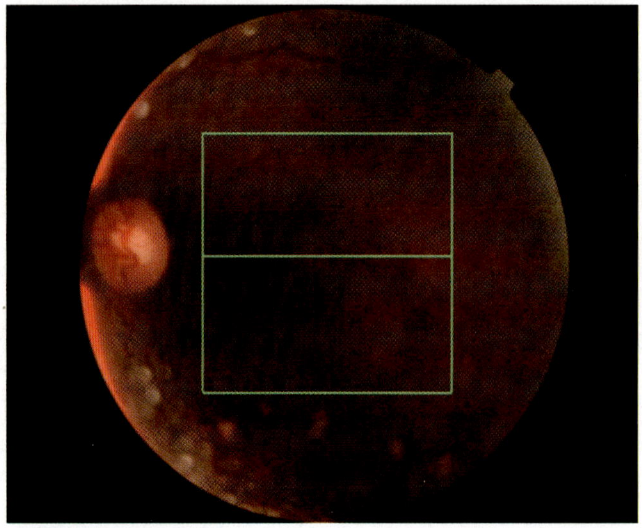

Figure 23.2.3A: Color fundus photograph showing the horizontal line scan through the fovea

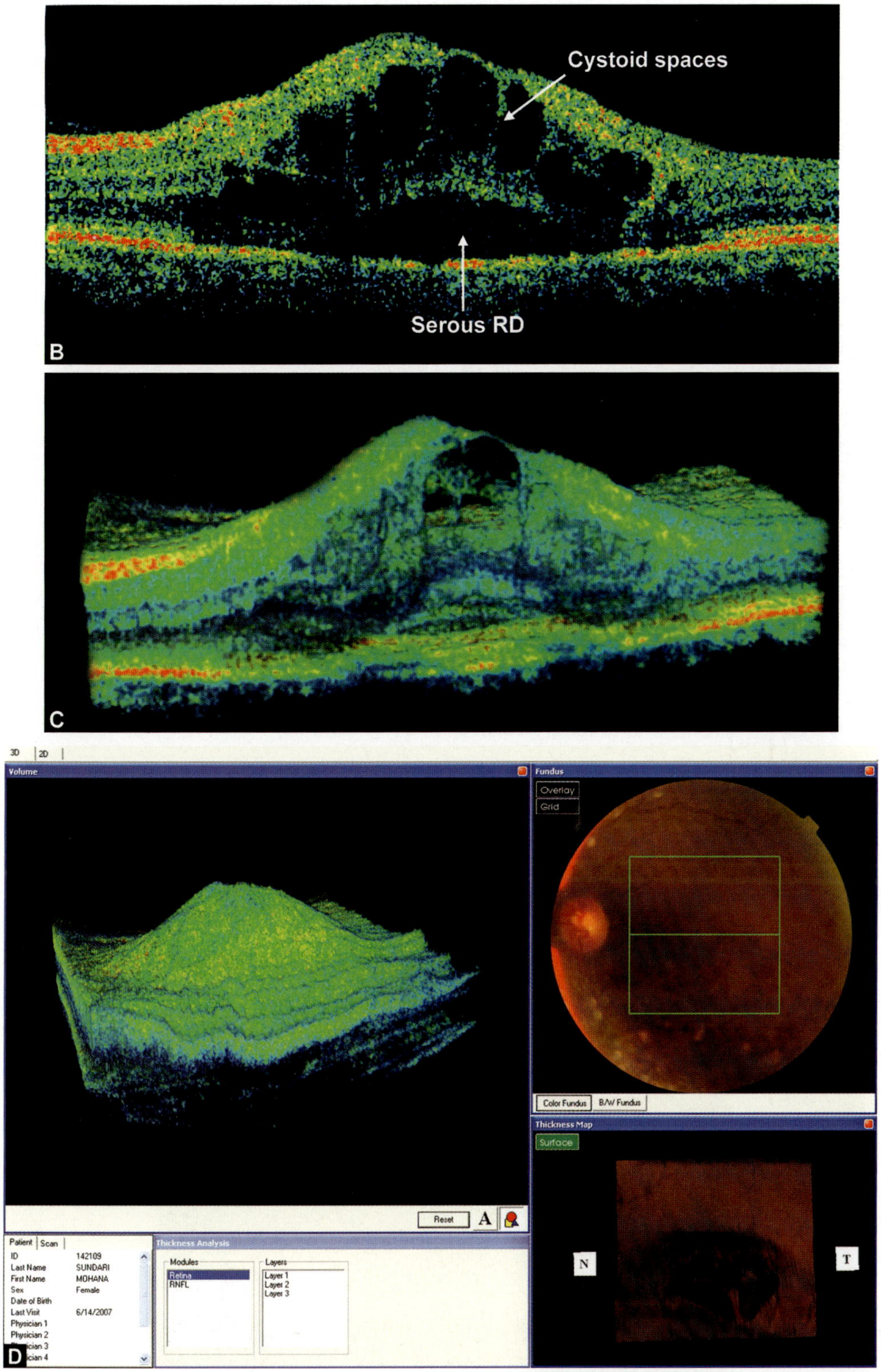

Figures 23.2.3B to D: (B) Horizontal line scan, 2D image showing loss of foveal contour, central retinal thickening and multiple hyporeflective areas with intervening hyper-reflective septae consistent with cystoid macular edema. Another hyporeflective area under the fovea is suggestive of serous retinal detachment. (C) Cropped 3D image showing loss of foveal contour, central retinal thickening and multiple hyporeflective areas with intervening hyper-reflective septae consistent with cystoid macular edema. Another hyporeflective area under the fovea is suggestive of serous retinal detachment. (D) 3D image of Case 23.2

CASE 23.3: INFERIOR HEMI BRANCH VEIN OCCLUSION

Case Summary

A 72-year-old man was seen with decreased vision in the right eye of two months duration. His best-corrected visual acuity in this eye was 6/18. Fluorescein angiography showed inferior hemi branch vein occlusion with leakage of dye in the fovea (Figures 23.3.1 and 23.3.2).

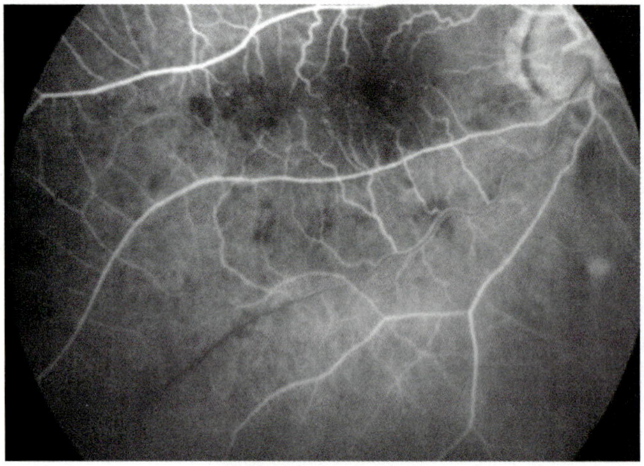

Figure 23.3.1: Early phase angiogram shows inferior hemi branch retinal vein occlusion

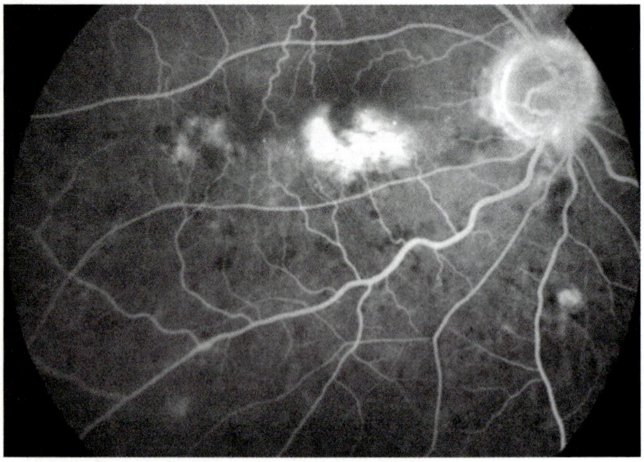

Figure 23.3.2: Late phase shows dilated leaking capillaries

Optical Coherence Tomography

Horizontal line scan showed loss of foveal contour, central retinal thickening and multiple hyporeflective spaces in the neurosensory retina suggestive of cystoid macular edema. In addition, there was a hyper-reflective membrane on the retinal surface (Figures 23.3.3A to D).

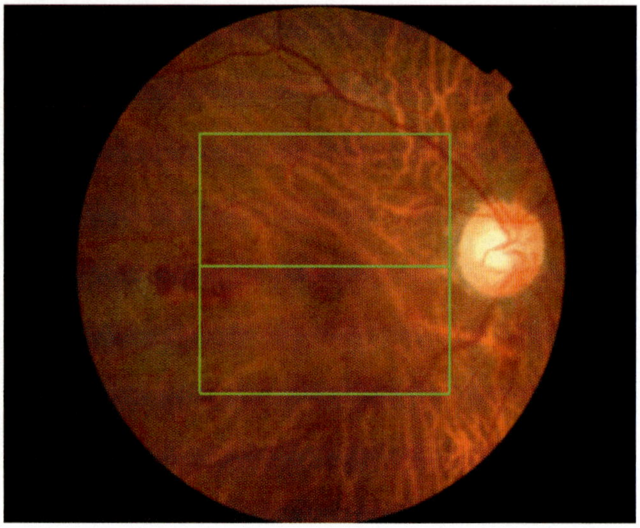

Figure 23.3.3A: Color fundus photograph showing the horizontal line scan through the fovea

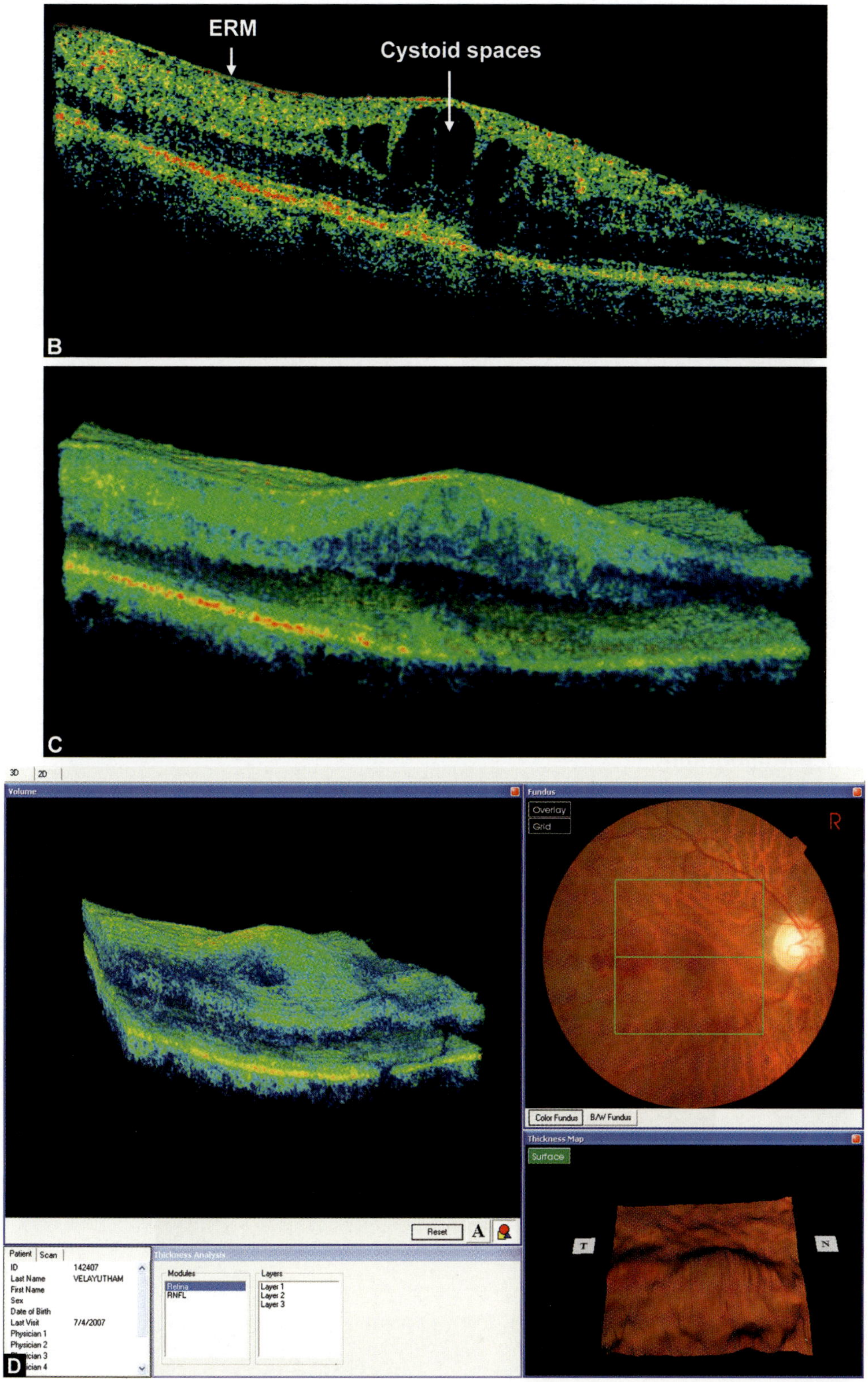

Figures 23.3.3B to D: (B) Horizontal line scan 2D image showing loss of foveal contour, central retinal thickening and multiple hypo-reflective spaces in the neurosensory retina suggestive of cystoid macular edema. ERM is visible. (C) Cropped 3D image showing loss of foveal contour, central retinal thickening and multiple hyporeflective spaces in the neurosensory retina suggestive of cystoid macular edema. ERM is visible. (D) 3D image of Case 23.3

CASE 23.4: SUPERIOR TEMPORAL BRANCH VEIN OCCLUSION

Case Summary

A 45-year-old woman was seen for a routine eye examination. Her best-corrected visual acuity in the right eye was 6/9. Fluorescein angiography showed superior temporal branch retinal vein occlusion with leakage of dye in the fovea (Figures 23.4.1 and 23.4.2).

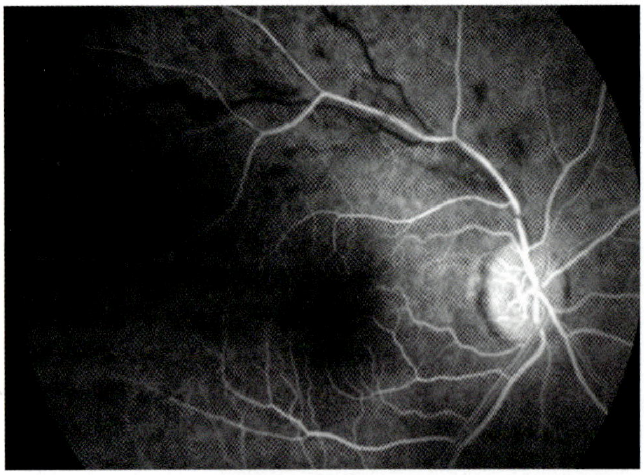

Figure 23.4.1: Early phase angiogram shows superior temporal branch vein occlusion

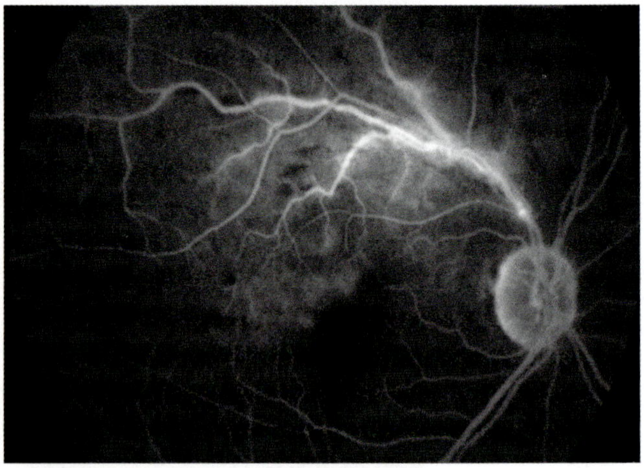

Figure 23.4.2: Late phase angiogram shows dilated leaking capillaries

Optical Coherence Tomography

Horizontal line scan showed hyporeflective cyst like spaces in the outer retina suggestive of retinal edema (Figures 23.4.3A to D).

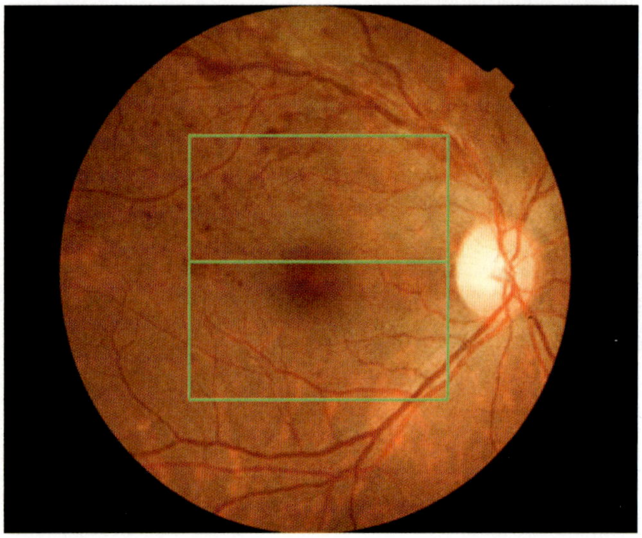

Figure 23.4.3A: Color fundus photograph showing the horizontal line scan through the fovea

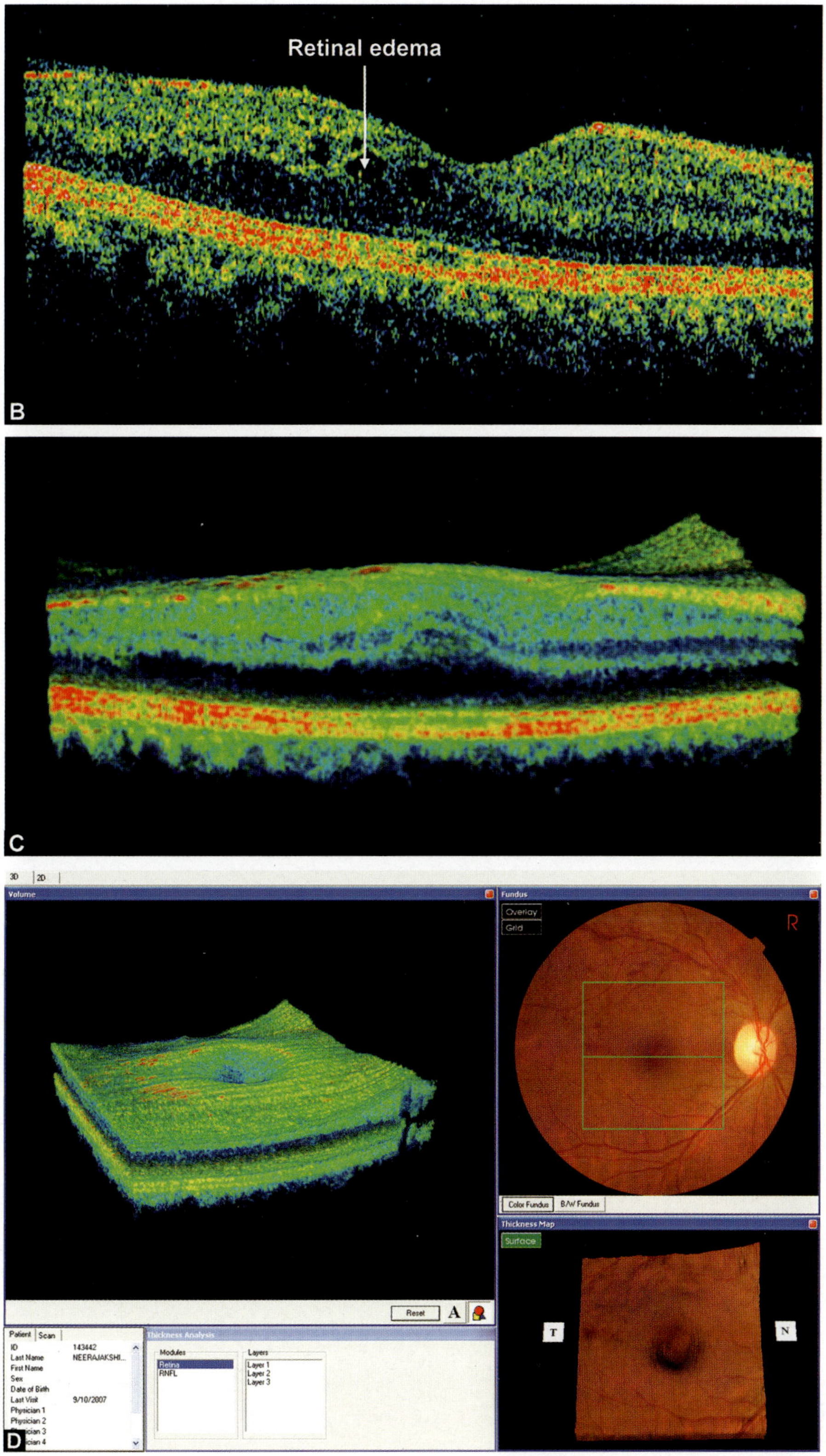

Figures 23.4.3B to D: (B) Horizontal line scan 2D image showing hyporeflective cyst like spaces in the outer retina suggestive of retinal edema. (C) Cropped 3D image showing hyporeflective cyst like spaces in the outer retina suggestive of retinal edema. (D) 3D image of Case 23.4

SUGGESTED READING

1. Spaide RF, Lee JK, Klancnik JK Jr, Gross NE. Optical coherence tomography of branch retinal vein occlusion. Retina. 2003; 23(3):343-7.
2. Ozdemir H, Karacorlu M, Karacorlu S. Serous macular detachment in central retinal vein occlusion. Retina. 2005;25(5):561-3.
3. Shroff D, Mehta DK, Arora R, Narula R, Chauhan D. Natural history of macular status in recent–onset branch retinal vein occlusion: an optical coherence tomography study. Int Ophthalmo. 2007 [Epub ahead of print].
4. Yamaike N, Tsujikawa A, Ota M, Sakamoto A, Kotera Y, Kita M, et al. Three-dimensional imaging of cystoid macular edema in retinal vein occlusion. Ophthalmology 2007 [Epub ahead of print].

Index

S

T

U

V

W

X